Second Edition

Medical Language

ACCELERATED

Steven L. Jones, PhD
Rice University

Andrew Cavanagh, MD
Texas A&M College of Medicine

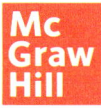

Mc
Graw
Hill

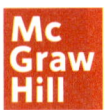

MEDICAL LANGUAGE ACCELERATED, SECOND EDITION

Published by McGraw-Hill Education, 2 Penn Plaza, New York, NY 10121. Copyright © 2021 by McGraw-Hill Education. All rights reserved. Printed in the United States of America. Previous edition © 2017. No part of this publication may be reproduced or distributed in any form or by any means, or stored in a database or retrieval system, without the prior written consent of McGraw-Hill Education, including, but not limited to, in any network or other electronic storage or transmission, or broadcast for distance learning.

Some ancillaries, including electronic and print components, may not be available to customers outside the United States.

This book is printed on acid-free paper.

1 2 3 4 5 6 7 8 9 LCR 24 23 22 21 20

ISBN 978-1-260-01773-1 (bound edition)
MHID 1-260-01773-7 (bound edition)
ISBN 978-1-260-47161-8 (loose-leaf edition)
MHID 1-260-47161-6 (loose-leaf edition)

Executive Portfolio Manager: *William Lawrensen*
Marketing Manager: *James Connely*
Senior Product Developer: *Christine Scheid*
Content Project Managers: *Ann Courtney/Brent dela Cruz*
Buyer: *Susan K. Culbertson*
Designer: *David W. Hash*
Content Licensing Specialist: *Lorraine Buczek*
Cover Image: *Frank Rohde*
Compositor: *SPi Global*

All credits appearing on page are considered to be an extension of the copyright page.

Library of Congress Cataloging-in-Publication Data

Names: Jones, Steven L., 1975- , author. | Cavanagh, Andrew, author.
Title: Medical language accelerated / Steven L. Jones, Andrew Cavanagh.
Description: Second edition. | New York, NY : McGraw-Hill Education, 2020.
  | Includes index. | Audience: Ages 18
Identifiers: LCCN 2019035881 | ISBN 9781260017731 (bound edition : alk. paper)
  | ISBN 9781260471618 (loose-leaf edition : alk. paper)
Subjects: MESH: Terminology as Topic | Problems and Exercises
Classification: LCC R123 | NLM W 18.2 | DDC 610.1/4—dc23
LC record available at https://lccn.loc.gov/2019035881

The Internet addresses listed in the text were accurate at the time of publication. The inclusion of a website does not indicate an endorsement by the authors or McGraw-Hill Education, and McGraw-Hill Education does not guarantee the accuracy of the information presented at these sites.

mheducation.com/highered

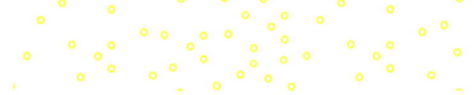

To our wives:

Tamber Jones

and

Ashley Cavanagh.

Your devotion, support, encouragement,

and assistance made this book possible.

brief contents

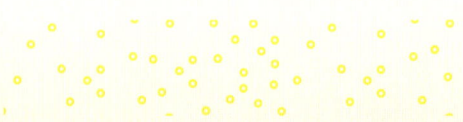

Steven L. Jones, PhD

Steve holds a BA in Greek and Latin from Baylor University, an MA in Greek, Latin, and Classical Studies from Bryn Mawr College, and a PhD in Classics from the University of Texas at Austin. Steve currently teaches Medical Terminology at Rice University in Houston, TX. He has held previous faculty appointments at Trinity University, the University of Texas at Austin, Baylor University, and Houston Baptist University. In addition to Medical Terminology, he teaches courses on Latin, Greek, Mythology, Classical Civilization, and Early Christianity.

When not breaking down medical words, Steve enjoys taking road trips with his wife and six children, watching baseball, eating tacos, drinking ice-cold Dr Pepper, and showing off his parallel-parking skills.

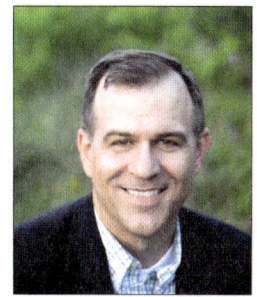
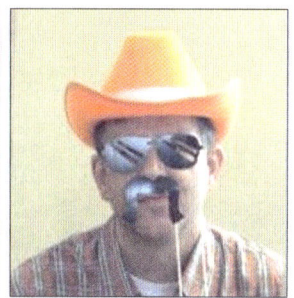
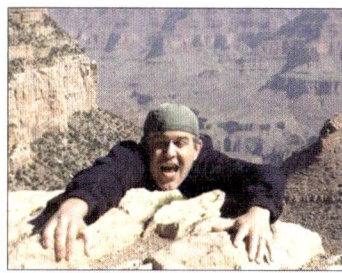

(top-left): Steve L. Jones; (top-right and bottom): Tamber Jones

Andrew Cavanagh, MD

Andy holds a BS in genetics from Texas A&M University and an MD from Texas A&M College of Medicine. After completing his residency at Palmetto Health Children's Hospital, he moved to the Austin area. He is currently owner and Chief Medical Officer of Chisholm Trail Pediatrics in Georgetown, TX. In addition to being board certified in pediatrics, Andy has served as the pediatric specialty chief for Dell Children's Medical Center and on the board of Dell Children's Medical Center Executive Committee. He is currently clinical assistant professor of pediatrics at the Texas A&M College of Medicine.

When not comforting sick children at work or wrestling with his own three kids at home, Andy enjoys powerlifting, hiking, and making his wife laugh.

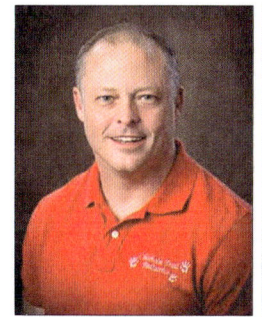
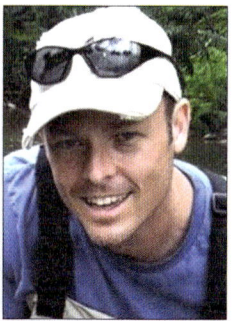
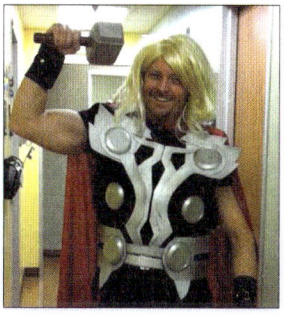

(top-left): Shane Littleton; (top-right): Ashley Cavanagh; (bottom): Andy Cavanagh

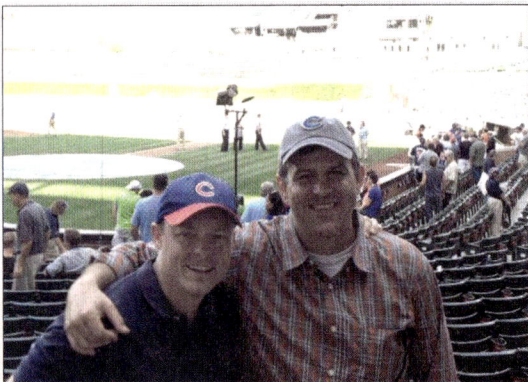

Courtesy Steve L. Jones

A Note from the Authors on Why They Wrote This Book

This book has its beginning in the friendship that Andy and Steve developed while they both lived in Austin. Andy was beginning his pediatric practice. Steve was completing his doctorate at UT. They had kids the same age and attended the same church. One evening after dinner, while sitting on Andy's back porch, Steve mentioned a new course he had been assigned to teach: Medical Terminology. What started as Steve complaining ended in a game where Andy tried to stump Steve by asking him what various medical words meant. Andy was amazed at how much Steve could figure out just by breaking down words. Steve was astonished to realize that most people—from medical assistants to medical doctors—weren't taught medical language this way. Through this conversation and others like it, Steve and Andy realized three things:

1. Understanding how to break down medical language is an essential skill in the medical field.
2. Having a basic knowledge of the Greek and Latin roots made medical language radically transparent.
3. The current market is lacking a textbook that teaches medical language this way.

This book is their attempt to meet those needs.

New to the Second Edition

1. Body system chapters have word tables focusing on radiology, oncology, and pharmacology.
2. Overview of burns (Chapter 3)
3. Expanded coverage of sexual transmitted infections (Chapter 12)

How to Use the Book

The Approach

Medical Language Accelerated approaches medical terminology not as words to be memorized but as a language to be learned. If you treat medical terminology as a language and learn how to read terms like sentences, you will be able to communicate clearly as a health care professional and will be a full participant in the culture of medicine. Memorizing definitions is equal to a traveler memorizing a few phrases in another language to help during a brief vacation: It will help a traveler survive for a few days. But if one is going to live in another culture for an extended period of time, learning to speak and understand the language becomes essential.

Medical Language Accelerated teaches students to **break down words into their composite word parts.** Instead of a dictionary full of terms that need to be memorized, a student equipped with groups of roots, prefixes, and suffixes can easily understand a vast amount of medical terminology.

Medical Language Accelerated bridges the gap between the two somewhat disparate fields that make up medical terminology—medicine and second-language acquisition—by providing assistance in language skills to equip health care professionals with the ability to learn and apply a useful skill and not lists of words. It will also equip language professionals with real-world examples that make their knowledge of languages applicable to working in the world of health care.

The process is best illustrated by considering the following word: pneumonoultramicroscopicsilicovolcanoconiosis. Memorizing the definition to words like this would seem like an intimidating task. If you break it into its composite parts, you get:

pneumono / ultra   / micro / scopic / silico
lung   / *extremely* / *small* / *looking* / *sand*

/ volcano / coni / osis
/ *volcanic* / *dust* / *condition*

Through knowledge of roots and word formation, the meaning becomes transparent: "A condition of the lungs caused by extremely small bits of volcanic sand." Instead of having to memorize a long list of even longer words, a student equipped with the knowledge of roots and how to break apart words can tackle—and not be intimidated by—the most complicated sounding medical terms.

The approach to medical terminology presented in this book was originally developed for *Acquiring Medical Language*. We adapted the methodology for use in an accelerated format hence the new title: *Medical Terminology Accelerated*. The approach is unchanged. The principle difference between the two books deals with the coverage of terms included in each text. *Medical Terminology Accelerated* emphasizes the terms that readily breakdown according to the principles taught in this book. Every word reinforces the roots associated with each body system and reiterates prefixes and suffixes. The result is a book that allows students to adopt an accelerated approach to learning medical terminology.

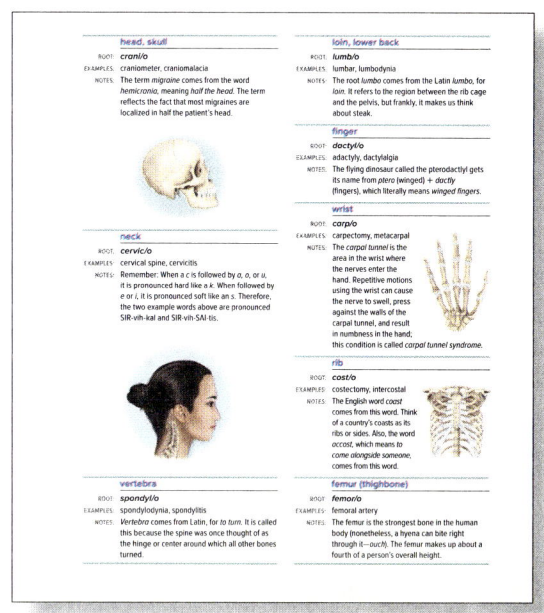

Organization and Key Features

Medical Language Accelerated begins with two introductory chapters: Chapter 1, Introduction to Medical Language; and Chapter 2, Introduction to Health Records. Chapters 3 through 13 are dedicated to individual systems of the body and review common roots, words, and abbreviations for each system.

1. **"Card-Based" Approach:** Each chapter opens with a section on word parts for that particular body system. Students are introduced to roots via pages with illustrations of body systems surrounded by "cards" containing the names of body parts, specific word roots related to those parts, a few examples containing the roots, as well as some interesting facts to make the information more memorable. The student is exposed to all relevant information (the root, its meaning, its use) and sees how each root relates to the other roots in the context of the body system, without ever needing to turn the page.

2. **SOAP Note Organization:** After the student is introduced to the important roots for the chapter using "cards," the medical terms relevant to the body system are presented using the SOAP note as an organizational framework. *SOAP* is an acronym used by many health care professionals to help organize the diagnostic process (SOAP is explained more fully in Chapter 2). The terms will be divided under the following headings:

 Subjective: Patient History, Problems, Complaints

 Objective: Observation and Discovery

 Assessment: Diagnosis and Pathology

 Plan: Treatments and Therapies

The SOAP note method is a fundamental way of thinking about the language of health care. By building this approach into the framework of the pedagogy, *Medical Language Accelerated* prepares future health care professionals to speak the language of medicine.

3. **Realistic Medical Histories:** *Medical Language Accelerated* incorporates realistic medical histories in reviewing each chapter's material to expose students to what they can expect in the real world. The student is given an example of an electronic health care record and is asked a series of questions. Though it is not expected that

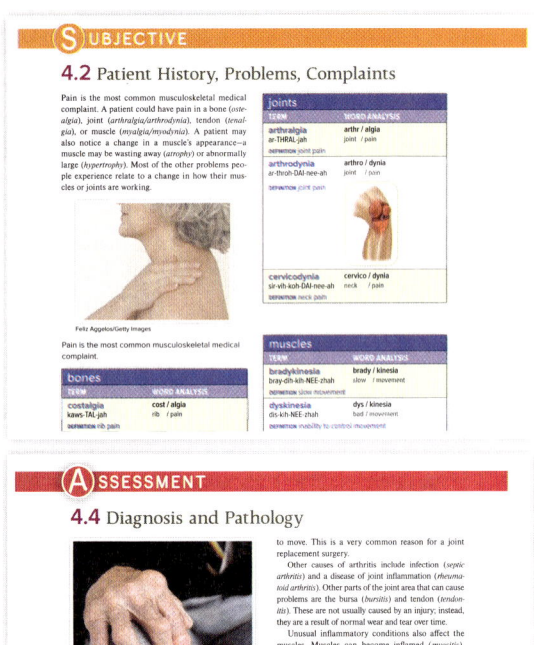

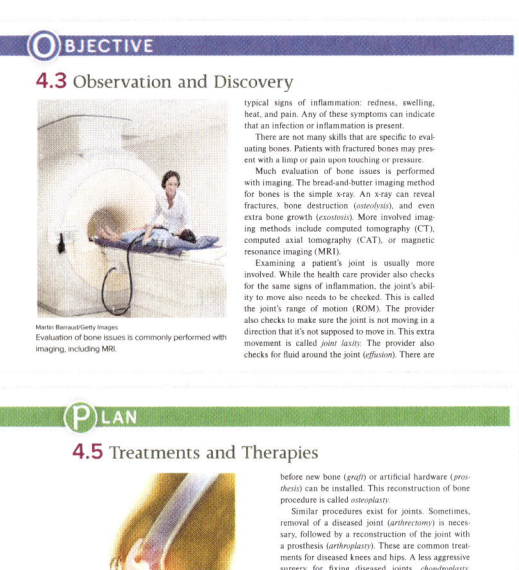

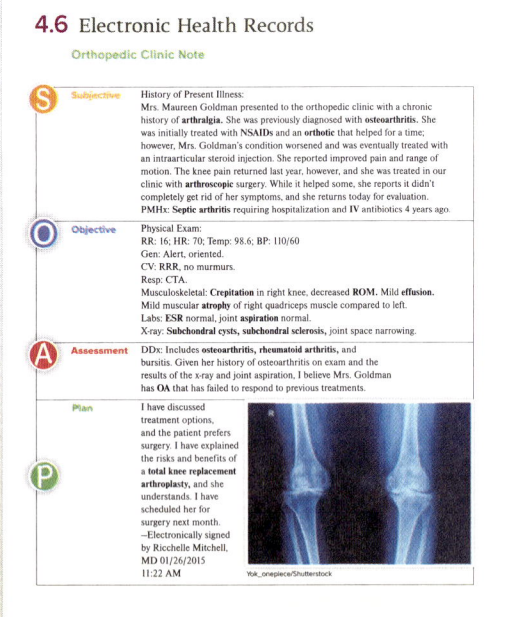

4.2 Patient History, Problems, Complaints

SUBJECTIVE

Pain is the most common musculoskeletal medical complaint. A patient could have pain in a bone (*ostealgia*), joint (*arthralgia/arthrodynia*), tendon (*tenalgia*), or muscle (*myalgia/myodynia*). A patient may also notice a change in a muscle's appearance—a muscle may be wasting away (*atrophy*) or abnormally large (*hypertrophy*). Most of the other problems people experience relate to a change in how their muscles or joints are working.

Pain is the most common musculoskeletal medical complaint.

Felix Aggelos/Getty Images

joints

TERM	WORD ANALYSIS
arthralgia ar-THRAL-jah	arthr / algia joint / pain
DEFINITION joint pain	
arthrodynia ar-throh-DAI-nee-ah	arthro / dynia joint / pain
DEFINITION joint pain	
cervicodynia sir-vih-koh-DAI-nee-ah	cervico / dynia neck / pain
DEFINITION neck pain	

bones

TERM	WORD ANALYSIS
costalgia kaws-TAL-jah	cost / algia rib / pain
DEFINITION rib pain	

muscles

TERM	WORD ANALYSIS
bradykinesia bray-dih-kih-NEE-zhah	brady / kinesia slow / movement
DEFINITION slow movement	
dyskinesia dis-kih-NEE-zhah	dys / kinesia bad / movement
DEFINITION inability to control movement	

4.4 Diagnosis and Pathology

ASSESSMENT

Image Source/Getty Images

to move. This is a very common reason for a joint replacement surgery.

Other causes of arthritis include infection (*septic arthritis*) and a disease of joint inflammation (*rheumatoid arthritis*). Other parts of the joint area that can cause problems are the bursa (*bursitis*) and tendon (*tendonitis*). These are not usually caused by an injury; instead, they are a result of normal wear and tear over time.

Unusual inflammatory conditions also affect the muscles. Muscles can become inflamed (*myositis*). Sometimes this can involve the skin as well (*dermatomyositis*). General problems with all the muscles are called *myopathies. Myasthenia gravis* and *muscular dystrophy* are two of the most common types of myopathy.

4.3 Observation and Discovery

OBJECTIVE

Martin Barraud/Getty Images
Evaluation of bone issues is commonly performed with imaging, including MRI.

typical signs of inflammation: redness, swelling, heat, and pain. Any of these symptoms can indicate that an infection or inflammation is present.

There are not many skills that are specific to evaluating bones. Patients with fractured bones may present with a limp or pain upon touching or pressure.

Much evaluation of bone issues is performed with imaging. The bread-and-butter imaging method for bones is the simple x-ray. An x-ray can reveal fractures, bone destruction (*osteolysis*), and even extra bone growth (*exostosis*). More involved imaging methods include computed tomography (CT), computed axial tomography (CAT), or magnetic resonance imaging (MRI).

Examining a patient's joint is usually more involved. While the health care provider also checks for the same signs of inflammation, the joint's ability to move also needs to be checked. This is called the joint's range of motion (ROM). The provider also checks to make sure the joint is not moving in a direction that it's not supposed to move in. This extra movement is called *joint laxity*. The provider also checks for fluid around the joint (*effusion*). There are

4.5 Treatments and Therapies

PLAN

Dr. P. Marazzi/Science Photo Library/Getty Images
Common procedures for the musculoskeletal system include knee and hip replacements.

before new bone (*graft*) or artificial hardware (*prosthesis*) can be installed. This reconstruction of bone procedure is called *osteoplasty*.

Similar procedures exist for joints. Sometimes, removal of a diseased joint (*arthrectomy*) is necessary, followed by a reconstruction of the joint with a prosthesis (*arthroplasty*). These are common treatments for diseased knees and hips. A less aggressive surgery for fixing diseased joints, *chondroplasty*, involves fixing the bad cartilage of a joint. It is very common in athletes and older patients with chronic osteoarthritis.

Not all orthopedic surgery involves complete reconstruction of a bone or joint. Sometimes something that has snapped must be repaired, as in a tendon repair (*tenorrhaphy*) or a muscle repair (*myorrhaphy*). Other times, new attachments must be made. This can involve attaching leftover muscle to bone (*myodesis*) after an amputation or fixing two bones surrounding a joint (*arthrodesis*). While the latter procedure results in immobility of the joint, it may be necessary to relieve pain.

---

everything in the record will be intelligible to them, the goal is to expose students to the context in which they will see medical terminology. This process will encourage students not to feel

4.6 Electronic Health Records

Orthopedic Clinic Note

S Subjective
History of Present Illness:
Mrs. Maureen Goldman presented to the orthopedic clinic with a chronic history of **arthralgia**. She was previously diagnosed with **osteoarthritis**. She was initially treated with NSAIDs and an **orthotic** that helped for a time; however, Mrs. Goldman's condition worsened and was eventually treated with an intraarticular steroid injection. She reported improved pain and range of motion. The knee pain returned last year, however, and she was treated in our clinic with **arthroscopic** surgery. While it helped some, she reports it didn't completely get rid of her symptoms, and she returns today for evaluation.
PMHx: **Septic arthritis** requiring hospitalization and **IV** antibiotics 4 years ago.

O Objective
Physical Exam:
RR: 16; HR: 70; Temp: 98.6; BP: 110/60
Gen: Alert, oriented.
CV: RRR, no murmurs.
Resp: CTA.
Musculoskeletal: **Crepitation** in right knee, decreased **ROM**. Mild **effusion**. Mild muscular **atrophy** of right quadriceps muscle compared to left.
Labs: **ESR** normal, joint **aspiration** normal.
X-ray: **Subchondral cysts, subchondral sclerosis**, joint space narrowing.

A Assessment
DDx: Includes **osteoarthritis, rheumatoid arthritis,** and bursitis. Given her history of osteoarthritis on exam and the results of the x-ray and joint aspiration, I believe Mrs. Goldman has **OA** that has failed to respond to previous treatments.

P Plan
I have discussed treatment options, and the patient prefers surgery. I have explained the risks and benefits of a **total knee replacement arthroplasty**, and she understands. I have scheduled her for surgery next month.
—Electronically signed by Ricchelle Mitchell, MD 01/26/2015 11:22 AM

Yok_onepiece/Shutterstock

---

intimidated by the prospect of seeing words they are unfamiliar with. We have seen this help students glean information from the chart by using the skills they are acquiring in translating medical terminology.

4. **Practice Exercises:** Each section ends with an abundance of practice exercises, giving students the opportunity to practice and apply what they have just learned. Exercises are grouped into categories: Pronunciation, Translation, and Generation. This progression and repetition allows students to gradually build their skills—and their confidence—as they learn to apply their medical language skills. Abundant Chapter Review exercises, as well as additional labeling and audio exercises, are available through McGraw-Hill Connect®.

S Learning Outcome 5.2 Exercises

PRONUNCIATION

EXERCISE 1 Indicate which syllable is emphasized when pronounced.

EXAMPLE: bronchitis bron**chi**tis

1. paresis _____
2. neuralgia _____
3. aphasia _____
4. paralysis _____
5. dysphasia _____

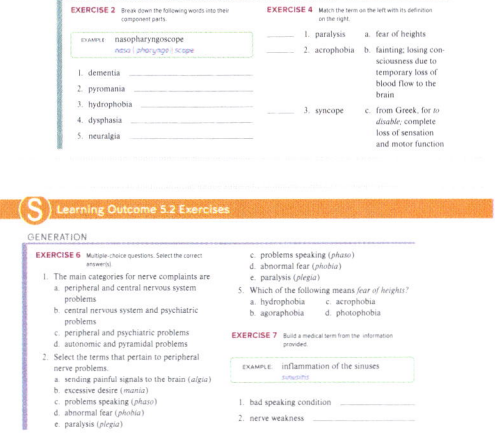

To the Instructor

To teach medical terminology as a language, we adopt techniques employed in second-language acquisition. This helps students not just learn the roots, but also adopt a way of thinking and speaking that enables them to communicate using the language of medicine. Cognitive and educational psychologists divide language instruction techniques into two primary categories: contextualized ("real-world" exercises) and decontextualized (academic/grammar exercises).

Using this framework, some of the techniques employed in *Medical Language Accelerated* include:

1. **Contextualized Language Techniques ("real-world" exercises)**

   a. *Link new language to old language.* Pointing out instances of medical terms or roots in everyday use enables the students to connect new information they are studying with information they already possess.

   b. *Use new language in context.* Using the "card" system to introduce the root words enables students to understand word parts in the context of larger body systems and in relation to other word parts. Using realistic medical charts enables students to see the terms they use not as lists but as parts of a system of communication.

2. **Decontextualized Language Techniques (academic/grammar exercises)**

   a. *Use repetition.* The students are exposed to roots, prefixes, and suffixes multiple times and in multiple ways. Roots are changed by the addition of prefixes or suffixes. Familiar prefixes and suffixes are applied to new roots. This way, the word components are continuously reinforced.

   b. *Use translation.* Students are asked to provide literal definitions of medical terms, which provides practice in breaking down words into their component parts and determining their meaning.

   c. *Use generation.* Students are asked to produce medical terms based on the literal definition provided. Though this is only an academic exercise, such practice reinforces material learned by reversing the cognitive process of translation.

As you use this text, here are some things to keep in mind:

1. **Breakdown Is the Key**—the goals of this approach to medical terminology are to help students internalize the word parts (roots, prefixes, suffixes) and to reinforce the concept that medical terms are not to be memorized but to be translated.

2. **Words Are Practice**—the words in each chapter are a chance to practice breaking down terms into their component parts, identifying the roots, and learning to define the terms using this translation method. Because of that, each chapter contains four classes of words.

   a. *Essential words that break down*—Each chapter contains words that are essential for students to know AND that break down easily using this method. The core of each chapter is words like this. The goal is to show students that the vast majority of medical terms are translatable using the method taught by this book.

b. *Non-essential words that break down—* Each chapter also contains words that are not necessarily essential for students to know or common in the medical field, but break down clearly and are easily translatable using the method taught by this book. We include them as chances to practice the concept of translating medical terms and to show how easy the method is to apply.

c. *Essential words that don't benefit from breakdown—* There are terms that can be broken down but the breakdown doesn't help you understand what the word means. This can happen for a variety of reasons, such as the term describes a symptom rather than the disease, reflects an outdated way of understanding the disease, is an ancient term than just means what it means, or is a very recent and technical term and so there are no other words to compare it to. In these cases, even though the method taught by this book may not be ideal in helping to learn these terms, we still provide breakdowns and other notes to help make the information stick in the student's memory.

d. *Essential words that don't break down—* We admit it. This method doesn't work for every word. Some words essential for students to know do not break into word components. They must be memorized. We include those words because they are crucial words for medical professionals to know. Our hope is that the inclusion of these words in the real-life health records and other contextualized learning environments in this book will support students in internalizing these essential terms.

3. **The Use of "Roots" in Place of "Combining Forms"—** We understand that it's common practice in medical terminology courses to teach students the difference between roots and combining forms. This is not a part of our approach, and you will see that in this book, the term *combining form* is absent and

the term *root* has been used in its place. Here are the reasons why we decided to do this.

a. In the real world of medical language, the classifications of "root" and "combining form" are nonexistent. The reason for this is that they mean virtually the same exact thing to healthcare professions in practice. The part of the term that is defined as a combining form can be used interchangeably with root without confusion. Also, word "roots" are more commonly used outside the world of medical terminology instruction. For our approach, using "root" instead of "combining form" prepares students better by presenting terminology as it is commonly used in broader health professions. If you were to hit "Ctrl+F" to find and replace all instances of the word *root* with *combining form* in our text, nothing . . . NOTHING . . . is changed, lost, or unclear to the student.

b. The importance of combining vowels and forms deals with how they impact pronunciation of terms, not definitions. Some instructors will argue, but there is only a minimal difference in meaning, if any. We feel that great confusion is created by insisting on and highlighting the difference as once a student completes the med term class, being able to identify a component part as root or combining form is no longer practical. We do recognize this difference between a root and a combining form in Chapter 1 as follows: "When we say that a word part such as *cardi/o* is a root, we aren't speaking precisely. Technically, *cardi/o* is called a combing form. A combining form is a combination of a root with a combining vowel."

c. The word *root* is shorter than *combining form* by more than a third of letters (4 letters vs. 13 letters). It may sound silly, but to us the purpose of teaching medical terminology is to streamline communication. The use of *combining form* is an unnecessary complication that doesn't bring value to the learner but may add potential confusion.

4. **Pronunciations are Challenging for Students.**

   a. *We all speak differently*—English is an incredibly diverse language with numerous dialects and accents from all over the globe. One consequence of this is that we all speak in slightly different ways. Some of us break words into syllables at slightly different places or pronounce certain syllables differently. With that in mind, the pronunciation guides given in the book should be viewed as guidelines or directions, not universal laws.

   b. *Phonetic* versus *non-phonetic syllable breakdowns*—In the exercises, we frequently ask students to break words into syllables. When that happens, students might ask for guidance in doing this. Though we didn't explicitly break words into syllables, the syllable breakdown can be determined by looking at the Phonetic Pronunciation guide provided for each word. Encourage students to use critical thinking skills to align letters in the term with syllables in the guides.

   c. *For example*—Consider the word salpingoscope. The phonetic pronunciation guide describes it as: sal-PING-goh-skohp. But how does that translate to syllable breakdown? Why is the "g" is used in two syllables? Shouldn't it be either "sal-pin-go-scope" or "sal-ping-o-scope"? Well, a case can be made for either of those two choices. The truth of the matter is that we all say the word slightly different. The word is most accurately pronounced by leaving a little bit of the "g" in both syllables. Admit it, when you drop the G from PIN, you end up saying PIN a little bit differently. We say this not to complicate things but to encourage you to be flexible. We acknowledge that our pronunciation guides aren't etched in stone . . . more like etched in Silly Putty.

In addition to providing innovative approaches to learning medical terminology, McGraw-Hill Education knows how much effort it takes to prepare for a new course. Through focus groups, symposia, reviews, and conversations with instructors like you, we have gathered information about the materials you need to facilitate successful courses. We are committed to providing you with high-quality, accurate instructor support.

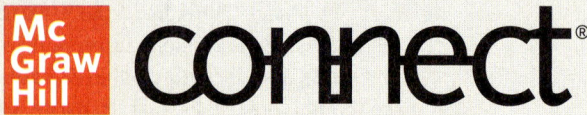

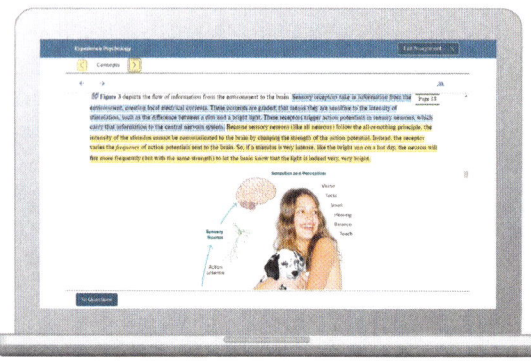

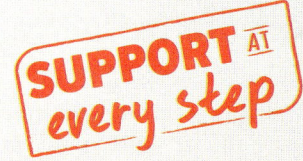

FOR STUDENTS

Effective, efficient studying.

Connect helps you be more productive with your study time and get better grades using tools like SmartBook 2.0, which highlights key concepts and creates a personalized study plan. Connect sets you up for success, so you walk into class with confidence and walk out with better grades.

Study anytime, anywhere.

Download the free ReadAnywhere app and access your online eBook or SmartBook 2.0 assignments when it's convenient, even if you're offline. And since the app automatically syncs with your eBook and SmartBook 2.0 assignments in Connect, all of your work is available every time you open it. Find out more at **www.mheducation.com/readanywhere**

"I really liked this app—it made it easy to study when you don't have your text- book in front of you."

- Jordan Cunningham, Eastern Washington University

Calendar: pwettaphotos/Getty Images

No surprises.

The Connect Calendar and Reports tools keep you on track with the work you need to get done and your assignment scores. Life gets busy; Connect tools help you keep learning through it all.

Learning for everyone.

McGraw-Hill works directly with Accessibility Services Departments and faculty to meet the learning needs of all students. Please contact your Accessibility Services office and ask them to email accessibility@mheducation.com, or visit **www.mheducation.com/about/accessibility** for more information.

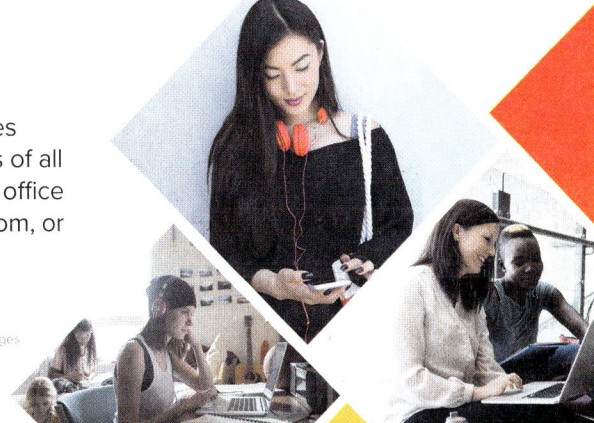

Top: Jenner Images/Getty Images. Left: Hero Images/Getty Images. Right: Hero Images/Getty Images

A Note from the Authors: To the Student

The purpose of this program is to equip you with foundational skills as you prepare for a career in health and medicine. As you enter the culture of medicine, you will need to speak the language to understand what is going on around you and to be understood by your colleagues and patients. Though learning medical language can seem a daunting task, it is our hope that this program reduces some of the anxiety that accompanies learning any new language. We hope this program shows you how clear the language of medicine is to understand as you begin to master some key concepts. As you get started, here are some helpful words of advice:

1. *Don't panic.* Immersing yourself in any new language can be intimidating. On occasion, you will probably feel overwhelmed, like you are being bombarded with information you don't understand and don't know how to make sense of. Start by trying not to panic. Things always look intimidating when you begin. The water is always coldest when you first jump in. You will get used to it. Be patient. Follow the steps.

2. *Eat the elephant.* Do you know how to eat an elephant? One bite at a time. One of the easiest ways to keep from panicking is to break down things into easily digestible chunks. Don't focus on the total amount of information you have to learn; rather, focus on the bite in front of you.

3. *Practice makes permanent.* The easiest way to master medical language is to practice. You readily absorb what you are repeatedly exposed to. So practice. Repeat. Do it again. The more you do it, the more you will be able to do it, and the more you will enjoy doing it.

4. *Build bridges.* Medical language is everywhere: on TV shows, in the news, in your own life. Look for it. See if you can figure out the meaning of words you hear. Build connections between what you are learning and the world you live in. See how often you encounter these words. The more you practice it, the more it will be burned into your memory.

Acknowledgments

Suggestions have been received from faculty and students throughout the country. This is vital feedback that is relied on for product development. Each person who has offered comments and suggestions has our thanks. The efforts of many people are needed to develop and improve a product. Among these people are the reviewers and consultants who point out areas of concern, cite areas of strength, and make recommendations for change. In this regard, the following instructors provided feedback that was enormously helpful in preparing the book and related products.

Reviewers
We'd like to thank the many reviewers and SMEs who have helped us with the first, and now this second edition.

Dora P. Bailey, BS
Durham Technical Community College

Mark Beck, BA, MA, PhD
University of South
Carolina at Columbia

Ranelle Brew, EdD, CHES
Grand Valley State University

Mauri Brueggeman, MEd, MLS (ASCP)^{CM}
Northcentral Technical College

Gina Capitano MS, RT(R)
Misericordia University

Alice Clegg, MHEd, BS
Dixie State University

Colleen L. Croxall, PhD
Eastern Michigan University

Teresa Diana
Cape Fear Community College

Stephanie Duncan, MSN, RN, CCRN
Marygrove College

Mary Fabick, MSN,
MEd, RN-BC, CEN
Milligan College

Sandra Flynn, AS
Guilford Technical Community
College

Kenneth D. Franks
Bossier Parish Community College

Dr. Joel Gluck, DPM
Community College of
Rhode Island

M.J. Hilliard BS, CST
Healthcare Preparatory Institute

Amy Johns
Moberly Area Community College

Judith Karls, RN, BSN, MSE
Madison Area Technical College

Tonya Kendrix, MSN,
MBA, HCM, RN
South Arkansas Community College

Tricia Leggett, DHEd, RT(R)(QM)
Zane State College

Kathryn R. Maxwell, MA BSN RN
The Ohio State University
College of Medicine

Tammy McClish, MEd,
CMA (AAMA)
The University of Akron

Tabitha Mocilan
ECPI University

Cynthia K. (Cindy) Moore, PhD, RDN
R & D Wellness & Nutrition,
Tyson Foods, Inc.

Mirella Pardee, MSN, MA, RN
University of Toledo

Constance Phillips, MA, MPH
Boston University

Mary M. Prorok, RN, MSN
South Hills School of
Business & Technology

Amy Bolinger Snow, MS
Greenville Technical College

Charlene Thiessen, MEd,
BA, CMT, AHDI-F
GateWay Community College

Dr. Mimi Vaassen, PT,
DPT, GCS, CLT
Assistant Professor of Physical Therapy
Clarke University

Amy Way, PhD
Lock Haven University of
Pennsylvania

Kari Williams, BS, DC
Front Range Community College

Charles K. Williston, MS, BA, CPC
Traviss Career Center

Luisa L. Zirkle, BS Medical
Technology, BS Biology,
Master Ed
Tidewater Community College

Digital Tool Development

Special thanks to the instructors who helped with the development of Connect, LearnSmart, and SmartBook.

Judith Karls, RN, BSN, MSE
Madison Area Technical College

Amy Kennedy, MSN, RN

Rhonna Krouse, MS.,
ACSM-EP-C, CISSN
College of Western Idaho

Jocelyn Lewis, PT, DPT, MS
Community College of Philadelphia

Dr. Vicky Navaroli, PhD
Goodwin College

Mirella Pardee, MSN, MA, RN
University of Toledo

Lorie Sablad, ARNP, MSN
Valencia Community College

Acknowledgments from the Authors

We would like to thank the following individuals who helped develop, critique, and shape our textbook, our digital materials, and our other ancillaries. We are grateful for the efforts of our team at McGraw-Hill Education who made all of this come together. We would especially like to thank Michelle Vogler, Director; William Lawrensen, Executive Portfolio Manager; Christine "Chipper" Scheid, Senior Product Developer; Roxan Kinsey, Executive Marketing Manager; Ann Courtney, Senior Content Project Manager; Brent dela Cruz, Lead Content Project Manager; David Hash, Lead Designer; and Lorraine Buczek, Content Licensing Specialist.

Acknowledgments from Steven L. Jones

Above all, I am grateful for the love and support of my family: my wife, Tamber, and our six children, I am also thankful for the support of my colleagues at the universities where I worked while completing this project. At Rice University: Nicholas K. Iammarino, Chair of the Department of Kinesiology; and Jennifer Zinn-Winkler, the program administrator. At Houston Baptist University: President Robert Sloan,

Christopher Hammons, Micah Mattix, Timothy A. Brookins, Evan J. Getz, Gary Hartenburg, Randy Hatchett, and Jerry Walls. In addition, I am deeply indebted to my friends for their encouragement: Daniel Benton, Michael Bordelon, Michael Czapla, Nathan Cook, Russell Thompson, Dan Euhus, and Brad Flurry.

Acknowledgments from Andrew Cavanagh

I am most thankful for the loving support of my wife, Ashley, and children, Katie, Nathaniel, and Jack. I owe a great debt of gratitude to my mother, Katherine Cavanagh, who worked tirelessly to provide for me as I grew up and passed on to me her admirable work ethic. I would also like to thank John Blevins for fostering my love of medicine and pediatrics and for being a great role model. I would like to thank Caughman Taylor and the entire residency training program at Palmetto Health Richland, University of South Carolina, for their amazing teaching and dedication to the lives of the residents. I am grateful for Chisholm Trail Pediatrics. It is a joy to practice medicine in such a positive environment.

Introduction to Medical Language

1

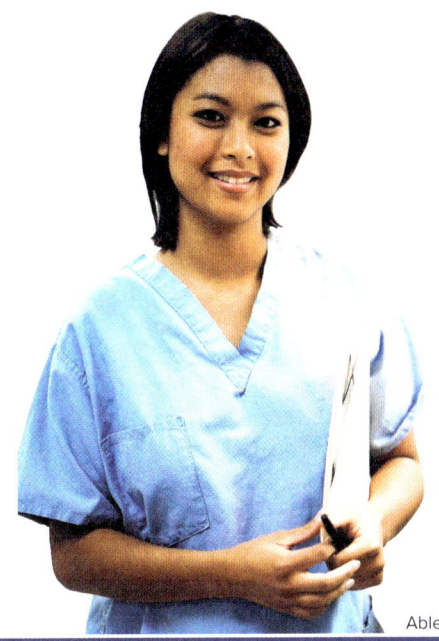

Introduction

You've probably had conversations with people who like to use big words. Maybe you've responded with a blank expression and a sarcastic phrase—something like, "Say it in English, please!" This happens all the time in health care practices.

When a patient comes in for treatment, he or she is often bombarded with unfamiliar words. The patient leaves bewildered, wondering what the health care professional just said. Sometimes patients do get up the courage to ask what it all means, and health care professionals explain in simpler terms. And patients wonder, "Well, why couldn't you have just said that in the first place? Why did you have to use all those big words?"

Ablestock.com/Getty Images

Learning Outcomes

Upon completion of this chapter, you will be able to:

1.1 Summarize the purpose of **medical language.**

1.2 Summarize the origins of **medical language.**

1.3 Summarize the principles of **medical language.**

1.4 Summarize how to pronounce terms associated with **medical language.**

1.5 Identify the parts used to build **medical language.**

1.6 Summarize how to put together **medical terms.**

1.7 Describe how **medical terms** are translated.

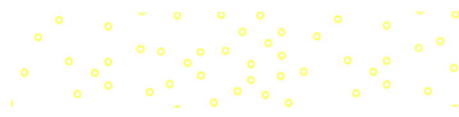

1.1 The Purpose of Medical Language

Why Is Medical Language Necessary?

"Why did you have to use all those big words?" is a good question. Why is medical language necessary? Following are a few reasons why medical language is both necessary and useful.

First, medical language allows health care professionals to be **clear.** Ours is a multicultural society. Many languages are spoken, each with their own words for illnesses and body parts. By using medical language, health care professionals are able to communicate and understand one another clearly, no matter what their first language is.

Second, medical language allows health care professionals to communicate **quickly.** Think about how this works in English. Instead of saying "a tall thing in the yard with green leaves," we just use the word "*tree.*" Instead of saying "a meal made up of a few slices of meat and cheese, topped with lettuce, mustard, and mayonnaise, and placed between two slices of bread," we just say "*sandwich.*" Instead of having to use valuable time describing the symptoms of a disease or the findings of an examination, a health care professional uses medical language in order to be clear and easily understandable to other health care professionals.

Third, medical language allows health care professionals to **comfort** patients. This reason might seem kind of odd, but it is true. When patients first enter a health care facility, they often don't feel well and are a little confused and worried about what is going on. Using medical language reassures patients that the health care professionals know what is going on and are in control. Sometimes a patient can be calmed and reassured that everything is OK by a health care professional repeating the same symptoms the patient reported—in medical language.

For example, one of us once saw a doctor about a rapid heart rate. The doctor was very reassuring—it was just "tachycardia." The doctor, however, didn't know he was talking to someone who was familiar with medical language. *Tachycardia* breaks down to *tachy* (fast, as in a car's *tachometer* reports the engine's revolutions per minute) + *card* (heart) + *ia* (condition). It literally means *fast heart condition.* The doctor was just repeating what he had heard.

Here's another example. Once, a young boy was sick and his doctors performed a series of tests to find out what was wrong. After receiving the test reports, the boy's parents were reassured. The doctors had diagnosed their child with an "idiopathic blood disorder." The diagnosis was enough for them.

Because the doctors had attached a fancy medical term to their son's condition, the parents figured the doctors knew what was wrong and how to treat it. In truth, the doctors hadn't told them anything. *Idiopathic* breaks down to *idio* (private or alone) + *pathic* (disease or suffering). It literally means *suffering alone.* The boy's condition was something the doctors had never seen before.

Medical language enables health care professionals to communicate quickly and easily no matter what their specific specialty or native language.
Jupiterimages/Getty Images

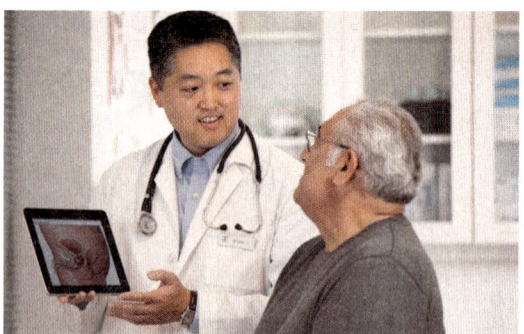
Medical language is able to reassure patients that health care professionals know what is going on and are in control.
Ariel Skelley/Blend Images LLC

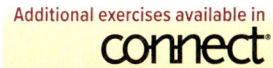
EXERCISE 1 Multiple-choice questions. Select the correct answer.

1. Which of the following is NOT a reason why medical language is necessary and useful?
   a. Medical language allows health care professionals to be clear.
   b. Medical language allows health care professionals to comfort patients.
   c. Medical language allows health care professionals to communicate quickly.
   d. Medical language allows health care professionals to intimidate their patients.

2. Medical language allows health care professionals to be clear because
   a. few people really understand medical terminology, so at least everyone is speaking the same way
   b. health care professionals are in control of the situation and don't want to scare patients with a language that they could understand
   c. we live in a multicultural society with a variety of languages, and medical language is a way of speaking the same way about the same thing despite your native language
   d. none of these

3. Medical language allows health care professionals to communicate quickly because
   a. it is a quick way to speak to other health care professionals without taking the time to describe symptoms or examine findings
   b. the patients are usually baffled by the terminology and do not ask additional questions
   c. words with many syllables always communicate more information than words with few syllables
   d. none of these

4. Medical language allows health care professionals to comfort patients because
   a. it communicates a sense that the health care professionals are in control of the situation
   b. it lets the patients know that the health care professionals are not caught off guard by the symptoms at hand
   c. it lets the patients know that the health care professionals know what is going on
   d. all of these

1.2 The Origins of Medical Language

Where Does It Come From?

Medical language is made up primarily (but not exclusively) of words taken from two ancient languages: Greek and Latin. Other words creep in from other sources, but Greek and Latin serve as the foundation of medical language.

Some of these other sources include:

Eponyms. The word *eponym* is derived from the Greek words *epi* (upon) + *onyma* (name). It literally means *to put your name on something.* Thus, an eponym is a word formed by including the name of the person who discovered or invented whatever is being described. Sometimes, in the case of diseases, an eponym is named in honor of the disease's first or most noteworthy diagnosed victim.

This reminds us of a great old joke.

A doctor says to a patient, "I have good news and bad news. Which do you want first?"

The patient responds, "The good news."

The doctor replies, "Well, you are about to have a disease named after you."

One famous eponym is Lou Gehrig's disease. The neurological disease was named after the famous New York Yankees first baseman who suffered from the disease. The disease's scientific name is *amyotrophic lateral sclerosis.*

Acronyms. The word *acronym* is derived from the Greek words *acro* (high, end) + *onyma* (name). It literally means *to make a name with the ends.* Thus, an acronym is a word made up of the first letters of each of the words that make up a phrase. One example is the diagnostic imaging process called *magnetic resonance imaging,* or MRI. Remember that acronyms are just shorthand—you still need to know what the words mean.

Modern languages. Frequently, words from modern languages creep into the vocabulary of health care professionals. These words tend to come from whatever language happens to be most commonly spoken by the majority of health care professionals. In centuries past, German or French were the most common languages, so they were the foundation of many medical terms. Currently, the fastest-growing and most-used language in the world is English. Thus, English has also contributed a fair number of medical terms.

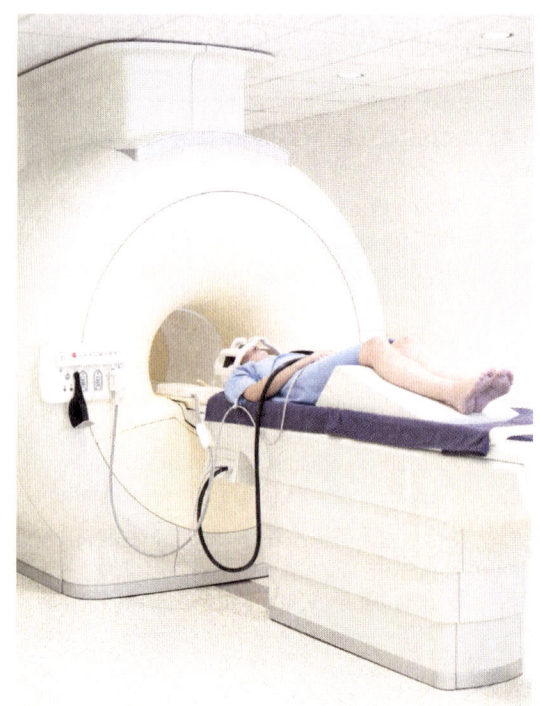

MRI, which stands for *magnetic resonance imaging,* is an example of an acronym.

Martin Barraud/Getty Images

Why Greek and Latin?

Although the three previously mentioned sources have contributed a significant number of words to the language of medicine, Greek and Latin make up its foundation and backbone. Even *eponym* and *acronym* were derived from Greek! But why are Greek and Latin so prevalent? There are at least three reasons why.

Reason 1: The foundations of Western medicine were in ancient Greece and Rome. The first people to systematically study the human body and develop theories about health and disease were the ancient Greeks. The Hippocratic Oath, the foundation of modern medical ethical codes, is named after and was possibly composed by a man named Hippocrates who lived in Greece from about 460 BC to about 370 BC. Hippocrates is widely considered to be the father of Western medicine.

The development of the health care profession began in ancient Greece and continued in ancient Rome. There, Galen, who lived from AD 129 to about AD 217, made some of the greatest advancements of our understanding of the human body, how disease affects it, and how drugs work.

Medical advances began to occur with greater frequency during the scientific revolution, adding to an already existing body of knowledge based on ancient Greek and Latin. In fact, some of the oldest terms have been in use for more than 2,000 years, such as terms for the skin, because these body parts were more easily viewed and studied.

Reason 2: Latin was the global language of the scientific revolution. The scientific revolution took place from the 16th through the 18th century. It was a time of enormous discoveries in physics, biology, chemistry, and human anatomy. This period saw a rapid increase in human knowledge thanks to the scientific method, which is a set of techniques developed in this period and still in use today using observation and experimentation for developing, testing, and proving or disproving hypotheses.

Medical research involving many different subjects, peoples, and places occurred all over Europe.

To allow people from England, Italy, Spain, Poland, and elsewhere to talk with one another, Latin became the language of scholarly discussion. It was already the common language of the Holy Roman Empire and Catholic Church, so many people already knew it well.

By using Latin to record and spread news of their discoveries, scientists of this time were able to share their new knowledge beyond the borders of their countries. At the same time, the number of medical words that sprang from Latin grew.

Reason 3: Dead languages don't change. "Fine," you think. "The language of medicine is based on Greek and Latin. But why do we keep using it? No one speaks either of these languages anymore. Why don't we just use English?"

The reason we keep using Greek and Latin is exactly that—no one speaks them anymore. All spoken languages change over time. Take the English word *green,* for instance, and its non-color-related meaning. In the past 20 or so years, the word *green* has become understood to mean *environmentally responsible,* as in the phrase *green energy.* Before that, the term was widely understood to mean something different: *immature* or *inexperienced,* such as "I just started this job, so I am still a little *green.*" Dead languages, which aren't spoken anymore, have an advantage because they don't change. There is no worry that words will change their meaning over time.

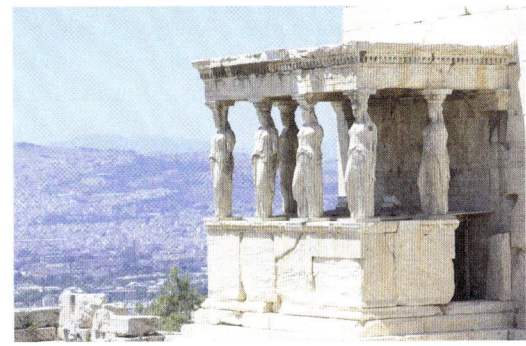

The foundations of Western medicine were laid in Greece and Rome.
Marco Simoni/Getty Images

Learning Outcome 1.2 Exercises

EXERCISE 1 True or false questions. Indicate true answers with a T and false answers with an F.

1. Medical language is made up primarily, but not exclusively, of words taken from two ancient languages: Greek and Latin. _____

2. Some other sources of medical language include eponyms, acronyms, and modern languages. _____

3. An example of an eponym is a medical term named after a famous patient who had the disease. _____

4. *MRI* is an example of an eponym. _____

5. Acronyms are used to say things more quickly. _____

6. Greek and Latin provide the basis of the language of medicine because Western medicine has its foundations in the Greek and Roman cultures. _____

7. The first people to systematically study the human body and develop theories about health and disease were the ancient Greeks. _____

8. Even though German was the global language of the scientific revolution, the Catholic Church forced all academics to use Latin, a language unknown to most people. _____

9. During the scientific revolution, Latin was used as the language of scholarly discussion in order to allow people across Europe to share their knowledge more quickly despite their different native languages. _____

10. A dead language is a language that people do not like to hear or speak anymore because it is no longer useful to a society. _____

11. Latin and Greek provide an excellent basis for medical terminology because dead languages do not change. _____

1.3 The Principles of Medical Language

How Does It Work?

Don't think of medical language as words to be memorized. Instead, they are sentences to be translated.[1]

Each medical word is a description of some aspect of health care. Think of it this way: If you were taking a trip to another country, you might try to memorize a few key words or phrases. It might be useful to know how to say common things such as "Where is the bathroom?" or "How much does this cost?" But if you were going to live in that country for a while, you wouldn't just try to memorize a few stock phrases, you would try to learn the language so you could understand what other people were saying.

The same is true of medical language. If you understand the way the language works, you will be able not only to know the meaning of a few individual words but also to break down and understand words you have never seen before, and even generate words on your own.

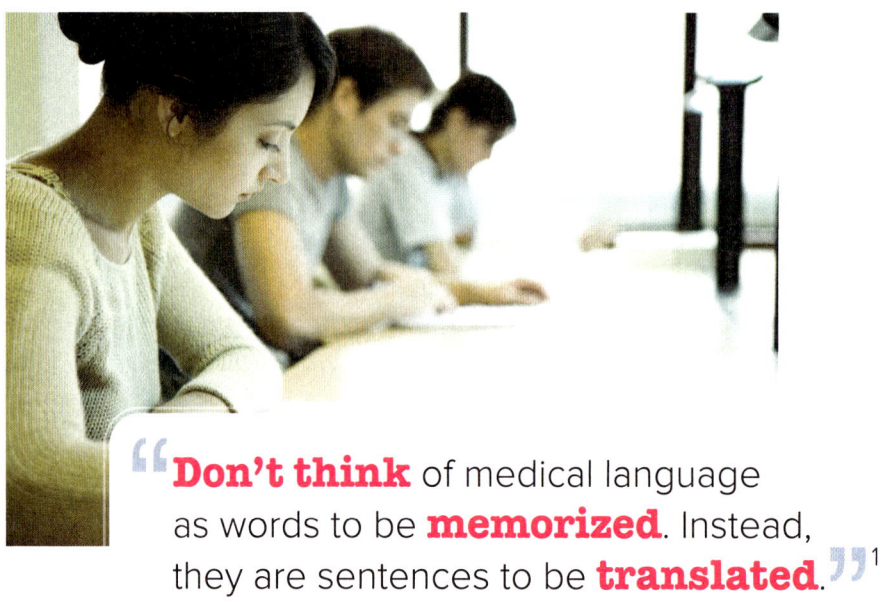

"**Don't think** of medical language as words to be **memorized**. Instead, they are sentences to be **translated**."[1]

S. Olsson/PhotoAlto

1.4 How to Pronounce Terms Associated with Medical Language

The first step in learning any language is learning correct pronunciation. Like any other language, knowing and understanding medical terminology is useless unless you pronounce the terms correctly. With medical terms, the matter is complicated by two facts: First, many of the words come from foreign languages (and not just any foreign languages, but foreign languages no one speaks anymore). Second, some of the words are really long.

You probably have noticed the way native speakers of other languages pronounce certain letters differently. Think of the word *tortilla*. It takes a

---

[1] For more on this concept, see Lesley A. Dean-Jones, "Teaching Medical Terminology as a Classics Course," *Classical Journal* 93 (1998), pp. 290–96.

bit of experience with Spanish to know that two *l*s placed together (*ll*) are pronounced like a *y*. You say *tor-TEE-yah,* not *tor-TILL-ah.* The Spanish word for yellow, *amarillo,* follows this rule. It is pronounced ah-mah-REE-yoh. But the Texas town of the same name is pronounced very differently: am-ah-RIL-oh.

The same is true for medical language. The best way to learn terms is by encountering them in context. Once you get a little experience with the language, you will pick up the unique ways that certain letters are pronounced. In the meantime, refer to the accompanying chart of some commonly mispronounced letters.

LETTER	SOUND	EXAMPLE
c (before *a, o, u*)	k	*cardiac* (KAR-dee-ak) *contra* (KON-trah) *cut* (KUT)
c (before *e, i, y*)	s	*cephalic* (seh-FAL-ik) *cilium* (SIL-ee-um) *cyst* (SIST)
ch	k	*chiropractor* (KAI-roh-PRAK-tor)
g (before *a, o, u*)	g	*gamma* (GAM-ah) *goiter* (GOI-ter) *gutta* (GUT-tah)
g (before *e, i, y*)	j	*genetic* (jeh-NEH-tik) *giant* (JAI-int) *biology* (bai-AW-loh-jee)
ph	f	*pharmacy* (FAR-mah-see)
pn	n	*pneumonia* (noo-MOHN-yah)
pt (initial)	t	*pterigium* (tir-IH-jee-um)
rh, rrh	r	*rhinoplasty* (RAI-noh-PLAS-tee) *hemorrhage* (HEH-moh-rij)
x (initial)	z	*xeroderma* (ZER-oh-DER-mah)

Syllable Emphasis

Every medical term is constructed from syllables. Another thing that can affect the way words are pronounced is which syllable or syllables should be stressed, or emphasized. You must always make sure to put the emphasis on the correct syllable.

For example, consider that last phrase: *Put the emphasis on the right syllable.* The correct way to pronounce it would be:

> PUT the EM-fah-sis on the RAIT SIL-ah-bul.

It would sound funny to say:

> PUT the em-FAH-sis on the RAIT si-LAH-bul.

Knowing which syllable to emphasize can seem tricky but is actually pretty easy. Usually, for the sake of emphasis, the only syllables that you need to focus on are the last three syllables. So, starting at the end of the word, count back three syllables.

When it comes to emphasizing the correct syllable, the basic rule is this: In most words, the emphasis usually falls on the third-to-last syllable (the *antepenult,* if you are keeping track).

Cardiac is split into three syllables: car / di / ac.

Count backward three syllables from the end of the word to figure out which syllable gets emphasized: *car.*

Therefore, the word is pronounced **KAR** / dee / ak.

Cardiology is split into five syllables: car / di / o / lo / gy.

Count backward three syllables from the end of the word to figure out which syllable gets emphasized: *o.*

Therefore, the word is pronounced kar / dee / **AW** / loh / jee.

It gets tricky when a word remains unchanged except for the addition or subtraction of only a few letters.

Two good examples are the words *colonoscopy* and *colonoscope.*

Colonoscopy is split into five syllables: co / lon / o / sco / py.

Count backward three syllables from the end of the word to figure out which syllable gets emphasized: *o.*

Therefore, the word is pronounced koh / lon / **AW** / skoh / pee.

Colonoscope is split into four syllables: co / lon / o / scope.

Count backward three syllables from the end of the word to figure out which syllable gets emphasized: *lon.*

Therefore, the word is pronounced koh / **LAWN** / oh / skohp.

Notice how easy it is to spot the pronunciation change if you focus on counting backward from the end of the word?

As with any rule, there are countless exceptions and technicalities. That said, the easiest way to master pronunciation is not to learn countless rules, but instead to *practice pronouncing words.* Learn this one rule—let's call it the three-syllable rule—and make sure you take note of the pronunciations offered throughout the chapters. Don't just read them silently! Pronounce the words out loud. The more times you practice saying a word, the more comfortable and natural you will feel when you have to use it for real.

But make sure you are pronouncing correctly. Practice does *not* make perfect; practice makes permanent. Whatever you do over and over will be cemented in your brain, so make sure you do it right. *Perfect* practice makes perfect.

Learning Outcome 1.4 Exercises

EXERCISE 1   Identify the correct pronunciation for the underlined syllable.

EXAMPLE: thoracocentesis   *answer: koh (the c is hard because it is followed by an o)*

thoracentesis   *answer: sin (the c is soft because it is followed by an i)*

_____	1. **gut**	a. jut	b. gut
_____	2. di**git**	a. jit	b. git
_____	3. **gag** reflex	a. jag	b. gag
_____	4. dermatolo**gy**	a. jee	b. gee
_____	5. **gen**eticist	a. jen	b. gen
_____	6. **go**nad	a. joh	b. goh
_____	7. colla**gen**	a. jen	b. gen
_____	8. **phar**macist	a. par	b. far
_____	9. **cu**ticle	a. kyoo	b. suh
_____	10. **cor**nea	a. kor	b. sor
_____	11. **cath**eter	a. kath	b. sath
_____	12. on**co**logy	a. kaw	b. saw

_____	13. genet**icist**	a. kist	b. sist
_____	14. pharma**cist**	a. kist	b. sist
_____	15. **cyst**ic fibrosis	a. kis	b. sis
_____	16. **chol**era	a. kawl	b. chohl
_____	17. psy**chos**is	a. koh	b. choh
_____	18. pneumato**cele**	a. keel	b. seel
_____	19. **rheu**matoid arthritis	a. roo	b. rhee-yoo
_____	20. **pneu**matocele	a. noo	b. puh-noo
_____	21. **pter**ion	a. tir	b. puh-tir
_____	22. **xer**osis	a. zer	b. ex-er
_____	23. en**ceph**alitis	a. kep	b. sef
_____	24. **cirrho**sis	a. kir-hoh	b. sir-oh

EXERCISE 2   Indicate which syllable(s) is emphasized when pronounced.

> EXAMPLE: bronchitis bron**chi**tis

1. cholera _____
2. cornea _____
3. cuticle _____
4. catheter _____
5. collagen _____
6. anemia _____
7. oncology _____
8. optometry _____
9. rheumatoid _____
10. geneticist _____
11. dermatology _____
12. psychotherapist _____

1.5 Parts Used to Build Medical Language

Just as any language has nouns, verbs, and adjectives, the language of medicine is made up of three main building blocks: roots, suffixes, and prefixes. Medical language is constructed by combining a root with a suffix and often a prefix.

> Root—foundation or subject of the term
>
> Suffix—ending that gives essential meaning to the term
>
> Prefix—added to the beginning of a term when needed to further modify the root

Common Roots

A root is the foundation of any medical term. Roots function like nouns in the language of medicine. It is the base, or subject, of a word—it is what the word is about. Most roots refer to things such as body parts, organs, and fluids.

There are a few types of roots in medical language. In the roots that follow, notice that a slash divides the last letter from the rest of the word (as in *arthr/o*). The final letter in these roots is called a *combining vowel;* these are discussed in detail later in the chapter. For now, just know that the final letter occurs in some words and not in others. Whenever possible, the examples provided include some words that have, and some that don't have, the combining vowel. Don't worry about what the example words mean. This is just to get you used to seeing the roots in context.

Some meanings have only one potential root.

ROOT	DEFINITION	EXAMPLES
cardi/o KAR-dee-oh	heart	*cardiology, pericardium*
gastr/o GAS-tro	stomach	*gastrointestinal, gastritis*

Some meanings have a few similar-sounding potential roots. Why? Some suffixes just sound better when attached to another root. Look at the examples in the chart below and switch the roots around—*hematorrhage* and *hemoma.* The meanings are the same, but they sure sound funny.

ROOT	DEFINITION	EXAMPLES
hem/o HEE-moh	blood	*hemorrhage*
hemat/o heh-MAH-toh		*hematoma*

Some meanings have a couple of potential roots that are completely different but mean the same thing. This is because one word comes from Greek and the other comes from Latin. Normally, however, one of the

ROOT	DEFINITION	EXAMPLES
arthr/o AR-throh	joint	*arthroscope, arthritis*

roots is much more commonly used than the other. Of the roots below, *myo* is used much more often than *musculo*.

ROOT	DEFINITION	EXAMPLES
my/o MAI-oh	muscle	*myocardial, myalgia*
muscul/o MUS-kyoo-loh		*musculoskeletal, muscular*

Some meanings have several potential roots that mean the same thing. Some are similar, and some are completely different. These are basically a combination of the two previous categories. These meanings each have a couple of similar roots *as well as* at least one root from Greek and one from Latin.

ROOT	DEFINITION	EXAMPLES
derm/o DER-moh	skin	*dermoscopy, dermis*
dermat/o der-MAT-oh		*dermatology, dermatitis*
cutane/o kyoo-TAY-nee-oh		*subcutaneous*
pneum/o NOO-moh	lung	*pneumotomy*

ROOT	DEFINITION	EXAMPLES
pneumon/o noo-MAW-noh	lung	*pneumonia, pneumonitis*
pulmon/o PUL-maw-noh		*pulmonologist, cardiopulmonary*

Question: Why doesn't each meaning have only one potential root?

Answer: The main reason multiple roots are available is to provide *options*. Some suffixes simply sound better or are easier to say when they are combined with one root rather than another.

GENERAL PURPOSE ROOTS

This list contains roots that will recur often in subsequent chapters. It is important to learn these roots now.

ROOT	DEFINITION	EXAMPLES
gen/o JIN-oh	creation, cause	*pathogenic*
hydr/o HAI-droh	water	*hydrophobia, dehydration* Brand X Pictures/ Getty Images
morph/o MOR-foh	shape, change	*morphology*
myc/o MAI-koh	fungus	*dermatomycosis*
necr/o NEK-roh	death	*necrosis*
orth/o OR-thoh	straight	*orthodontist*
path/o PAH-thoh	suffering, disease	*pathology*
phag/o FAY-goh	eat	*aphagia*
plas/o PLAS-oh	formation	*hyperplasia*
py/o PAI-oh	pus	*pyorrhea, pyemia*
scler/o SKLEH-roh	hard	*scleroderma*

ROOT	DEFINITION	EXAMPLES
sten/o STIH-noh	narrowing	stenosis kalus/Getty Images
troph/o TROH-foh	nourishment, development	trophology, hypertrophy
xen/o ZEE-noh	foreign	xenograft
xer/o ZEH-roh	dry	xerosis, xerasia

SUFFIX	DEFINITION	EXAMPLES
-ic ik		medic
-ous us		subcutaneous
-tic tik		neurotic

Noun. All these suffixes turn the root they are added to into nouns.

SUFFIX	DEFINITION	EXAMPLES
-ia ee-ah	condition	pneumonia
-ism iz-um		autism
-ium ee-um	tissue, structure	pericardium
-y ee	condition, procedure, process	hypertrophy

Diminutive. When added to a root, these suffixes transform a term's meaning to a smaller version of the root. In English, for example, the suffix *-let* is diminutive. A *booklet* is a *little book.* In Spanish, the suffix *-ita* is diminutive. *Señora* is the Spanish word for *lady,* so *señorita* therefore means *little lady.*

SUFFIX	DEFINITION	EXAMPLES
-icle ik-el	small	ventricle
-ole ohl		arteriole
-ula yoo-lah		uvula
-ule yool		pustule

Common Suffixes

A *suffix* is a word part placed at the end of a word. The word *suffix* literally means *to attach (fix) after or below (sub,* which if you say it fast starts to sound like *suff).* As roots function as nouns, so suffixes function as verbs in the language of medicine. They describe something the root is doing or something that is happening to the root.

There are many types of suffixes in medical language. In general, they can be divided into two basic groups: simple and complex.

SIMPLE SUFFIXES

These suffixes (as their name suggests) are basic and are used to turn a root into a complete word.

Adjective. These suffixes turn the root they follow into an adjective. Thus, they all mean *pertaining to* or something similar to that.

SUFFIX	DEFINITION	EXAMPLES
-ac ak	pertaining to	cardiac
-al al		skeletal
-ar ar		muscular
-ary ar-ee		pulmonary
-eal ee-al		esophageal

COMPLEX SUFFIXES

Complex suffixes aren't necessarily more difficult to understand than simple suffixes. They just have more parts. Sometimes, these suffixes are referred to as compound or combination suffixes because the suffixes themselves are put together from other suffixes, roots, and prefixes.

Following is an example.

The suffix -y means *condition, process*, or *procedure*. When combined with *tom/o*, a root meaning *to cut*, the result is the complex suffix -*tomy*, which means *a cutting procedure* or *incision*.

tom/o (cut) + -*y* (process, procedure) = -*tomy* = a cutting procedure or incision

But you can take it a step further. If you add the prefix *ec-* to -*tomy*, you will create the complex suffix -*ectomy*, which means *to cut out* or *to surgically remove something*.

ec- (out) + *tom/o* (cut) + -*y* (process, procedure) = -*ectomy* = a cutting out procedure or surgical removal

Following are some lists of some categories of complex suffixes. Some complex suffixes are professional terms.

SUFFIX	DEFINITION	EXAMPLES
-iatrics ee-AH-triks	medical science	*pediatrics*
		 pediatrics Rido/Shutterstock
-iatry AI-ah-tree		*psychiatry*
-iatrist AI-ah-trist	specialist in medicine of	*psychiatrist*
-ist ist	specialist	*dentist*
-logist loh-jist	specialist in the study of	*psychologist*
		 psychologist Don Hammond/ Design Pics
-logy loh-jee	study of	*psychology*

Some complex suffixes describe symptoms, diseases, or conditions that are either mentioned by patients or diagnosed by health professionals.

symptoms, diseases, and conditions

SUFFIX	DEFINITION	EXAMPLES
-algia AL-jah	pain	*myalgia*
-dynia DAI-nee-ah		*gastrodynia*
-cele SEEL	hernia (a bulging of tissue into an area where it doesn't belong)	*hydrocele*
-emia EE-mee-ah	blood condition	*leukemia* **leukemia** Steve Gschmeissner/ Science Source
-iasis AI-ah-sis	presence of	*lithiasis*
-itis AI-tis	inflammation	*arthritis*
-lysis lih-sis	loosen, break down	*hemolysis*
-malacia mah-LAY-shah	abnormal softening	*osteomalacia*
-megaly MEH-gah-lee	enlargement	*hepatomegaly*
-oid OYD	resembling	*keloid*
-oma OH-mah	tumor	*melanoma* **melanoma** Source: National Cancer Institute (NCI)
-osis OH-sis	condition	*thrombosis*

symptoms, diseases, and conditions *continued*

SUFFIX	DEFINITION	EXAMPLES
-pathy pah-thee	disease	myopathy
-penia PEE-nee-ah	deficiency	leukopenia
-ptosis puh-TOH-sis	drooping	nephroptosis
-rrhage RIJ	excessive flow	hemorrhage
-rrhagia RAY-jee-ah		menorrhagia
-rrhea REE-ah	flow	diarrhea
-rrhexis REK-sis	rupture	metrorrhexis
-spasm SPAZ-um	involuntary contraction	myospasm

Some complex suffixes describe tests and treatments performed by health professionals. Although it is convenient to place tests and treatments in the same category and label them as "procedures," it is important to distinguish between the two. A *test* is a *procedure done to gain more information in order to diagnose a problem.* A *treatment* is a *process done after a diagnosis to fix a problem.*

tests

SUFFIX	DEFINITION	EXAMPLES
-centesis sin-TEE-sis	puncture	amniocentesis
-gram gram	written record	cardiogram
		Stockbyte/Getty Images
-graph graf	instrument used to produce a record	cardiograph
-graphy grah-fee	process of recording	cardiography
-meter mee-ter	instrument used to measure	cephalometer

tests *continued*

SUFFIX	DEFINITION	EXAMPLES
-metry meh-tree	process of measuring	cephalometry
-scope skohp	instrument used to look	arthroscope
-scopy skoh-pee	process of looking	arthroscopy

treatments

SUFFIX	DEFINITION	EXAMPLES
-desis DEE-sis	binding, fixation	arthrodesis
-ectomy EK-toh-mee	removal	vasectomy
-pexy PEK-see	surgical fixation	retinopexy
-plasty PLAS-tee	reconstruction	rhinoplasty
-rrhaphy rah-fee	suture	herniorrhaphy
-stomy stoh-mee	creation of an opening	colostomy
-tomy toh-mee	incision	dermotomy

SINGULARS AND PLURALS

In English, the most common way to turn a word from singular to plural is to add an "s." The plural of *bag* is *bags,* for example. But there are other ways too. The plural of *goose* is *geese.* The plural of *mouse* is *mice.* The plural of *ox* is *oxen.* The plural of *sheep* is *sheep.*

The same is true for medical terms. Because medical words come from different languages, singular words become plural in a variety of ways.

SINGULAR	PLURAL	EXAMPLES	
-a	-ae	vertebra larva	vertebrae larvae
-ax	-aces	thorax	thoraces
-ex	-ices	cortex	cortices
-ix	-ices	appendix	appendices
-is	-es	neurosis diagnosis	neuroses diagnoses
-ma	-mata	sarcoma carcinoma	sarcomata carcinomata
-on	-a	spermatozoon ganglion	spermatozoa ganglia
-um	-a	datum bacterium ovum	data bacteria ova
-us	-i	nucleus alveolus thrombus	nuclei alveoli thrombi
-y	-ies	biopsy myopathy	biopsies myopathies

Common Prefixes

A *prefix* is a word part placed at the beginning of a word. The word *prefix* literally means *to attach (fix) before (pre)*. Prefixes function like adjectives in the language of medicine. They supply additional information as needed. In the same way that not every sentence has an adjective, not every medical term has a prefix.

There are many types of prefixes in medical language. Following are a few examples.

NEGATION PREFIXES
Some prefixes negate things:

negation		
PREFIX	**MEANING**	**EXAMPLES**
a- ay	not	aphasia
an- an		anemia
anti- AN-tee	against	antibiotics

negation *continued*		
PREFIX	**MEANING**	**EXAMPLES**
contra- KON-trah	against	contraceptive
de- dee	down, away from	dehydration

TIME OR SPEED PREFIXES
Some prefixes describe time or speed:

time/speed		
PREFIX	**MEANING**	**EXAMPLES**
ante- an-tee	before	antepartum
pre- pree		precondition
pro- proh	before, on behalf of	probiotic

probiotic

Bob Coyle/
McGraw-Hill Higher
Education

post- pohst	after	postpartum
brady- brah-dih	slow	bradycardia
tachy- tak-ih	fast	tachycardia
re- ree	again	rehabilitation

DIRECTION OR POSITION PREFIXES
Some prefixes describe direction or position:

direction/position		
PREFIX	**MEANING**	**EXAMPLES**
ab- ab	away	abduct
ad- ad	toward	adrenaline
circum- sir-kum	around	circumcision
peri- per-ee		pericardium

direction/position *continued*

PREFIX	MEANING	EXAMPLES
dia- dai-ah	through	*diagnostic*
trans- tranz		*translate*
e- eh	out	*evoke*
ec- ek		*ectopic*
ex- eks		*exhale*
ecto- ek-toh	outside	*ectoderm*
exo- ek-soh		*exoskeleton*
extra- eks-trah		*extracorporeal*
en- en	in, inside	*enema*
endo- en-doh		*endocrine*
intra- in-trah		*intravenous*

intravenous

mmmx/123RF

PREFIX	MEANING	EXAMPLES
epi- eh-pee	upon	*epididymus*
inter- in-ter	between	*intercostal*
sub- sub	beneath	*subcutaneous*

SIZE OR QUANTITY PREFIXES

Some prefixes describe size or quantity:

size/quantity

PREFIX	MEANING	EXAMPLES
bi- bai	two	*bilateral*
hemi- heh-mee	half	*hemiplegia*
semi- seh-mee		*semilunar*

size/quantity *continued*

PREFIX	MEANING	EXAMPLES
hyper- hai-per	over	*hyperthermia*
hypo- hai-poh	under	*hypothermia*
macro- mak-roh	large	*macrotia*
micro- mai-kroh	small	*microdontia*
mono- maw-noh	one	*monocyte*
uni- yoo-nee		*unisex*
oligo- aw-lih-goh	few	*oligomenorrhea*
pan- pan	all	*pancytopenia*
poly- pawlee	many	*polygraph*
multi- mul-tee		*multicellular*

GENERAL PREFIXES

Some prefixes are general:

general

PREFIX	MEANING	EXAMPLES
con- kon	with, together	*congestion*

congestion

iStockphoto/Getty Images

PREFIX	MEANING	EXAMPLES
sym- sim		*symmetry*
syn- sin		*syndrome*
dys- dis	bad	*dysentery*
eu- yoo	good	*euphoria*

EXERCISE 1 Match the root on the left with its definition on the right.

_____ 1. gen/o   a. shape, change

_____ 2. necr/o   b. creation, cause

_____ 3. xer/o   c. death

_____ 4. morph/o   d. dry

_____ 5. troph/o   e. eat

_____ 6. plas/o   f. foreign

_____ 7. sten/o   g. formation

_____ 8. phag/o   h. narrowing

_____ 9. xen/o   i. nourishment, development

EXERCISE 2 Translate the following roots.

1. hydr/o _____

2. orth/o _____

3. necr/o _____

4. myc/o _____

5. py/o _____

6. xer/o _____

7. path/o _____

8. scler/o _____

9. phag/o _____

10. xen/o _____

EXERCISE 3 Underline and define the roots in the following terms.

1. morphology _____

2. dysplasia _____

3. hypertrophic _____

4. teratogenic _____

5. mycosis _____

6. craniostenosis _____

EXER...

1. water _____

2. creation, cause _____

3. pus _____

4. straight _____

5. fungus _____

6. suffering, disease _____

7. hard _____

8. formation _____

EXERCISE 5 Match the suffix on the left with its definition on the right. Some definitions will be used more than once.

_____ 1. -ium   a. condition

_____ 2. -icle   b. pertaining to

_____ 3. -ous   c. tissue, structure

_____ 4. -ac   d. small

_____ 5. -ia

_____ 6. -eal

EXERCISE 6 Translate the following suffixes.

1. -y _____

2. -ism _____

3. -al _____

4. -ic, -tic _____

5. -ar, -ary _____

6. -ole, -ule, -ula _____

EXERCISE 7 Underline and define the suffix in the following terms.

1. cardiac _____

2. gastric _____

_____

3. nei _____

4. sl _____

5. _____

6ular _____

.eous _____

.rteriole _____

11. ventricle _____

12. pustule _____

13. uvula _____

14. pneumonia _____

15. autism _____

16. pericardium _____

17. hypertrophy _____

EXERCISE 8 Match the suffix on the left with its definition on the right. Some definitions will be used more than once.

_____ 1. -logy

_____ 2. -logist

_____ 3. -ist

_____ 4. -iatrist

_____ 5. -iatry

a. medical science

b. specialist

c. specialist in the medicine of

d. specialist in the study of

e. study of

EXERCISE 9 Identify the suffixes for the following definitions.

1. tissue, structure _____

2. condition, process, procedure _____

3. condition (3 possible options) _____

4. small or any suffix that makes the root a diminutive, or smaller, version of the root (choose 3 of the 4 possible options)

_____

5. pertaining to (or any suffix that makes a root into an adjective) (choose 4 of the 8 possible options) _____

EXERCISE 10 Translate the following suffixes.

1. -logy _____

2. -logist _____

3. -ist _____

4. -iatrist _____

5. -iatry _____

6. -iatrics _____

EXERCISE 11 Underline and define the suffix in the following terms.

1. cardiology _____

2. cardiologist _____

3. pathology _____

4. pathologist _____

5. psychology _____

6. psychologist _____

7. dentist _____

8. psychiatry _____

9. psychiatrist _____

10. pediatrics _____

EXERCISE 12 Identify the suffixes for the following definitions.

1. specialist _____

2. specialist in the study of _____

3. study of _____

4. specialist in the medicine of _____

5. medical science (2 suffixes) _____

EXERCISE 13 Match the suffix on the left with its definition on the right. Some definitions will be used more than once.

_____ 1. -oid   a. deficiency

_____ 2. -iasis   b. drooping

_____ 3. -cele   c. flow

_____ 4. -penia   d. hernia

_____ 5. -rrhea   e. loosen, break down

_____ 6. -lysis   f. presence of

_____ 7. -ptosis   g. resembling

_____ 8. -rrhexis   h. rupture

EXERCISE 14 Translate the following suffixes.

1. -spasm _____

2. -megaly _____

3. -oma _____

4. -emia _____

5. -itis _____

6. -osis _____

7. -pathy _____

8. -algia _____

9. -dynia _____

10. -malacia _____

11. -rrhage, -rrhagia _____

EXERCISE 15 Underline and define the suffix in the following terms.

1. myospasm _____

2. myopathy _____

3. cardiomegaly _____

4. gastritis _____

5. gastralgia _____

6. gastrodynia _____

7. gastromalacia _____

8. hematoma _____

9. melanoma _____

10. hemolysis _____

11. hemorrhage _____

12. hydrocele _____

13. leukopenia _____

14. stenosis _____

EXERCISE 16 Identify the suffixes for the following definitions.

1. tumor _____

2. resembling _____

3. blood condition _____

4. presence of _____

5. deficiency _____

6. hernia _____

7. drooping _____

8. flow _____

9. rupture _____

EXERCISE 17 Match the suffix on the left with its definition on the right. Some definitions will be used more than once.

_____ 1. -meter   a. instrument used to look

_____ 2. -metry   b. instrument used to measure

_____ 3. -scope   c. instrument used to produce a record

_____ 4. -scopy   d. process of looking

_____ 5. -graph   e. process of measuring

_____ 6. -graphy   f. process of recording

_____ 7. -gram   g. puncture

_____ 8. -centesis   h. written record

Learning Outcome 1.5 Exercises

EXERCISE 18   Translate the following suffixes.

1. -meter _____

2. -metry _____

3. -scope _____

4. -scopy _____

5. -graph _____

6. -graphy _____

7. -gram _____

8. -centesis _____

EXERCISE 19   Underline and define the suffix in the following terms.

1. audiogram _____

2. audiograph _____

3. audiometer _____

4. gastroscope _____

5. audiography _____

6. audiometry _____

7. gastroscopy _____

8. ovariocentesis _____

EXERCISE 20   Identify the suffixes for the following definitions.

1. instrument used to look _____

2. process of looking _____

3. instrument used to measure _____

_____

4. process of measuring _____

5. written record _____

6. instrument used to produce a record _____

_____

7. process of recording _____

8. puncture _____

EXERCISE 21   Match the suffix on the left with its definition on the right.

_____ 1. -plasty   a. binding

_____ 2. -tomy   b. creation of an opening

_____ 3. -ectomy   c. incision

_____ 4. -stomy   d. reconstruction

_____ 5. -pexy   e. removal

_____ 6. -desis   f. surgical fixation

_____ 7. -rrhaphy   g. suture

EXERCISE 22   Translate the following suffixes.

1. -plasty _____

2. -tomy _____

3. -ectomy _____

4. -stomy _____

5. -pexy _____

6. -desis _____

7. -rrhaphy _____

EXERCISE 23   Underline and define the suffix in the following terms.

1. myoplasty _____

2. tracheotomy _____

3. tracheostomy _____

4. gastrectomy _____

5. gastropexy _____

6. myodesis _____

7. myorrhaphy _____

EXERCISE 24   Identify the suffixes for the following definitions.

1. reconstruction _____

2. removal _____

3. incision _____

4. creation of an opening _____

5. surgical fixation _____

6. binding _____

7. suture _____

EXERCISE 25 Match the singular suffix on the left with the suffix that will make the same term plural on the right. Some plural suffixes will be used more than once.

Singular		**Plural**	
_____	1. -ax	a. -a	
_____	2. -ix	b. -aces	
_____	3. -ex	c. -ae	
_____	4. -ma	d. -es	
_____	5. -is	e. -i	
_____	6. -a	f. -ices	
_____	7. -um	g. -ies	
_____	8. -on	h. -mata	
_____	9. -y		
_____	10. -us		

EXERCISE 26 Match the prefix on the left with its definition on the right. Some definitions will be used more than once.

_____	1. pre-	a. after	
_____	2. post-	b. again	
_____	3. re-	c. against	
_____	4. contra-	d. before	
_____	5. anti-	e. before, on behalf of	
_____	6. pro-	f. down, away from	
_____	7. de-	g. fast	
_____	8. a-	h. not	
_____	9. an-	i. slow	
_____	10. ante-		
_____	11. tachy-		
_____	12. brady-		

EXERCISE 27 Translate the following prefixes.

1. pre- _____

2. post- _____

3. re- _____

4. contra- _____

5. anti- _____

6. pro- _____

7. de- _____

8. a- _____

9. an- _____

10. ante- _____

11. tachy- _____

12. brady- _____

EXERCISE 28 Underline and define the prefix in the following terms.

1. prenatal _____

2. postnatal _____

3. antepartum _____

4. probiotic _____

5. antibiotic _____

6. contraceptive _____

7. dehydration _____

8. rehabilitation _____

9. bradypnea _____

10. tachypnea _____

11. apnea _____

EXERCISE 29 Identify the prefixes for the following definitions.

1. again _____

2. after _____

3. slow _____

4. fast _____

5. down, away from _____

6. before, on behalf of _____

7. before (2 prefixes) _____

8. not (2 prefixes) _____

9. against (2 prefixes) _____

EXERCISE 30 Match the prefix on the left with its definition on the right. Some definitions will be used more than once.

_____ 1. ab-   a. out

_____ 2. ad-   b. around

_____ 3. peri-   c. upon

_____ 4. trans-   d. beneath

_____ 5. ec-   e. away

_____ 6. ecto-   f. between

_____ 7. extra-   g. in, inside

_____ 8. en-   h. toward

_____ 9. intra-   i. through

_____ 10. epi-   j. outside

_____ 11. sub-

_____ 12. inter-

EXERCISE 31 Translate the following prefixes.

1. sub- _____

2. inter- _____

3. circum- _____

4. dia- _____

5. ab- _____

6. ad- _____

7. epi- _____

8. e-, ec-, ex- _____

9. ecto-, exo-, extra- _____

10. en-, endo-, intra- _____

EXERCISE 32 Underline and define the prefix in the following terms.

1. transdermal _____

2. exhale _____

3. extravascular _____

4. circumcision _____

5. pericardium _____

6. pericarditis _____

7. subcutaneous _____

8. exoskeleton _____

9. ectoderm _____

10. ectopic _____

11. intercostal _____

12. intravenous _____

13. intradermal _____

14. epidermal _____

15. epicardium _____

16. endometrium _____

17. abduct _____

18. evoke _____

19. diarrhea _____

20. enuresis _____

EXERCISE 33 Identify the prefixes for the following definitions.

1. beneath _____

2. between _____

3. upon _____

4. away _____

5. toward _____

6. around (2 prefixes) _____

7. through (2 prefixes) _____

8. in, inside (3 prefixes) _____

9. out (3 prefixes) _____

10. outside (3 prefixes) _____

EXERCISE 34 Match the prefix on the left with its definition on the right. Some definitions will be used more than once.

_____ 1. bi-   a. all

_____ 2. uni-   b. few

_____ 3. multi-   c. half

_____ 4. micro-   d. large

_____ 5. macro-   e. many

_____ 6. mono-   f. one

_____ 7. poly-   g. over

_____ 8. hyper-   h. small

_____ 9. hemi-   i. two

_____ 10. hypo-   j. under

_____ 11. pan-

_____ 12. oligo-

EXERCISE 35 Translate the following prefixes.

1. bi- _____

2. uni- _____

3. multi- _____

4. micro- _____

5. macro- _____

6. mono- _____

7. poly- _____

8. hyper- _____

9. hemi- _____

10. hypo- _____

11. pan- _____

12. oligo- _____

EXERCISE 36 Underline and define the prefixes in the following terms.

1. unilateral _____

2. bilateral _____

3. monocyte _____

4. oliguria _____

5. polyuria _____

6. polygraph _____

7. hyperpnea _____

8. hypopnea _____

9. macrocephaly _____

10. microcephaly _____

11. pancytopenia _____

12. heminephrectomy _____

13. panhypopituitarism (two prefixes) _____

EXERCISE 37 Identify the prefixes for the following definitions.

1. large _____

2. small _____

3. over _____

4. under _____

5. two _____

6. all _____

7. few _____

8. one (2 prefixes) _____

9. many (2 prefixes) _____

10. half (2 prefixes) _____

EXERCISE 38 Match the prefix on the left with its definition on the right. Some definitions will be used more than once.

_____ 1. syn-   a. bad

_____ 2. sym-   b. good

_____ 3. con-   c. with, together

_____ 4. dys-

_____ 5. eu-

EXERCISE 39 Translate the following prefixes.

1. syn- _____

2. sym- _____

3. con- _____

4. dys- _____

5. eu- _____

EXERCISE 40 Underline and define the prefix in the following terms.

1. congenital _____

2. congestion _____

3. dysuria _____

4. dyspnea _____

5. eupnea _____

6. euthyroid _____

7. syndrome _____

8. symmetry _____

EXERCISE 41 Identify the prefixes for the following definitions.

1. bad _____

2. good _____

3. with, together (3 prefixes) _____

1.6 How to Put Together Medical Terms

Putting It All Together

Now you know about roots, suffixes, and prefixes. There's an additional piece that often goes unnoticed: the *combining vowel (CV)*. Take the root *cardio,* which means *heart.* That *o* on the end is optional. It is used when needed to make it easier to combine this root with other word parts. But if it is not needed, it can go away.

So when we say that a word part like *cardio* is a root, we're not speaking precisely. Technically, *cardio* is called a *combining form.* A combining form is a combination of a root with a combining vowel.

So in the example above:

cardi would be the root (which doesn't change)

o would be the combining vowel (which can come or go as needed)

cardi/o would be the combining form (the slash is there to help you tell the difference between the root and combining vowel)

Note: O is by far the most common combining vowel. The letter *i* is a distant second.

Do Use a Combining Vowel

To join a root to any suffix beginning with a consonant:

splen/o   spleen
-megaly   enlargement

ROOT	CV	SUFFIX	WORD	DEFINITION
splen	o	-megaly	splenomegaly	enlargement of the spleen

To join two roots together:

hepat/o	liver
splen/o	spleen
-megaly	enlargement

ROOT	CV	ROOT	CV	SUFFIX	WORD	DEFINITION
hepat	o	splen	o	-megaly	hepatosplenomegaly	enlargement of the liver and spleen

To join two roots together, ***even when*** *the second root begins with a vowel:*

gastr/o	stomach
enter/o	intestine
-logy	study of

ROOT	CV	ROOT	CV	SUFFIX	WORD	DEFINITION
gastr	o	enter	o	-logy	gastroenterology	study of the stomach and intestine

Don't Use a Combining Vowel

To join a root to a suffix that begins with a vowel:

hepat/o	liver
splen/o	spleen
cardi/o	heart
-ectomy	surgical removal
-itis	inflammation

ROOT	CV	SUFFIX	WORD	DEFINITION
hepat		-itis	hepatitis	inflammation of the liver
splen		-ectomy	splenectomy	surgical removal of the spleen
cardi		-itis	carditis	inflammation of the heart

Note: In the last word, the root ends with the same letter that begins the suffix (*cardi + itis*). In cases like this, you do not use a combining vowel, and you also drop the final vowel of the root.

EXERCISE 1 Indicate whether a combining vowel is necessary, and explain why or why not.

EXAMPLE:	Root	Suffix	Combining Vowel?
	splen/o	-megaly	☒ Yes (suffix begins with a consonant)
			☐ No

ROOT	SUFFIX	COMBINING VOWEL?
1. cardi/o	-gram	☐ Yes _____
		☐ No _____
2. gastr/o	-scope	☐ Yes _____
		☐ No _____
3. cardi/o	-logist	☐ Yes _____
		☐ No _____
4. cardi/o	-megaly	☐ Yes _____
		☐ No _____
5. gastr/o	-ic	☐ Yes _____
		☐ No _____
6. cardi/o	-itis	☐ Yes _____
		☐ No _____
7. gastr/o	-itis	☐ Yes _____
		☐ No _____
8. cardi/o + my/o	-tomy	☐ Yes _____
		☐ No _____

EXERCISE 2 Build a medical term from the information provided.

EXAMPLE:	Root	Suffix	Term
	splen/o	-megaly	splenomegaly

ROOT	SUFFIX	TERM
1. cardi/o	-gram	
2. gastr/o	-scope	
3. cardi/o	-logist	
4. cardi/o	-megaly	
5. gastr/o	-dynia	
6. gastr/o	-itis	
7. gastr/o + esophag/o	-eal	

1.7 How Medical Terms Are Translated

Think of Medical Terms as Sentences

You can usually figure out the definition of a term by interpreting the

- suffix first
- then the prefix (if one is present)
- then the root or roots

How to translate:

1. Read the word.
2. Say the word out loud.
3. Break the word into parts (suffixes, roots, and prefixes).
4. Translate the parts.
5. Reassemble the pieces into a statement.

Example:

arthritis

1. Read the word: arthritis
2. Say the word out loud: ar-THRAI-tis
3. Break the word into parts (suffixes, roots, and prefixes):   arthr / itis
4. Translate the parts: joint / inflammation
5. Reassemble the pieces into one statement: inflammation of the joint

Here's how this would look in a chart:

TERM	WORD ANALYSIS
1. arthritis	**3.** arthr / itis
2. ar-THRAI-tis	**4.** joint/inflammation
5. DEFINITION inflammation of the joint	

Some examples are shown to allow you to see the process at work. Don't worry about trying to learn the words themselves right now. They will be taught in later chapters. Right now, focus on getting comfortable with looking at medical terms, breaking them down, and then translating them. The biggest problem people have with medical terms is that they are intimidated by how long or how foreign they look. But if you don't panic and follow these five simple steps, you will be surprised at how quickly you will become comfortable with the language.

Group 1. This group is made up of relatively simple words. Most have just one root and one suffix, and the definition is easily deduced from the word analysis.

TERM	WORD ANALYSIS
arthritis ar-THRAI-tis	arthr / itis joint / inflammation
DEFINITION inflammation of the joint	
cardiology kar-dee-AW-loh-jee	cardio / logy heart / study of
DEFINITION study of the heart	
myalgia mai-AL-jah	my / algia muscle / pain
DEFINITION pain of muscle	

Group 2. This group of words contains slightly more complex words. The words in this section are made up of at least three parts—either multiple roots or a prefix, root, and suffix.

TERM	WORD ANALYSIS
cardiopulmonary KAR-dee-oh-PUL-mon-AR-ee	cardio / pulmon / ary heart / lung / pertaining to
DEFINITION pertaining to the heart and lungs	
dermatomycosis der-MAH-toh-mai-KOH-sis	dermato / myc / osis skin / fungus / condition
DEFINITION skin condition caused by fungus	
hyperplasia hai-per-PLAY-zhah	hyper / plas / ia over / formation / condition
DEFINITION overformation condition	
pericardium peh-ree-KAR-dee-um	peri / card / ium around / heart / tissue
DEFINITION tissue around the heart	

EXERCISE 1 Underline and define the root in the following terms.

1. cardiology _____

2. arthritis _____

3. carditis _____

4. hepatitis _____

5. arthralgia _____

6. myalgia _____

7. myotomy _____

8. arthrectomy _____

9. myectomy _____

EXERCISE 2 Underline and define the suffix in the following terms.

1. cardiology _____

2. arthritis _____

3. carditis _____

4. hepatitis _____

5. arthralgia _____

6. myalgia _____

7. myotomy _____

8. arthrectomy _____

9. myectomy _____

EXERCISE 3 Translate the following terms.

> **EXAMPLE:** sinusitis *inflammation of the sinuses*

1. cardiology _____

2. arthritis _____

3. carditis _____

4. hepatitis _____

5. arthralgia _____

6. myalgia _____

7. myotomy _____

8. arthrectomy _____

9. myectomy _____

Additional exercises available in **connect**

Chapter Review exercises, along with additional practice items, are available in Connect!

review of prefixes, roots, and suffixes

PREFIXES	ROOTS	SUFFIXES
a- = not	**arthr/o** = joint	**-ac** = pertaining to
ab- = away	**cardi/o** = heart	**-al** = pertaining to
ad- = toward	**derm/o, dermat/o** = skin	**-algia** = pain
an- = not	**enter/o** = small intestine	**-ar, -ary** = pertaining to
ante- = before	**gastr/o** = stomach	**-cele** = hernia
anti- = against	**gen/o** = generation, cause	**-centesis** = puncture
bi- = two	**hem/o, hemat/o** = blood	**-desis** = binding
brady- = slow	**hepat/o** = liver	**-dynia** = pain
circum- = around	**hydr/o** = water	**-eal** = pertaining to
con- = with, together	**morph/o** = shape, change	**-ectomy** = removal
contra- = against	**muscul/o** = muscle	**-emia** = blood condition
de- = down, away from	**my/o** = muscle	**-gram** = written record
dia- = through	**myc/o** = fungus	**-graph** = instrument used to produce a record
dys- = bad	**necr/o** = death	**-graphy** = process of recording
e- = out	**neur/o** = nerve	**-ia** = condition
ec- = out	**orth/o** = straight	**-iasis** = presence of
ecto- = outside	**path/o** = suffering, disease	**-iatrics** = medical science
en- = in, inside	**phag/o** = eat	**-iatrist** = specialist in medicine of
endo- = in, inside	**plas/o** = formation	**-iatry** = medical science
epi- = upon	**pneum/o, pneumon/o** = lung	**-ic** = pertaining to
eu- = good	**pulmon/o** = lung	**-icle** = small
ex- = out	**py/o** = pus	**-ism** = condition
exo- = outside	**scler/o** = hard	**-ist** = specialist
extra- = outside	**sten/o** = narrowing	**-itis** = inflammation
hemi- = half	**troph/o** = nourishment, development	**-ium** = tissue, structure
hyper- = over	**vas/o, vascul/o** = blood vessel	**-logist** = specialist in the study of
hypo- = under	**xen/o** = foreign	**-logy** = study of
inter- = between	**xer/o** = dry	**-lysis** = loosen, break down
intra- = in, inside		**-malacia** = abnormal softening
macro- = large		**-megaly** = enlargement
micro- = small		**-meter** = instrument used to measure
mono- = one		**-metry** = process of measuring
multi- = many		**-oid** = resembling
oligo- = few		**-ole** = small
pan- = all		**-oma** = tumor
peri- = around		**-osis** = condition
poly- = many		**-ous** = pertaining to
post- = after		**-pathy** = disease
pre- = before		**-penia** = deficiency
pro- = before, on behalf of		**-pexy** = surgical fixation
re- = again		**-plasty** = reconstruction

review of prefixes, roots, and suffixes *continued*

PREFIXES	ROOTS	SUFFIXES
semi- = half		**-ptosis** = drooping
sub- = beneath		**-rrhage, -rrhagia** = excessive flow
sym- = with, together		**-rrhaphy** = suture
syn- = with, together		**-rrhea** = flow
tachy- = fast		**-rrhexis** = rupture
trans- = through		**-scope** = instrument used to look
uni- = one		**-scopy** = process of looking
		-spasm = involuntary contraction
		-stomy = creation of an opening
		-tic = pertaining to
		-tomy = incision
		-ula, -ule = small
		-y = condition, procedure, process

Introduction to Health Records

2

Introduction

Medical records save lives. The information they contain can be critical in patient care. For example, documentation of a patient's allergy to a medication can prevent an adverse, potentially fatal, outcome. Whether found in a paper chart or an electronic health record (EHR), the information contained in a patient's records serves as a road map to his or her health history, detailing previous illnesses and treatments, continuing medical problems, history of family illnesses, and any current medications. These data provide a clearer picture of the best route to take in future treatment of the patient. With an increasingly busy and time-constrained patient culture, seeking care in multiple places, such as emergency departments (EDs) and urgent care clinics, has become more commonplace. This further fuels the need for thorough documentation because it is the bedrock of solid communication among health care providers.

Medical records are an indispensable component of medicine, so it is prudent to be well acquainted with their general layout. There are countless types of medical documents or records in medicine, from routine wellness visit notes to hospital discharge summaries. Even x-ray reports are medical notes.

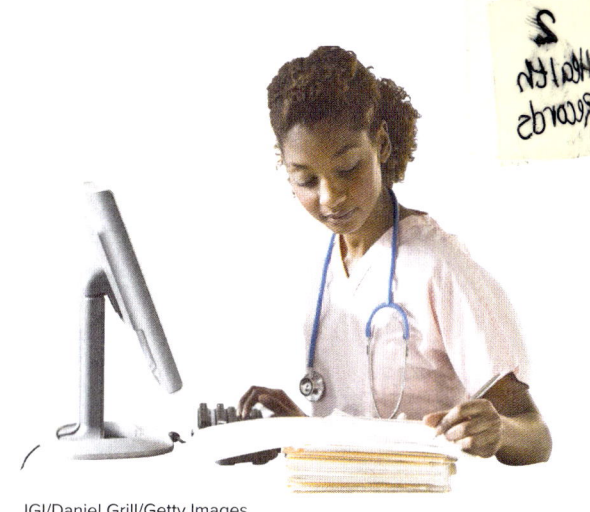

JGI/Daniel Grill/Getty Images

To the untrained eye, the layout or sheer volume of information of a medical note may be intimidating. In reality, most medical notes share a consistent, logical organization or layout as well as characteristic language. We addressed the concept of medical language in the first chapter, and it will be the main focus of this textbook. In this chapter, we discuss the organization or layout of medical documents. Having a good grasp on the general flow of medical notes allows for successful navigation through the different elements of a patient's chart so you may find any relevant details you seek.

Learning Outcomes

Upon completion of this chapter, you will be able to:

2.1 Summarize the **SOAP method.**

2.2 Identify the types of **health records.**

2.3 Use common terms on **health records.**

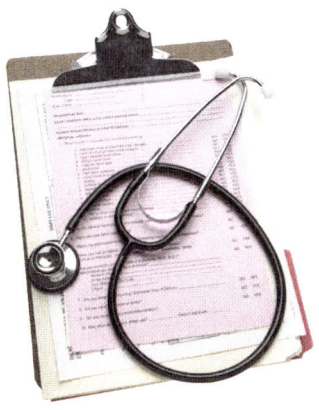

Creatas/Getty Images

2.1 The SOAP Method

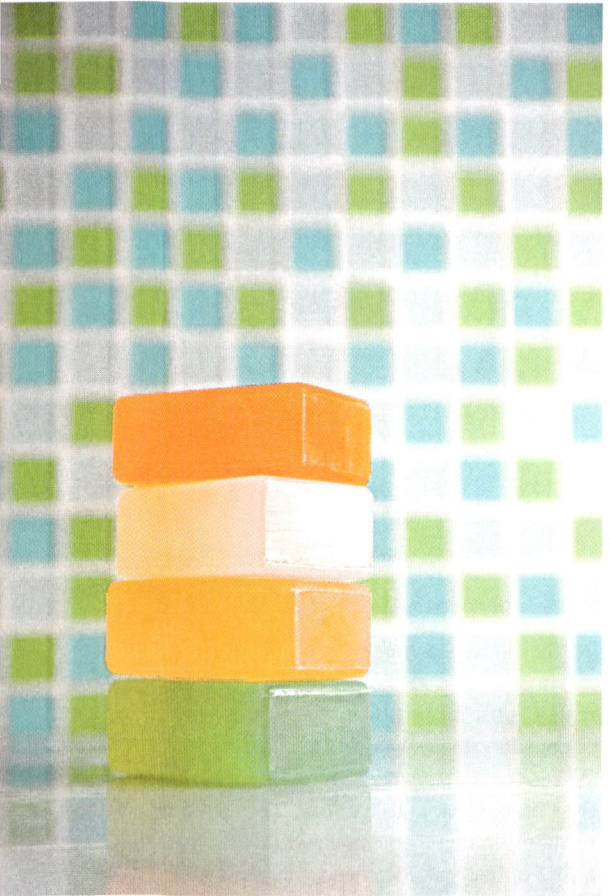

Fuse/Getty Images

 The first part of the note is the **subjective** part. It is subject to how a patient experiences and personally describes his or her problem as well as personal and family medical histories. Put simply, it is the problem in the patient's own words. The subjective data include the duration of the problem, the quality of the problem, and any exacerbating or relieving factors for that problem.

 The next step in the investigative process involves collecting **objective** data. Objective data comprise the patient's physical exam, any laboratory findings, and imaging studies performed at the visit.

 Upon gathering all the pertinent information, the health care provider formulates a logical analysis. This is known as the **assessment.** An assessment could be a diagnosis, an identification of a problem, or a list of possibilities for the diagnosis, which is known as a *differential diagnosis.*

 The provider then formulates a **plan,** or a course of action consistent with his or her assessment. The plan could be a treatment with medicine or a procedure. It could also consist of collecting further data to help arrive at a more accurate diagnosis.

The process of collecting subjective history, gathering objective data, formulating an assessment, and developing an action plan is repeated in every health care visit across all disciplines of medicine. It is the baseline of thought in medicine. Consequently, health care records reflect this thought process.

Medical notes share a consistent pattern in their organization and layout. This pattern reflects the thought process of health professionals in general. Patient visits typically revolve around addressing a problem. Providers employ a logical approach to solving these problems. In its most rudimentary form, this pattern is presented as what is known as a *SOAP note. SOAP* is an acronym that stands for the four general parts of a medical note: **s**ubjective, **o**bjective, **a**ssessment, and **p**lan.

Diagnostic work in medicine is very similar to the investigative work of a detective. By collecting data and using deductive reasoning, a health care provider can make the most accurate assessment of the patient's problem.

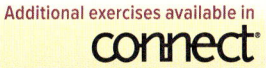
EXERCISE 1 Match the part of the medical SOAP note on the left with its description on the right.

_____ 1. subjective   a. cause of the problem

_____ 2. objective   b. treatment with medicine or a procedure

_____ 3. assessment   c. a description of the problem in the patient's own words

_____ 4. plan   d. data collected to assist in understanding the nature of the problem

EXERCISE 2 Multiple-choice questions. Select the correct answer.

1. The *S* in *SOAP* stands for
   a. scrutinize   c. subjective
   b. studies   d. survey

2. The *O* in *SOAP* stands for
   a. objective   c. order
   b. opinion   d. outline

3. The *A* in *SOAP* stands for
   a. action   c. arrangement
   b. appraisal   d. assessment

4. The *P* in *SOAP* stands for
   a. plan   c. prognosis
   b. procedure   d. purpose

5. A SOAP note is
   a. a pattern used in writing medical notes
   b. a way of thinking
   c. all of these
   d. none of these

6. A *diagnosis* is
   a. a list of possible causes of the patient's problem or complaint
   b. ordering more labs
   c. the identification of the actual problem
   d. treatment with medicine or a procedure

7. A *differential diagnosis* is
   a. a list of possible causes of the patient's problem or complaint
   b. ordering more labs
   c. the identification of the actual problem
   d. treatment with medicine or a procedure

EXERCISE 3 Identify the part of the SOAP note in which the following information would be found.

> EXAMPLE: Ordering additional lab work to help arrive at the cause   *P (Plan)*

1. Scheduling surgery _____

2. Past medical history, family history _____

3. A diagnosis _____

4. Patient's description of the problem or complaint _____

5. Treatment with medicine _____

6. An identification of the cause of the problem or complaint _____

7. Lab results _____

8. Determination of how long the patient has suffered from the same complaint _____

9. Information forms provided by the patient prior to the appointment _____

10. Initial imaging studies (for example, an x-ray) _____

11. Differential diagnosis _____

12. Ordering more tests or images _____

13. The patient's exam _____

14. List of possible causes that fit the description of the patient's problem _____

EXERCISE 4 Give an example of what would be found in each part of the SOAP note.

1. S—Subjective _____

2. O—Objective _____

3. A—Assessment _____

4. P—Plan _____

2.2 Types of Health Records

From an office setting to the hospital to the operating room, patients receive medical care in many different environments. Consequently, medical documentation of these visits demonstrates differences in their length and format. Regardless of these differences, medical notes continue to follow the same progression, starting from the subjective and ending with the plan. Even radiology and pathology reports exhibit this trend.

Medical records are routinely scoured to find specific information, such as:

- "What medicine did the cardiologist prescribe for the patient?"
- "When is the patient supposed to follow up?"
- "What did the patient have?"

In these instances, subheadings can serve as helpful guideposts. The following table features some common subheadings and their meanings.

The following are descriptions and examples of common types of health care records. As you will notice, they are not complete. The intention is to illustrate how charts are organized. Do not allow yourself to be distracted by any medical terms you have yet to learn. The notes are purposefully color-coded to help emphasize their segment in the SOAP format. The different sections of each note are color-coded in the following manner:

- Subjective: blue
- Objective: red
- Assessment: yellow
- Plan: green (*Note:* Sometimes assessment and plan run together; these instances appear in light green.)

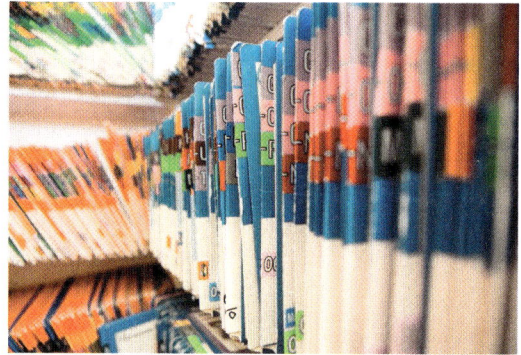

Health records play a vital role in helping organize and document a patient's medical history.
MarkLevant/Getty Images

sections of a health record	description
Chief complaint	The main reason for the patient's visit
History of present illness	The story of the patient's problem
Review of systems	Description of individual body systems in order to discover any symptoms not directly related to the main problem
Past medical history	Other significant past illnesses, such as high blood pressure, asthma, or diabetes
Past surgical history	Any of the patient's past surgeries
Family history	Any significant illnesses that run in the patient's family
Social history	A record of habits such as smoking, drinking, drug abuse, and sexual practices that can impact health

Example Note #1: Clinic Note

Anytime a health care professional sees a patient in an office setting, he or she must document the visit. These notes can be handwritten, dictated, or electronic, or they may involve simply circling the correct words or checking boxes on a template. Regardless of how they are done, these notes always follow the SOAP method. For new patients, there is generally more information in the chart. The SOAP notes for subsequent visits are often more streamlined.

The following is an example of a doctor's office SOAP note.

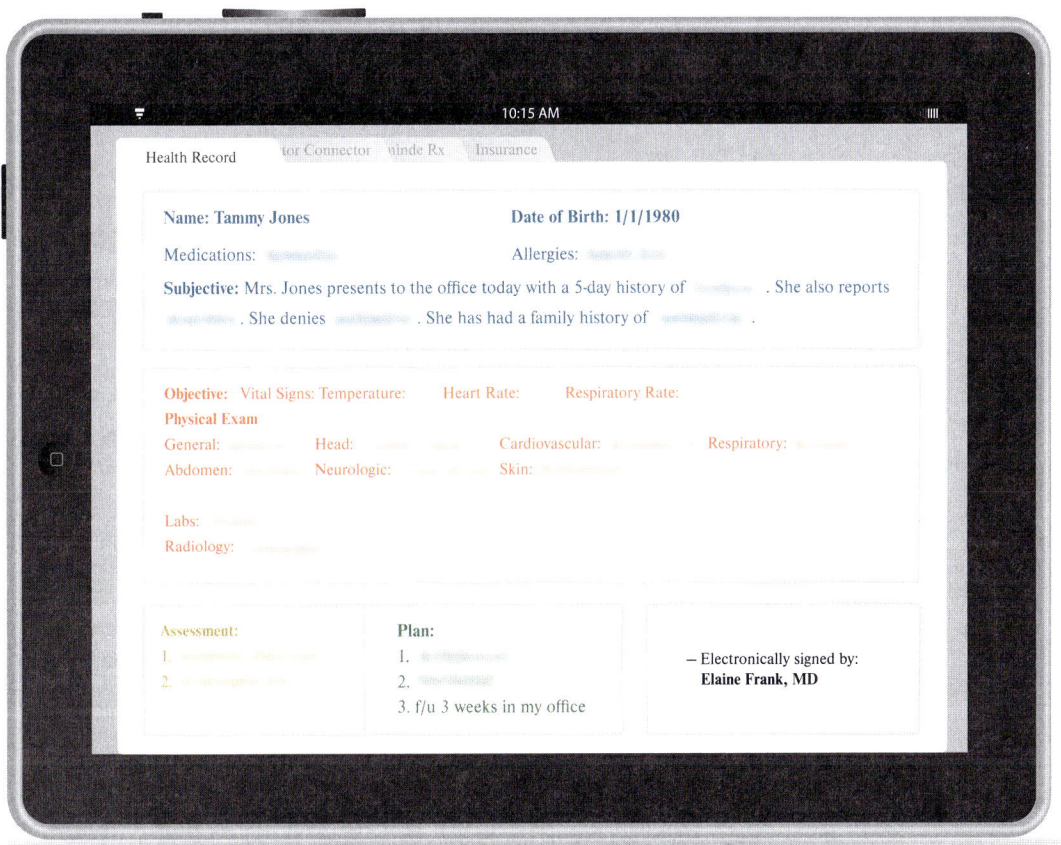

Example Note #2: Emergency Department Note

Patients seen in EDs and urgent care clinics are almost always new to the medical staff. Obtaining a good patient history from an ED patient is very important, as information about that patient's past is critical to getting a correct diagnosis in the present. One unique part of these notes is the ED course, which explains what happened to the patient during his or her stay in the ED. The ED course is a mixture of any completed diagnostic tests, the patient assessment, and a plan for the patient that unfolds over time.

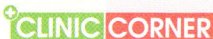

Chief Complaint: Cough.
History of Present Illness: Mr. Stephen Dufresne is a 43-year-old male with a 3-day history of cough with ▓▓▓ .
Past Medical History: Asthma.
Past Surgical History: None.
Social History: Lives with his wife and two children. Nonsmoker. Drinks 4 glasses of wine a week.

Family History:
Father: Deceased at 68 years of age from stroke.
Mother: Alive, high blood pressure.
Medications: Albuterol, prn.
Allergies: No known drug allergies.

Physical Exam:
Vital Signs: Temperature: ▓▓ Heart Rate: ▓ Respiratory Rate: ▓▓
General: ▓▓▓▓▓▓▓
Head: ▓▓▓▓▓
Cardiovascular: ▓▓▓▓▓▓▓
Respiratory: ▓▓▓▓▓▓▓▓
Abdomen: ▓▓▓▓▓▓
Neurologic: ▓▓▓▓▓▓
Skin: ▓▓▓▓▓▓▓

Emergency Department Course:
Mr. Dufresne arrived to the emergency department in no apparent distress. A chest x-ray showed ▓▓▓▓ . We treated him with oxygen and ▓▓▓▓ . After two treatments of albuterol, he improved. He was diagnosed with ▓▓▓▓ and treated with ▓▓▓▓▓ .

Disposition:
Discharged to home, with follow-up in 3 days with his PCP.

—Christine Christenson, MD

Example Note #3: Admission Summary

Upon admittance to the hospital, patients must provide a medical history and receive a physical exam. Afterward, the attending medical professional writes a detailed admission summary. Detailed admission summaries are usually thorough notes that are very heavy on the subjective and objective parts because the idea of the summary is to assemble all the facts in one place to help direct the entire hospital course.

- The assessment, which usually describes the thought process behind a patient's diagnosis and a list of possible causes for the patient's problem, is known as a *differential diagnosis.*

- The plan portion of the summary usually involves further testing, as well as care for the patient.

In a problem-based approach, the assessment and plan portions of the summary will be placed together. In such an approach, the patient's problems are numbered. After each number, the problems are described. The description is followed with a plan of what will be done about the problems.

Occasionally, a hospital team will send a courtesy letter to the patient's primary care provider (PCP). This letter can be similar to an admission note but is usually briefer.

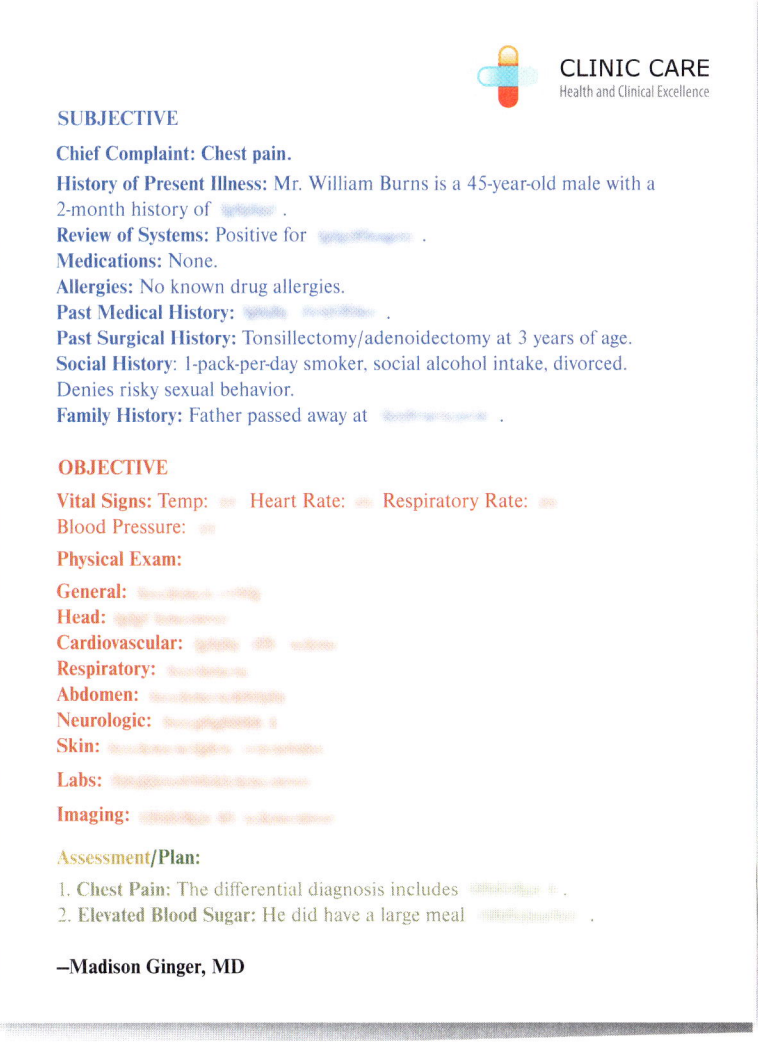

CLINIC CARE
Health and Clinical Excellence

SUBJECTIVE

Chief Complaint: Chest pain.

History of Present Illness: Mr. William Burns is a 45-year-old male with a 2-month history of ▨▨▨ .

Review of Systems: Positive for ▨▨▨ .

Medications: None.

Allergies: No known drug allergies.

Past Medical History: ▨▨▨ .

Past Surgical History: Tonsillectomy/adenoidectomy at 3 years of age.

Social History: 1-pack-per-day smoker, social alcohol intake, divorced. Denies risky sexual behavior.

Family History: Father passed away at ▨▨▨ .

OBJECTIVE

Vital Signs: Temp: ▨ Heart Rate: ▨ Respiratory Rate: ▨ Blood Pressure: ▨

Physical Exam:

General: ▨▨▨

Head: ▨▨▨

Cardiovascular: ▨▨▨

Respiratory: ▨▨▨

Abdomen: ▨▨▨

Neurologic: ▨▨▨

Skin: ▨▨▨

Labs: ▨▨▨

Imaging: ▨▨▨

Assessment/Plan:

1. **Chest Pain:** The differential diagnosis includes ▨▨▨ .
2. **Elevated Blood Sugar:** He did have a large meal ▨▨▨ .

—Madison Ginger, MD

summary of health record notes

	AUTHOR	LOCATION	PURPOSE	FORMAT AND ORDER	UNIQUE FEATURES
Clinic note	Medical professional	Clinic	Documents a visit	SOAP	New patient: Includes more history, separate form Repeat patient: Streamlined note
Consult note	Physician; usually a specialist	Clinic or hospital	Provides an expert opinion on a more challenging problem	SOAP	Can be in the form of a letter to the PCP
Emergency department note	ED medical staff	Emergency department	Documents an emergency department visit	SOAP	The A includes the ED course
Admission summary	Hospital medical professional	Hospital	Documents the admission of a patient to the hospital	SO A/P	S, O = Very thorough A = Differential diagnosis P = Further testing and care A + P = Problem-based approach
Discharge summary	Medical professional	Hospital	Describes when and why the patient was admitted; documents a longer stay	ASOP	Starts with A
Operative report	Surgeon		Documents a surgery in detail	ASOP	
Daily hospital note/progress note	Medical professional	Inpatient health care facility	Documents daily hospital visit	SO A/P	S—Focuses on how patient's condition has changed since the previous note A—Sometimes includes a differential diagnosis
Radiology report	Radiologist		Explains reason for image, how image was performed, what was seen on image, and radiologist's assessment; sometimes includes a recommendation	SOA	Usually includes only S, O, and A, but may include a P if it recommends that further studies should be performed
Pathology report	Pathologist		Provides reasons for test, what was seen on the test, and an assessment	SOA	
Prescription	Medical professional		Provides directions for a medication	P	1. Medicine's name 2. Instructions for patient 3. How much medicine should be given 4. Refills, if any 5. Health care professional's signature and whether generic substitution is allowed

2.3 Common Terms on Health Records

Your Future Second-Nature Words

Just as various sports have their own special words, such as *rebound, home run,* and *touchdown,* health records have special words that are essential to know. While the main purpose of this book is to help you use the roots of ancient words to break down medical words, you must also know many commonly used medical words that are not necessarily based on ancient languages.

When you have been working in the medical field long enough, these words will become second nature to you. You will use them so often that they will become part of your normal vocabulary. This chapter will introduce you to those terms so you will be better able to understand the stories told in health records.

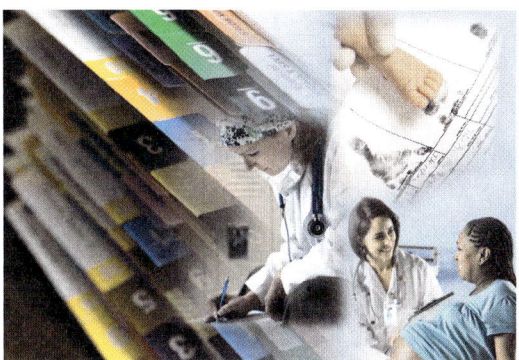

Just like any other specialized field, medicine has a whole host of words that sound strange the first time but become second nature the more you use them.

(doctor) Fuse/Getty Images; (infant foot) Comstock Images/ PictureQuest; (files) Antenna/Getty Images; (female doctor/patient) Terry Vine/Blend Images LLC

Subjective

As you recall, the subjective section of a health record tells the patient's personal story of his or her health issue. It includes things such as:

- the main reason for the health visit
- the description of his or her problem
- the timing of the problem
- previous medical problems or surgeries
- family health problems that might relate
- current medications and allergies

In describing the chief concern, you may include when the problem began, the severity, any associated problems, and whether anything seems to make the problem better or worse.

general subjective terms

TERM	DEFINITION
abrupt ah-BRUPT	all of a sudden
acute ah-KYOOT	it just started recently or is a sharp, severe symptom
afebrile AY-FEH-brail	to not have a fever

general subjective terms *continued*

TERM	DEFINITION
chronic KRAH-nik	it has been going on for a while now
exacerbation ek-SAS-er-BAY-shun	it is getting worse
febrile FEH-brail	to have a fever
genetic/hereditary jih-NEH-tik, hah-REH-dih-TEH-ree	runs in the family
lethargic lah-THAR-jik	a decrease in level of consciousness; in a medical record, this is generally an indication that the patient is really sick
malaise mah-LAYZ	not feeling well
noncontributory NON-kon-TRIH-byoo-TOR-ee	not related to this specific problem
progressive proh-GREH-siv	more and more each day
symptom SIM-tom	something a patient feels

PRONUNCIATION

EXERCISE 1 Indicate which syllable(s) is emphasized when pronounced.

EXAMPLE: bronchitis   bronchitis

1. progressive _____
2. lethargic _____
3. genetic _____
4. febrile _____

EXERCISE 2 Match the term on the left with its definition on the right.

_____ 1. symptom   a. something a patient feels

_____ 2. progressive   b. a decrease in the level of consciousness

_____ 3. chronic   c. symptoms recently began

_____ 4. febrile   d. symptoms have been present for a while

_____ 5. afebrile   e. to have a fever

_____ 6. acute   f. not feeling well

_____ 7. malaise   g. to not have a fever

_____ 8. lethargic   h. more and more each day

EXERCISE 3 Translate the following terms.

1. genetic _____
2. noncontributory _____
3. hereditary _____
4. abrupt _____
5. chronic _____
6. lethargic _____
7. exacerbation _____
8. malaise _____
9. afebrile _____

EXERCISE 4 Identify the medical term from the definition provided.

1. a problem that runs in the family _____
2. unrelated to the specific problem _____
3. a problem that recently began _____
4. all of a sudden _____
5. more and more each day _____
6. a problem that is getting worse _____
7. something a patient feels _____
8. to not have a fever _____

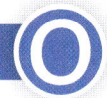

Objective

The objective part of a health record tells about the data collected during the health care provider's interaction with the patient. What does the provider notice about the patient when he or she examines the patient closely? How does the patient look, sound, feel, smell? It also includes any extra data obtained from tests done in a laboratory or from special images of the patient's body.

general objective terms	
TERM	**DEFINITION**
alert ah-LERT	able to answer questions; responsive; interactive
auscultation aw-skul-TAY-shun	to listen
marked MARKT	it really stands out
oriented OR-ee-EN-ted	being aware of who he or she is, where he or she is, and the current time; a patient who is aware of all three is "oriented × 3"
palpation pal-PAY-shun	to feel
percussion per-KUH-shun	to hit something and listen to the resulting sound or feel for the resulting vibration; drums are a percussion instrument
unremarkable un-ree-MARK-ah-bul	another way of saying normal

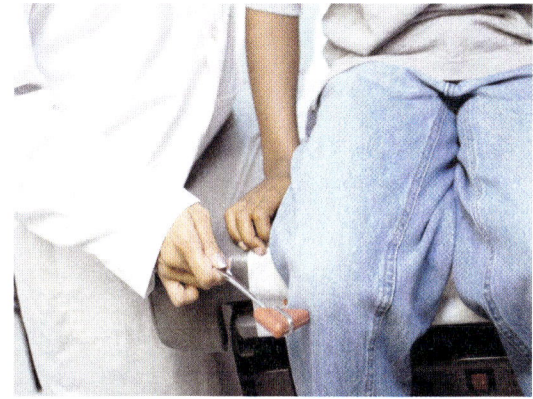

One piece of objective information is obtained by measuring a patient's muscle reflexes.

Getty Images

Learning Outcome 2.3 Exercises

EXERCISE 5 Indicate which syllable(s) is emphasized when pronounced.

> EXAMPLE: bronchitis   bronchitis

1. alert _____

2. unremarkable _____

3. palpation _____

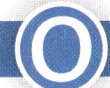

EXERCISE 6   Match the term on the left with its definition on the right.

_____ 1. unremarkable   a. able to answer questions; responsive; interactive

_____ 2. alert   b. able to identify one's name and location, the time of day, and the date

_____ 3. marked   c. something that really stands out

_____ 4. percussion   d. normal

_____ 5. oriented   e. to listen

_____ 6. auscultation   f. to feel

_____ 7. palpation   g. to hit something and listen to the sound or feel for the vibration

EXERCISE 7   Translate the following terms.

1. marked _____

2. unremarkable _____

3. percussion _____

4. oriented _____

5. auscultation _____

6. palpation _____

EXERCISE 8   Identify the medical term from the definition provided.

1. to listen _____

2. to feel _____

3. normal _____

4. something that really stands out _____

5. able to answer questions; responsive; interactive _____

6. to hit something and listen to the sound or feel for the vibration _____

Assessment

Once the facts from the patient are recorded and data about the patient are collected, it is time to put it all together to reach a conclusion on the nature of the problem. This is known as the *diagnosis*. Sometimes one exact problem is not so obvious at first. In these cases, a health care provider may list the most likely causes, called a *differential diagnosis*. In addition to a diagnosis, the provider may offer other opinions, such as severity of the problem and the chances for improvement.

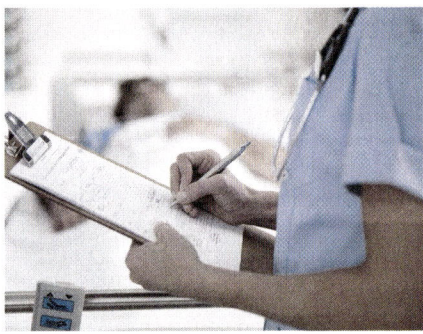

Martin Barraud/age fotostock

general assessment terms	
TERM	**DEFINITION**
impression im-PREH-shun	another way of saying assessment
diagnosis DAI-ag-NOH-sis	what the health care professional thinks the patient has
differential diagnosis dih-fer-EN-shal DAI-ag-NOH-sis	a list of conditions the patient may have based on the symptoms exhibited and the results of the exam
benign beh-NAIN	safe
malignant mah-LIG-nant	dangerous; a problem
degeneration dee-jin-er-AY-shun	to be getting worse
etiology ee-tee-AW-loh-jee	the cause
remission reh-MIH-shun	to get better or improve; most often used when discussing cancer; *remission* does not mean cure
idiopathic ih-dee-oh-PA-thik	no known specific cause; it just happens

general assessment terms *continued*	
TERM	**DEFINITION**
localized LOH-kah-LAIZD	stays in a certain part of the body
systemic/ generalized sih-STEM-ik, jin-er-ah- LAIZD	all over the body (or most of it)
morbidity mor-BID-ih-tee	the risk for being sick
mortality mor-TA-lih-tee	the risk for dying
prognosis prawg-NOH-sis	the chances for things getting better or worse
occult ah-KULT	hidden
pathogen PATH-oh-jin	the organism that causes the problem
lesion LEE-shun	diseased tissue
recurrent ree-KUR-ent	to have again
sequelae seh-KWEL-ah	a problem resulting from a disease or injury
pending PEN-ding	waiting for

 **A** **Learning Outcome 2.3 Exercises**

EXERCISE 9   Indicate which syllable(s) is emphasized when pronounced.

> EXAMPLE: bronchitis bron<u>chi</u>tis

1. impression _____
2. malignant _____
3. remission _____

4. systemic _____
5. morbidity _____
6. mortality _____
7. pathogen _____
8. prognosis _____
9. pending _____

EXERCISE 10   Match the term on the left with its definition on the right.

_____ 1. degeneration

_____ 2. differential diagnosis

_____ 3. diagnosis

_____ 4. impression

_____ 5. remission

_____ 6. mortality

_____ 7. prognosis

_____ 8. morbidity

_____ 9. pathogen

_____ 10. idiopathic

_____ 11. etiology

_____ 12. sequelae

a. assessment

b. what the health care professional thinks the patient has

c. a list of conditions the patient may have based on the symptoms exhibited and the results of the exam

d. to be getting worse

e. the cause

f. to get better or improve; most often used when discussing cancer; does not mean _cure_

g. no known specific cause; it just happens

h. the risk for being sick

i. the risk for dying

j. the chances for things getting better or worse

k. the organism that causes the problem

l. a problem resulting from a disease or injury

EXERCISE 11   Translate the following terms.

1. systematic _____

2. generalized _____

3. localized _____

4. occult _____

5. lesion _____

6. recurrent _____

7. pending _____

8. benign _____

9. malignant _____

10. impression _____

11. degeneration _____

12. remission _____

13. pathogen _____

14. sequelae _____

EXERCISE 12   Identify the medical term from the definition provided.

1. safe _____

2. dangerous; a problem _____

3. stays in a certain part of the body _____

4. all over the body _____

5. a list of things that the patient may have, based on symptoms and exam _____

6. what the medical professional thinks the patient may have _____

7. the cause _____

8. no known specific cause _____

9. the chances for things to get better or worse

_____

10. risk for being sick _____

11. risk for dying _____

12. hidden _____

13. diseased tissue _____

14. to have again _____

15. waiting for _____

Plan

In the health record, the plan lays out what the provider recommends to do about the patient's current health status. This may include medicine or home remedies, help from another health provider, surgery, or even waiting to see if the problem will improve on its own. Sometimes the plan is for more data collection to be done in the future to help figure out the true cause of the problem.

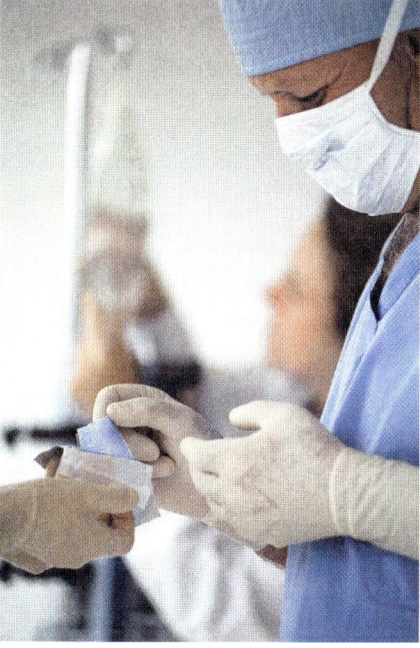

Once an assessment has been made, a course of action is decided upon. This plan can include everything from observation to medication and surgery.
Creatas/Getty Images

general plan terms	
TERM	**DEFINITION**
discharge DIS-charj	literally, to *unload*; it has two meanings: **1.** to send home (to unload the patient from the health care setting to home) **2.** fluid coming out of a part of the body (your body unloading a fluid)
disposition dis-poh-ZIH-shun	what happened to the patient at the end of the visit; often used at the end of ED notes to reference where the patient went after the visit (home, the intensive care unit or a normal hospital bed)
observation OB-zer-VAY-shun	watch, keep an eye on
palliative PA-lee-ah-tiv	treating the symptoms but not actually getting rid of the cause
prophylaxis PROH-fuh-LAK-sis	preventive treatment
reassurance ree-ah-SHUR-ants	to tell the patient that the problem is not serious or dangerous
sterile STEH-ril	extremely clean, germ-free conditions; especially important during medical procedures and surgery
supportive care suh-POR-tiv kehr	to treat the symptoms and make the patient feel better

 Learning Outcome 2.3 Exercises

EXERCISE 13 Indicate which syllable(s) is emphasized when pronounced.

EXAMPLE: bronchitis   bron<u>chi</u>tis

1. discharge _____

2. disposition _____

3. observation _____

4. reassurance _____

5. supportive care _____

EXERCISE 14   Match the term on the left with its definition on the right.

_____ 1. sterile

_____ 2. observation

_____ 3. disposition

_____ 4. discharge

_____ 5. reassurance

_____ 6. supportive care

_____ 7. prophylaxis

_____ 8. palliative

a. what happens to the patient at the end of the visit

b. to send home

c. preventive treatment

d. treating the symptoms but not actually getting rid of the cause

e. keep an eye on

f. to tell the patient that the problem is not serious or dangerous

g. to treat the symptoms and make the patient feel better

h. extremely clean, germ-free conditions; especially important during medical procedures and surgery

EXERCISE 15   Translate the following terms.

1. reassurance _____

2. sterile _____

3. discharge _____

4. observation _____

5. disposition _____

6. supportive care _____

7. palliative _____

8. prophylaxis _____

EXERCISE 16   Identify the medical term from the definition provided.

1. to send home _____

2. to keep an eye on _____

3. extremely clean, germ-free conditions _____ _____

4. what happens to the patient at the end of the visit _____

5. preventive treatment _____

6. to treat the symptoms to make the patient feel better _____

7. treating the symptoms but not actually getting rid of the cause _____

8. to tell the patient that the problem is not serious/dangerous _____

Body Planes and Orientation

In giving directions, being more specific leads to more accurate results. The same goes for describing parts of the body. Often, the words used to describe directions in the body are opposites, such as north and south. Following is more information about these body-specific opposites.

opposites	
TERM	**DEFINITION**
distal DIH-stal	farther away from the center *distal* and *distant* come from the same word and mean *far*
proximal PRAWK-sih-mal	closer in to the center *proximal* and *approximate* come from the same word and mean *close*

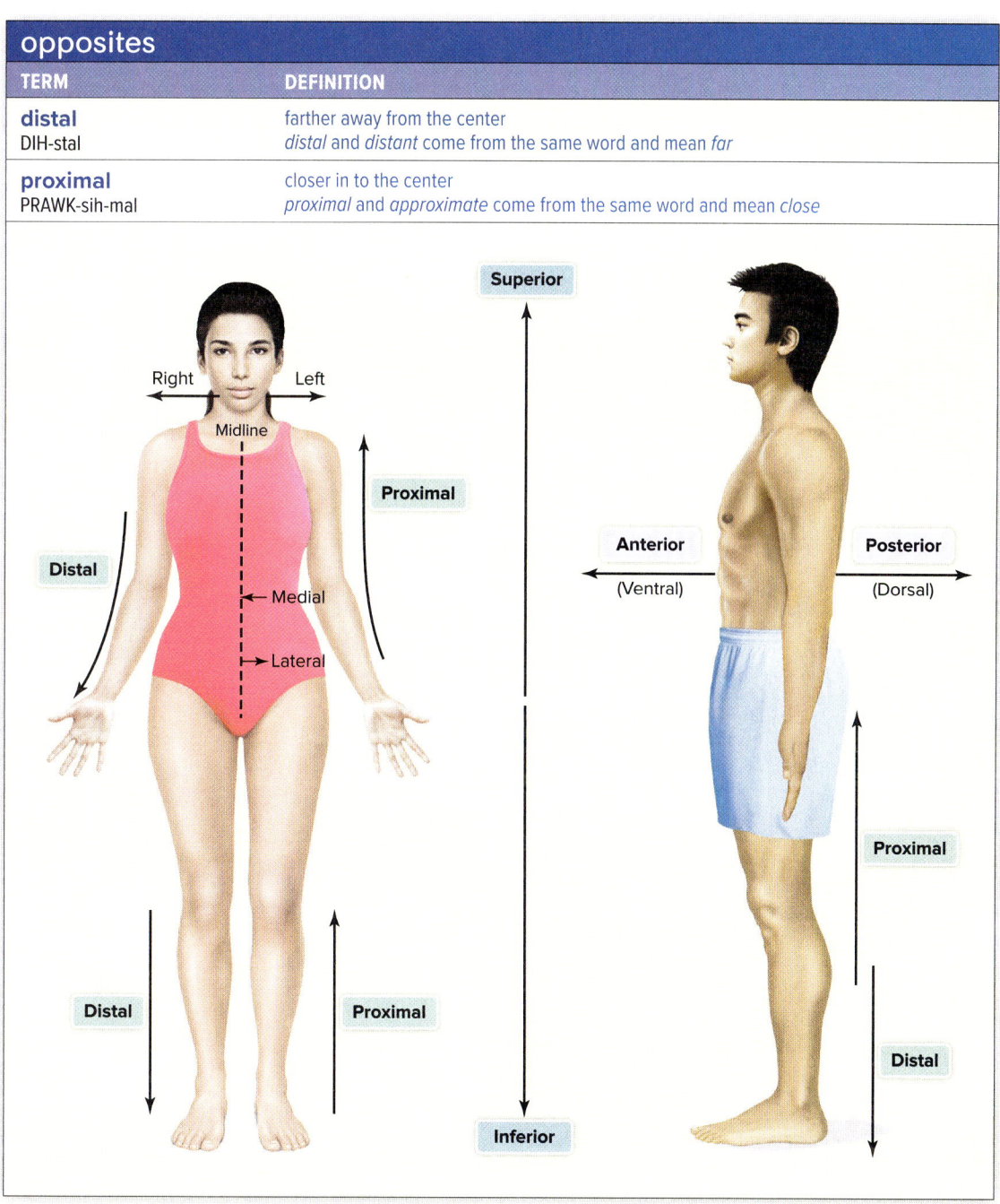

TERM	DEFINITION
lateral LA-ter-al	out to the side
	think of a quarterback lateraling a football to a running back
medial MEE-dee-al	toward the middle
	like the median of a highway
dorsal/posterior DOR-sal/ poh-STIH-ree-or	the back
	a dorsal fin on a shark is on its back
ventral/antral/ anterior VEN-tral/AN-tral/an-TIH-ree-or	the front
	the word *ventral* means *stomach*
caudal KOW-dal	toward the bottom
	from Latin, for *tail*
cranial KRAY-nee-al	toward the top
	from the Latin word *cranium*, which means *skull*

Cranial

Caudal

inferior in-FIH-ree-or	below
superior soo-PIH-ree-or	above

TERM	DEFINITION
prone PROHN	lying down on belly
supine SOO-pain	lying down on back

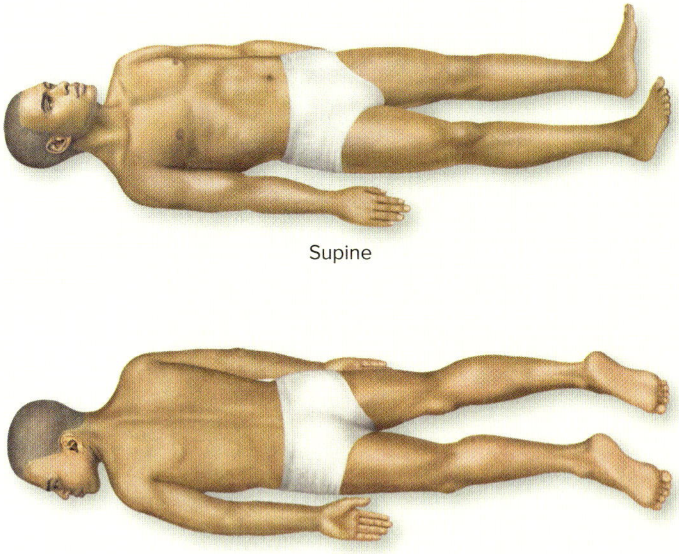

Supine

Prone

contralateral KON-trah-LA-ter-al	opposite side
ipsilateral IP-sih-LA-ter-al	same side

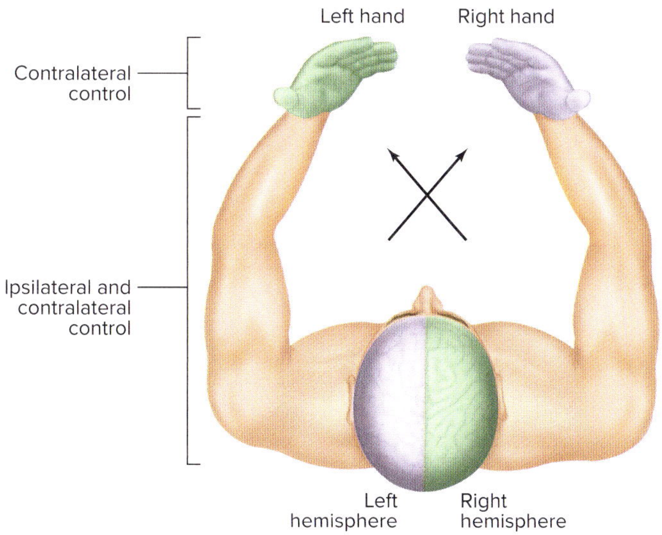

Left hand   Right hand

Contralateral control

Ipsilateral and contralateral control

Left hemisphere   Right hemisphere

TERM	DEFINITION
bilateral BAI-LA-ter-al	both sides
unilateral YOO-nih-LA-ter-al	one side

Unilateral   Bilateral

dorsum DOR-sum	the top of the hand or foot
palmar PAL-mar	the palm of the hand
plantar PLAN-tar	the sole of the foot

Palmar

Dorsum

Dorsum

Plantar

BODY PLANES

Another way of looking at the body is through the three dimensions: right to left (sagittal), front to back (coronal), and top to bottom (transverse). This is especially important in radiology. For instance, a computed tomography scan is actually a series of layered images along one of these dimensions.

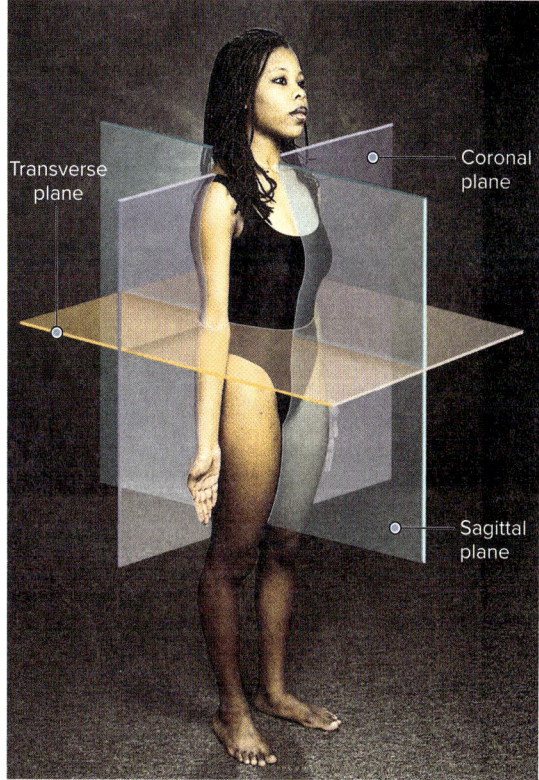

Joe DeGrandis/McGraw-Hill Education

body planes

TERM	DEFINITION
coronal kah-ROH-nal	divides the body into slices from front to back
	corona is Latin for *crown*; this plane divides the body in half from the top of the head down
sagittal SA-jih-tal	divides the body in slices right to left
	sagitta is Latin for *arrow*; think of this as dividing the body in half, as if someone shot an arrow through it.
transverse tranz-VERS	divides the body from top to bottom

Learning Outcome 2.3 Exercises

EXERCISE 17 Indicate which syllable(s) is emphasized when pronounced.

> EXAMPLE: bronchitis *bronchitis*

1. proximal _____
2. distal _____
3. ventral _____
4. antral _____

5. dorsal _____
6. dorsum _____
7. plantar _____
8. palmar _____
9. coronal _____
10. transverse _____

EXERCISE 18   Match the term on the left with its definition on the right.

_____ 1. bilateral
_____ 2. contralateral
_____ 3. ipsilateral

_____ 4. unilateral

_____ 5. transverse
_____ 6. dorsal
_____ 7. prone
_____ 8. coronal
_____ 9. supine

_____ 10. antral

_____ 11. sagittal

a. the back
b. the front
c. lying down on the belly

d. lying down on the back

e. opposite side
f. same side
g. one side
h. both sides
i. divides the body from top to bottom

j. divides the body in slices right to left

k. divides the body in slices from front to back

EXERCISE 19   Translate the following terms.

1. posterior _____
2. cranial _____
3. caudal _____
4. superior _____
5. plantar _____
6. palmar _____
7. transverse _____
8. sagittal _____

9. contralateral _____
10. ventral _____

EXERCISE 20   Identify the medical term from the definition provided.

1. farther away from the center _____
2. closer in to the center _____
3. out to the side _____
4. toward the middle _____
5. toward the top _____
6. the top of the hand or foot _____
7. one side _____
8. divides the body in slices from front to back

_____
9. lying down on the back _____
10. below _____

EXERCISE 21   Identify the opposite for the given term.

> **EXAMPLE:**   cranial   _caudal_

1. proximal _____
2. lateral _____
3. ventral _____
4. anterior _____
5. inferior _____
6. prone _____
7. ipsilateral _____
8. bilateral _____
9. palmar _____

The Integumentary System—Dermatology

3

Introduction and Overview of Dermatology

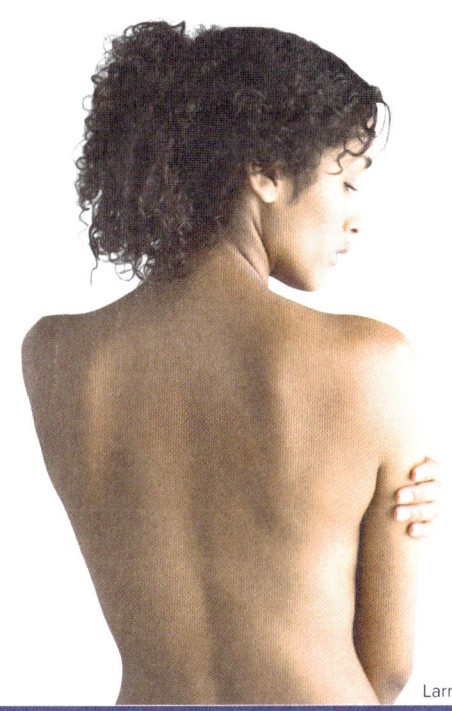

For thousands of years, walls of earth, wood, or stone surrounded cities. These outside walls defined the city boundaries. More importantly, they protected the city's inhabitants. By limiting access to the inside of the city and offering a strategic point of attack, walls deterred would-be invaders. In addition, walls provided a convenient vantage point to view the surrounding countryside. In effect, the walls offered protection and surveillance.

Skin serves a similar function as city walls. As an outer protective barrier, skin is the first line of defense from germs and irritants. It also serves as the body's first point of contact with its surroundings.

Larry Williams/Blend/Corbis

Learning Outcomes

Upon completion of this chapter, you will be able to:

3.1 Identify the **roots/word parts** associated with the **integumentary system.**

(S) 3.2 Translate the **Subjective** terms associated with the **integumentary system.**

(O) 3.3 Translate the **Objective** terms associated with the **integumentary system.**

(A) 3.4 Translate the **Assessment** terms associated with the **integumentary system.**

(P) 3.5 Translate the **Plan** terms associated with the **integumentary system.**

3.6 Distinguish terms associated with the **integumentary system** in the context of **electronic health records.**

3.1 Word Parts of the Integumentary System

Word Parts Associated with the Anatomy of the Integumentary System

At first glance, the skin appears to be very simple—just a thin layer of tissue covering our bodies. However, the truth is that the **integumentary system** (*the skin*) is very complex. Your skin (roots: *cutaneo/dermo*) has many structures, each of which has its own special job.

The outermost layer, the one that is visible, is the **epidermis**. Under the epidermis lies a deeper layer known as the **dermis**. This layer, which is much thicker than the epidermis, has fewer cells and a greater number of fibers to give the skin strength and flexibility. The dermis is also home to hair follicles, nerves, and glands.

- Hair follicles are the roots of your hair (*pilo/tricho*). The follicles anchor the hair to the skin and provide nourishment for the hair.
- The nerves of the dermis detect fine pressure, deep pressure, temperature, and pain. The vast network of nerves in your skin makes it the largest sensory organ in your body.
- The skin has two types of glands, which are groups of cells that release fluid. Sweat glands (*hidro*) release sweat to rid the body of waste and to cool the body. Sebaceous glands (*sebaceo*) secrete oil as a natural moisturizer for the skin and hair.

At the ends of your fingers and toes are nails, specialized tissue made of a hard substance (*keratin*). Your nails (*onycho/ungo*) protect your fingers and toes and provide a good base for movement.

fat

ROOTS: *adip/o, lip/o, steat/o*

EXAMPLES: adipocyte, lipoma, steatosis

NOTES: The next time you are offered a fatty food, you can tell the person who is offering it that you try to avoid *adipogenic* foods.

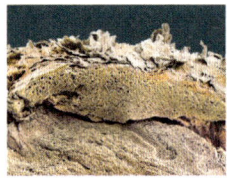
Science Photo Library/ Alamy Stock Photo

skin

ROOTS: *cutane/o, derm/o, dermat/o*

EXAMPLES: subcutaneous, epidermal, dermatology

NOTES: A patient once sought medical treatment for a rash around the mouth. When the health care professional diagnosed her with *perioral dermatitis,* the patient thought to herself, "Duh! You just said the same thing I said—just in a different language." Think about it: What does *perioral dermatitis* mean? You can break it down easily: *peri* = around, *oral* = mouth, *dermat* = skin, and *itis* = inflammation.

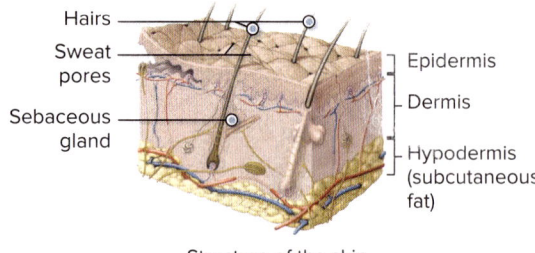

Hairs
Sweat pores
Sebaceous gland
Epidermis
Dermis
Hypodermis (subcutaneous fat)

Structure of the skin

hair

ROOTS: *pil/o, trich/o*

EXAMPLES: piloid, atrichosis

NOTES: The word *caterpillar* is believed to come from two Latin words: *catta,* meaning *cat,* and *pila,* meaning *hair;* thus, *caterpillar,* means *hairy cat.* Have you ever had split ends? If you do, you can always ask your hairstylist for a treatment for your *schizotrichia.*

sweat

ROOT: *hidr/o*

EXAMPLES: hyperhidrosis, hypohidrosis

NOTES: Humans have gone to great lengths to keep the environment cool—inventing air conditioning and fans, for example—which suggests that humans do not like to get sweaty. But if you didn't have the ability to sweat, your body would have a very hard time regulating its temperature. In fact, *anhidrosis,* which means a lack of sweat, can be a sign that something is wrong.

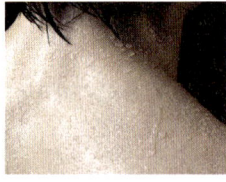
Scott Kleinman/The Image Bank/Getty Images

nail

ROOTS: *onych/o, ungu/o*

EXAMPLES: onychalgia, subungual

NOTES: Have you noticed that it is time to trim your nails? Excuse yourself to take care of that task by telling your friends you need to step outside to *exungulate*. If there is a broken nail, you can mention that you have diagnosed yourself with *onychoclasis*.

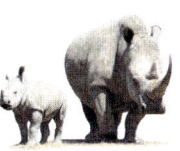

oil

ROOTS: *seb/o, sebace/o*

EXAMPLES: sebolith, pilosebaceous

NOTES: Later, when you learn more about the ears, you will learn the root *cerumen*, which refers to ear wax. Actually, *cerumen* is just sebum that is produced in the ears.

Word Parts Associated with Pathology—Change

Skin abnormalities are generally categorized into two groups: unusual skin texture and unusual skin color. Common problems with skin texture include hardness or horniness (*kerato-*) and dryness (*xero-*). Of course, skin tones differ from person to person and ethnicity to ethnicity, but certain prefixes are used to describe abnormal skin conditions: whiteness (*leuko-*), redness (*erythro-*), yellowness (*xantho-*), and blackness (*melano-*).

hard, horny

ROOT: *kerat/o*

EXAMPLES: keratosis, keratoderma

NOTES: The rhinoceros is so named because it has a horn on its nose. The dinosaur triceratops was so named because of the three (*tri*) horns (*kerat*) on its head.

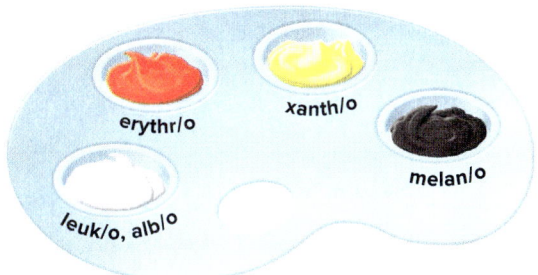

Volodymyr Burdiak/ Shutterstock

dry

ROOT: *xer/o*

EXAMPLE: xeroderma

NOTES: People who live in dry or desert regions often forgo lawns and instead use *xeriscaping,* which means landscaping using plants that require little water. Because grounds that are xeriscaped are typically rocky and brown, some think this type of landscaping is spelled *zeroscaping*— and the fact that the *x* is pronounced like a *z* probably does not help.

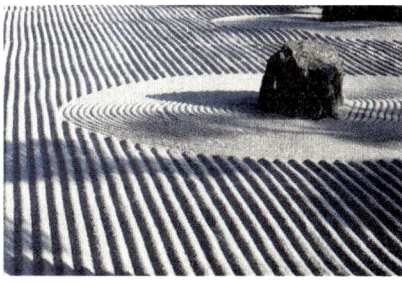

Akira Kaede/Getty Images

Word Parts Associated with Pathology—Skin Conditions Involving Color

One important aspect of diagnosing skin conditions is noting changes. This section gives the roots that refer to the most commonly occurring changes in skin color.

erythr/o

xanth/o

melan/o

leuk/o, alb/o

yellow

ROOT: *xanth/o*

EXAMPLE: xanthoderma

NOTES: If you are unable to see the color yellow, you may have *axanthopsia*.

red

ROOT: *erythr/o*

EXAMPLE: erythroderma

NOTES: *Erythroderma* is a redness of the skin. The Red Sea, a sea that separates Africa from Egypt, was originally called the Erythraen (or Red) Sea. The country Eritrea, which lies on the Red Sea between the Sudan and Ethiopia, gets its name from this ancient moniker for the sea.

white

ROOTS: *leuk/o, alb/o*

EXAMPLES: leukoderma, albinism

NOTES: A person with white hair has *leukotrichia*. A complete lack of skin pigment is known as *albinism*.

The *albatross* is a white seabird. Its name is derived in part from a need to distinguish it from a black seabird called the *frigate bird*.

black

ROOT: *melan/o*

EXAMPLE: melanoma

NOTES: Ancient Greeks thought that the human body was filled with four substances they called *humors:* bile (*chole*), black bile (*melan chole*), phlegm (*phlegma*), and blood (*sanguis*). According to this system, a healthy person must have all four humors in perfect balance. If a person was sick, an imbalance of the humors was to blame, and a physician's goal was to figure out which humor was too plentiful and which was insufficient. *Bloodletting* was developed to help rid the body of excess blood. The word *melancholy* also comes from belief in a balance of the humors because it was believed that a person who was sad or depressed had too much black bile.

Learning Outcome 3.1 Exercises

TRANSLATION

EXERCISE 1   Match the root on the left with its definition on the right. Some definitions will be used more than once.

_____	1. lip/o	a. fat
_____	2. derm/o	b. skin
_____	3. dermat/o	c. hair
_____	4. hidr/o	d. sweat
_____	5. adip/o	e. nail
_____	6. cutane/o	f. oil
_____	7. seb/o	g. hard, horny
_____	8. pil/o	h. dry
_____	9. steat/o	
_____	10. sebace/o	
_____	11. trich/o	
_____	12. onych/o	
_____	13. ungu/o	
_____	14. xer/o	
_____	15. kerat/o	

EXERCISE 2   Translate the following roots.

1. derm/o _____
2. lip/o _____
3. cutane/o _____
4. adip/o _____
5. dermat/o _____
6. seb/o _____
7. pil/o _____
8. hidr/o _____
9. ungu/o _____
10. steat/o _____
11. sebace/o _____
12. trich/o _____
13. onych/o _____

EXERCISE 3 Break down the following words into their component parts and translate.

> EXAMPLE: sinusitis   *sinus | itis*
> *inflammation of the sinuses*

1. dermatology _____
2. lipoma _____
3. steatosis _____
4. epidermal _____
5. subungual _____
6. subcutaneous _____
7. onychalgia _____
8. keratosis _____
9. xeroderma _____
10. leukoderma _____
11. erythroderma _____
12. melanoma _____

EXERCISE 4 Identify the roots for the following definitions.

1. dry _____
2. hard, horny _____
3. black _____
4. white _____

5. red _____
6. yellow _____

EXERCISE 5 Build a medical term from the information provided.

1. yellow skin _____
2. nail pain _____
3. dry conditions _____
4. inflammation of fat tissue _____
5. nail disease _____
6. pertaining to the skin _____
7. red skin _____
8. white skin _____

EXERCISE 6 Match the root on the left with its definition on the right. Some definitions will be used more than once.

_____ 1. alb/o   a. black
_____ 2. melan/o   b. red
_____ 3. leuk/o   c. white
_____ 4. erythr/o   d. yellow
_____ 5. xanth/o

GENERATION

EXERCISE 7 Identify the roots for the following definitions.

1. skin (3 roots) _____
2. fat (3 roots) _____
3. sweat (1 root) _____
4. oil (2 roots) _____
5. hair (2 roots) _____

6. nail (2 roots) _____
7. white (2 roots) _____
8. black (1 root) _____
9. red (1 root) _____
10. yellow (1 root) _____

3.2 Patient History, Problems, Complaints

The most common reason a person seeks medical care in relation to his or her skin is a new rash. The rash may be painful (*dermatalgia/dermatodynia*) or itchy (*pruritus*). The rash may appear as hives (*urticaria*) or as an oily secretion (*seborrhea*). The rash may be very dry (*xerosis*) or very wet (*macerate*). Patients may also notice that they are producing too much sweat (*hyperhidrosis*) or not enough sweat (*anhidrosis*).

Sometimes the patient's concern is change in normal skin color. These color changes may involve a loss of pigment (*depigmentation*) or darkening of the skin (*hypermelanosis*). Some people lack pigment altogether, as in *albinism*.

Another reason a patient might consult a dermatologist is problems with the hair. Hair falls under the responsibility of a dermatologist because the hair follicles are embedded in the skin. The most common hair complaint for men is hair loss (*alopecia*), but it occurs in women as well. Another hair problem is too much hair (*hypertrichosis*).

dermatological terms

TERM	WORD ANALYSIS
abrasion uh-BRAY-zhun	ab / rasion away / scrape
DEFINITION scraping away of skin	
albinism AL-bin-ism	albin / ism white / condition
DEFINITION lack of pigment in skin, causing patient to look white	
albino al-BAY-noh	albino
DEFINITION a person afflicted with albinism	
alopecia a-loh-PEE-sha	from Greek, for *fox*
DEFINITION baldness	Digital Vision/Getty Images
anhidrosis an-hi-DROH-sis	an / hidr / osis no / sweat / condition
DEFINITION lack of sweating	
dermatalgia der-mah-TAL-jah	dermat / algia skin / pain
DEFINITION skin pain	
dermatodynia der-MA-toh-DAI-nee-ah	dermato / dynia skin / pain
DEFINITION skin pain	

dermatological terms *continued*

TERM	WORD ANALYSIS
erythema eh-rih-THEE-ma	from Greek, for *redness*
DEFINITION redness	
erythroderma eh-RIH-throh-DER-ma	erythro / derma red / skin
DEFINITION red skin	
hidropoiesis hih-droh-poh-EE-sis	hidro / poiesis sweat / formation
DEFINITION the formation of sweat	
hyperhidrosis hai-per-hih-DROH-sis	hyper / hidr / osis over / sweat / condition
DEFINITION excessive sweating	
hyperkerotosis hai-per-ker-ah-TOH-sis	hyper / kerat / osis over / horny / condition
DEFINITION excessive growth of horny skin	
hypermelanosis hai-per-mel-an-OH-sis	hyper / melan / osis over / black / condition
DEFINITION excessive melanin in the skin	
hyperpigmentation hai-per-pig-men-TAY-shun	hyper / pigment / ation over / pigment / condition
DEFINITION excessive pigment in the skin	
hypohidrosis hai-poh-hih-DROH-sis	hypo / hidr / osis under / sweat / condition
DEFINITION diminished sweating	
hypomelanosis hai-poh-mel-an-OH-sis	hypo / melan / osis under / black / condition
DEFINITION diminished melanin in the skin	

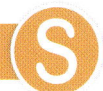

dermatological terms *continued*

TERM	WORD ANALYSIS
hypopigmentation hai-poh-pig-men-TAY-shun	hypo / pigment / ation under / pigment / condition
DEFINITION diminished pigment in the skin	
leukoderma loo-koh-DER-mah	leuko / derma white / skin
DEFINITION white skin	

Image Source/Getty Images

TERM	WORD ANALYSIS
onychophagia aw-nih-koh-FAY-jah	onycho / phag / ia nail / eat / condition
DEFINITION eating or biting the nails	

James Darell/Getty Images

TERM	WORD ANALYSIS
pruritus prur-AI-tis	from Latin, for *itching*
DEFINITION an itch	
NOTE: The ending on this word is easily confused with -*itis*.	

dermatological terms *continued*

TERM	WORD ANALYSIS
trichomegaly tri-koh-MEG-ah-lee	tricho / megaly hair / enlargement
DEFINITION abnormally thick hair	
urticaria ur-tih-KAR-ee-ah	from Latin, for *burning nettle*
DEFINITION swollen, raised, itchy areas of the skin	
xanthoderma zan-thoh-DER-mah	xantho / derma yellow / skin
DEFINITION yellow skin	

TERM	WORD ANALYSIS
xeroderma zeh-roh-DER-mah	xero / derma dry / skin
DEFINITION dry skin	
xerosis ze-ROH-sis	xer / osis dry / condition
DEFINITION condition of dryness	

S Learning Outcome 3.2 Exercises

TRANSLATION

EXERCISE 1 Match the term on the left with its definition on the right.

_____ 1. albino

_____ 2. alopecia

_____ 3. pruritus

_____ 4. urticaria

a. a person with a lack of skin pigment, causing the person to look completely white

b. baldness

c. an itch

d. swollen, raised, itchy areas of the skin

EXERCISE 2 Translate the following terms as literally as possible.

> EXAMPLE: nasopharyngoscope *an instrument for looking at the nose and throat*

1. albinism _____

2. xerosis _____

3. leukoderma _____

4. hypomelanosis _____

5. trichomegaly _____

6. erythroderma _____

7. hyperkeratosis _____

GENERATION

EXERCISE 3 Build a medical term from the information provided.

> EXAMPLE: inflammation of the sinuses *sinusitis*

1. yellow skin _____

2. dry skin _____

3. skin pain _____

4. no sweat condition _____

5. sweat formation _____

EXERCISE 4 Multiple-choice questions. Select the correct answer.

1. A person with albinism has what color skin?
   a. black   c. yellow
   b. red   d. white

2. *Pruritus* describes
   a. an itch   c. scraped skin
   b. soft skin   d. dry skin

3. Which term comes from the Latin, meaning *burning nettle,* and describes swollen, raised, itchy areas of the skin?
   a. pruritus   c. albinism
   b. urticaria   d. comedo

4. Select all terms below that have roots that mean *skin*.
   a. anhidrosis   e. leukoderma
   b. albinism   f. xeroderma
   c. erythema   g. xanthoderma
   d. hypohidrosis h. xerosis

5. Select all terms below that have roots meaning *sweat*.
   a. anhidrosis   e. leukoderma
   b. albinism   f. xanthoderma
   c. erythema   g. xeroderma
   d. hypohidrosis h. xerosis

6. Select all terms below that have roots meaning *white*.
   a. anhidrosis   e. leukoderma
   b. albinism   f. xanthoderma
   c. erythema   g. xeroderma
   d. hypohidrosis h. xerosis

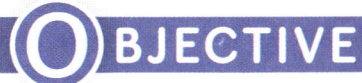

3.3 Observation and Discovery

A very specific language applies to rashes. This allows medical professionals to tell one another about rashes even when the patient is not present or no photo is available. These descriptions relate to the location, size, color, texture, and filling of the rash or its pustules, and they also describe whether the rash is flat or raised.

Usually, skin conditions are first described by their location. If the rash is limited to a specific area, it is *localized*. If the rash is all over the body, it is called a *generalized* rash. Some rashes begin in one area and spread to another. Rashes that start from the middle and work their way outward are *centrifugal*. Rashes that spread from the outside inward are *centripetal*.

Small bumps (under 1 cm) are called *papules*. When they become larger—specifically over 1 cm—they are called *nodules*. If they are large and flat, like a plateau, they are known as *plaques*.

What is inside the rash is important as well. Small bumps (less than 1 cm) filled with clear fluid are called *vesicles*. If the bumps are filled with pus, they are known as *pustules*. A larger vesicle, such as a blister, is called a *bulla,* and larger pustules are called *abscesses*. Small, flat spots, such as freckles, are known as *macules*. Larger macules are *patches*.

Some skin findings are actually caused by blood vessels of the skin or just below the skin. Small bruises under the skin are *petechiae*. Larger bruises are known as *ecchymosis*.

Diagnostic procedures in dermatology are limited. If the skin is being *cultured* for infection, it is being sampled to see if it harbors bacteria (C&S) [culture and sensitivity], a virus, or a fungus. The most common diagnostic procedure is a *skin biopsy*. Many skin conditions can only be clearly distinguished from one another when examined under a microscope. Thus, skin biopsy is a mainstay of dermatology.

Common skin conditions observed by doctors include periorbital hematoma (black eyes).
©Ingram Publishing

primary lesions

TERM	WORD ANALYSIS
Flat, Nonpalpable	
macule (freckle) MA-kyool, MAW-koo-lah **DEFINITION** small, flat, discolored area	from Latin, for *spot* or *stain* Tom Le Goff/Getty Images
patch pach **DEFINITION** larger, flat, discolored area	
Elevated, Palpable, Solid Mass	
papule PA-pyool **DEFINITION** a small solid mass	from Latin, for *pimple*

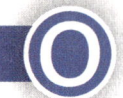

primary lesions *continued*

TERM	WORD ANALYSIS
Elevated, Palpable, Solid Mass	
plaque PLAK DEFINITION a solid mass on the surface of the skin	
Elevated, Fluid-Filled	
bulla BUL-lah DEFINITION a larger blister	from Latin, for *bubble*
pustule PUS-tyool DEFINITION a pus-filled blister	from Latin, for *little blister*
vesicle VEH-sih-kul DEFINITION a smaller blister	ves / icle bladder / little

secondary lesions

TERM	WORD ANALYSIS
Loss of Skin Surface	
ulcer UL-sir DEFINITION a sore	from Latin, for *sore*

Source: Dr Thomas F Sellers, Emory University, Atlanta GA/ CDC

secondary lesions *continued*

TERM	WORD ANALYSIS
Material on Skin Surface	
scale SKAYL DEFINITION skin flaking off	
crust krust DEFINITION a dried substance (i.e., blood, pus) on the skin	

vascular lesions

TERM	WORD ANALYSIS
ecchymosis eh-kih-MOH-sis DEFINITION a larger bruise	from Greek, for *to pour out*
petechia puh-TEE-kee-yah DEFINITION a small bruise	from Latin, for *freckle* or *spot*

©Ingram Publishing

scar formations

TERM	WORD ANALYSIS
cicatrix SIK-ah-triks DEFINITION scar	from Latin, for *scar*
keloid KEE-loid DEFINITION overgrowth of scar tissue	kel / oid tumor / resembling

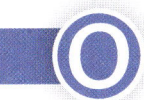

epidermal tumors

TERM	WORD ANALYSIS
nevus NEE-vus	from Latin, for *birthmark* or *mole*
DEFINITION mole	
verruca vah-ROO-kah	from Latin, for *wart*
DEFINITION wart	

Pathology

TERM	WORD ANALYSIS
biopsy (Bx) BAI-op-see	bi / ops / y two / eye / procedure
DEFINITION removal of tissue in order to examine it (with your own two eyes)	

Pathology *continued*

TERM	WORD ANALYSIS		
keratogenic keh-RA-toh-jen-ik	kerato / horny /	gen / creation /	ic pertaining to
DEFINITION causing horny tissue to develop			
keratosis KEH-rah-TOH-sis	kerat / osis horny / condition		
DEFINITION horny tissue condition			
onychocryptosis AW-nih-koh-krip-TOH-sis	onycho / nail /	crypt / hidden /	osis condition
DEFINITION an ingrown nail			
onychopathy aw-nik-AW-pah-thee	onycho / pathy nail / disease		
DEFINITION nail disease			
steatoma STEE-ah-TOH-ma	steat / oma fat / tumor		
DEFINITION a fatty tumor			

TRANSLATION

EXERCISE 1   Match the term on the left with its definition on the right.

_____   1. pustule   a. freckle; small, flat, discolored area

_____   2. patch   b. larger, flat, discolored area

_____   3. plaque   c. from Latin, for *pimple,* a small solid mass

_____   4. vesicle   d. a larger solid mass

_____   5. macule   e. a small blister

_____   6. papule   f. a large blister

_____   7. bulla   g. a pus-filled blister

EXERCISE 2   Match the term on the left with its definition on the right.

_____   1. ulcer   a. a small bruise

_____   2. petechia   b. a large bruise

_____   3. scale   c. skin flaking off

_____   4. crust   d. a sore

_____   5. keloid   e. dried substance (i.e., blood, pus) on the skin

_____   6. verruca   f. scar

_____   7. nevus   g. overgrowth of scar tissue

_____   8. cicatrix   h. mole

_____   9. ecchymosis   i. wart

EXERCISE 3   Translate the following terms as literally as possible.

EXAMPLE: **nasopharyngoscope**   *an instrument for looking at the nose and throat*

1. vesicle   _____

2. abscess   _____

3. keloid   _____

4. biopsy   _____

5. keratosis   _____

6. onychocryptosis   _____

GENERATION

EXERCISE 4   Build a medical term from the information provided.

EXAMPLE: inflammation of the sinuses   *sinusitis*

1. nail disease   _____

2. fat tumor   _____

3. pertaining to horny tissue creation   _____

EXERCISE 5   Multiple-choice questions. Select the correct answer(s).

1. Select all terms below that refer to flat, non-palpable lesions.

a. bulla   e. plaque

b. macule   f. pustule

c. papule   g. vesicle

d. patch

2. Select all terms below that refer to elevated, palpable, solid-mass lesions.
   a. bulla   e. plaque
   b. macule   f. pustule
   c. papule   g. vesicle
   d. patch

3. Select all terms below that refer to elevated, fluid-filled lesions.
   a. bulla   e. plaque
   b. macule   f. pustule
   c. papule   g. vesicle
   d. patch

4. Which elevated, fluid-filled lesion is pus-filled?
   a. bulla   c. pustule
   b. plaque   d. vesicle

5. Select all terms below that refer to lesions involving the loss of skin surface.
   a. crust   c. ulcer
   b. scale   d. macule

6. Select all terms below that refer to lesions involving material on the skin surface.
   a. crust   c. ulcer
   b. scale   d. macule

7. Select all terms below that refer to vascular lesions.
   a. cicatrix   d. nevus
   b. ecchymosis   e. petechia
   c. keloid   f. verruca

8. Select all terms below that refer to scar formation.
   a. cicatrix   d. nevus
   b. ecchymosis   e. petechia
   c. keloid   f. verruca

9. Select all terms below that refer to epidermal tumors.
   a. cicatrix   d. nevus
   b. ecchymosis   e. petechia
   c. keloid   f. verruca

10. Rashes that start from the middle and work their way outward are _____.
    a. centrifugal   c. generalized
    b. centripetal   d. localized

11. Rashes that spread from the outside inward are _____.
    a. centrifugal   c. generalized
    b. centripetal   d. localized

12. If the rash is limited to a specific area, it is a _____ rash.
    a. centrifugal   c. generalized
    b. centripetal   d. localized

13. If the rash is all over the body, it is a _____ rash.
    a. centrifugal   c. generalized
    b. centripetal   d. localized

EXERCISE 6   Define the following terms.

1. macule _____
2. patch _____
3. papule _____
4. plaque _____
5. bulla _____
6. pustule _____
7. ulcer _____
8. scale _____
9. crust _____
10. petechia _____
11. ecchymosis _____
12. cicatrix _____
13. verruca _____
14. nevus _____

3.4 Diagnosis and Pathology

Skin problems are fairly limited in variety. For the most part, skin problems are infections, inflammations, tumors, or changes in the skin. Bacterial infections of the skin can be a small yellow crust, such as *impetigo,* or a more extensive one, such as *cellulitis,* which invades deeper layers of skin.

Other skin structures may be infected by bacteria as well: *Hidradenitis* is an infection of the sweat glands in the skin. *Acne* is similar. It is an infection of the *sebaceous* glands that commonly occurs in puberty because of the increase in hormones. Skin can be infected with a fungus (*dermatomycosis*), and fingernails and toenails can also be infected with a fungus (*onychomycosis*). Nail infections typically require a long course of treatment.

Skin may be inflamed without being infected. *Dermatitis* is a general term for skin inflammation that does not indicate its cause.

Most tumors of the skin are related to ultraviolet (UV) exposure from the sun. As a result, dermatologists often spend at least part of their visits with their patients explaining how to avoid sun exposure.

- While *melanoma*, a cancer of the pigment-producing cells in the skin, is not the most common form of skin cancer, it is responsible for the most deaths. Melanomas are brown.

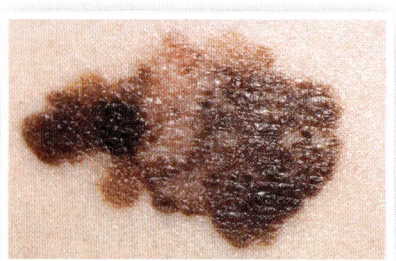

Malignant melanoma
Source: National Cancer Institute (NCI)

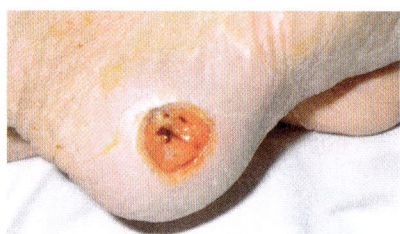

Decubitus ulcer
Mediscan/Alamy Stock Photo

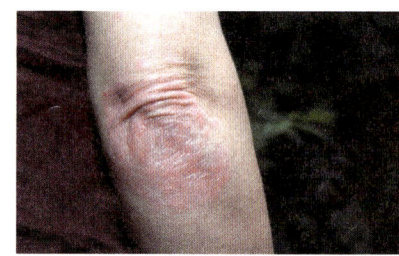

Dermatitis
Dave Bolton/Getty Images

dermatological terms

TERM	WORD ANALYSIS
acne vulgaris AK-nee vul-GAR-is	acne vulgaris acne common
DEFINITION inflammation of the skin follicles	
dermatitis der-mah-TAI-tis	dermat / itis skin / inflammation
DEFINITION inflammation of the skin	
dermatomycosis der-mah-toh-mai-KOH-sis	dermato / myc / osis skin / fungus / condition
DEFINITION a fungal skin condition	

Source: CDC

dermatological terms *continued*

TERM	WORD ANALYSIS
dermopathy der-MAW-pa-thee	dermo / pathy skin / disease
DEFINITION skin disease	
eczema EK-zeh-mah	from Greek, for *to boil over*
DEFINITION a red itchy rash that may weep or ooze, then become crusted and scaly	
hidradenitis hih-dra-deh-NAI-tis	hidr / aden / itis sweat / gland / inflammation
DEFINITION inflammation of the sweat glands	

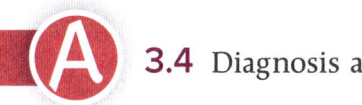
dermatological terms *continued*

TERM	WORD ANALYSIS
hypertrichosis HAI-per-trih-KOH-sis	hyper / trich / osis over / hair / condition
DEFINITION excessive growth of hair	
ichthyosis ik-thee-OH-sis	ichthy / osis fish scale / condiion
DEFINITION a condition in which the skin is dry and scaly and resembles fish scales	
impetigo im-peh-TAI-goh	from Latin, for *to attack*
DEFINITION a highly contagious bacterial infection of the skin	
mycodermatitis mai-koh-der-mah-TAI-tis	myco / dermat / itis fungus / skin / inflammation
DEFINITION inflammation of the skin caused by fungus	
onychomycosis AW-nih-koh-mai-KOH-sis	onycho / myc / osis nail / fungus / condition
DEFINITION a fungal condition of the nail	
sclerodermatitis skleh-roh-der-mah-TAI-tis	sclero / dermat / itis hard / skin / inflammation
DEFINITION inflammation of the skin accompanied by thickening and hardening	
scleronychia skleh-raw-NIH-kee-ah	scler / onych / ia hard / nail / condition
DEFINITION thickening and hardening of the nails	
seborrheic dermatitis se-boh-RAY-ik der-mah-TAI-tis	sebo / rrhe / ic oil / discharge / pertaining to dermat / itis skin / inflammation
DEFINITION inflammation of the skin caused by the discharge of oil (sebum)	
steatitis stay-ah-TAI-tis	steat / itis fat / inflammation
DEFINITION inflammation of fat tissue	
trichomycosis trik-koh-mai-KOH-sis	tricho / myc / osis hair / fungus / condition
DEFINITION a fungal condition of the hair	
xanthosis zan-THOH-sis	xanth / osis yellow / condition
DEFINITION yellowing of the skin	

burns

TERM	WORD ANALYSIS
first-degree burn first deh-GREE birn	
first-degree burn	
DEFINITION burn affecting only the epidermis or superficial layer of the skin	
second-degree burn SEH-kund deh-GREE birn	
second-degree burn	
DEFINITION deeper burn affecting both the epidermis and dermis	
third-degree burn third deh-GREE birn	
third-degree burn	
DEFINITION deep burn affecting the epidermis, dermis, and subcutaneous layer	
fourth-degree burn forth deh-GREE birn	
fourth-degree burn	
DEFINITION deep burn affecting not just all layers of the skin (epidermis, dermis, and subcutaneous layer) but also underlying tissues such as muscle, fascia, or bone	

oncology

TERM	WORD ANALYSIS
malignant melanoma ma-LIG-nant meh-lah-NOH-mah	malignant melan / oma bad black / tumor
DEFINITION a harmful tumor of melanin cells	

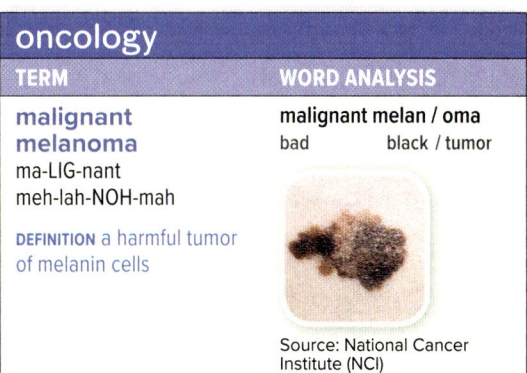

Source: National Cancer Institute (NCI)

TRANSLATION

EXERCISE 1 Underline and define the word parts from this chapter in the following terms.

1. hidradenitis (2 roots) _____

2. dermatomycosis (2 roots) _____

3. trichomycosis (2 roots) _____

4. seborrheic _____

5. steatitis _____

6. keratosis _____

7. scleronychia (2 roots) _____

8. xanthosis _____

EXERCISE 2 Match the term on the left with its definition on the right.

_____ 1. impetigo

_____ 2. acne vulgaris

_____ 3. eczema

_____ 4. ichthyosis

_____ 5. first-degree burn

_____ 6. second-degree burn

_____ 7. third-degree burn

_____ 8. fourth-degree burn

a. a burn affecting only the epidermis or superficial layer of the skin

b. a deeper burn affecting both the epidermis and dermis

c. a deep burn affecting the epidermis, dermis, and subcutaneous layer

d. a deep burn affecting not just all layers of the skin (epidermis, dermis, and subcutaneous layer) but also underlying tissues such as muscles, fascia, or bone

e. a highly contagious bacterial infection of the skin

f. a skin condition that is dry and scaly

g. a red, itchy rash that may weep or ooze and then become crusted and scaly

h. common acne

EXERCISE 3 Translate the following terms as literally as possible.

EXAMPLE: nasopharyngoscope *an instrument for looking at the nose and throat*

1. steatitis _____

2. mycodermatitis _____

3. sclerodermatitis _____

4. scleronychia _____

5. ichthyosis _____

6. malignant melanoma _____

GENERATION

EXERCISE 4 Build a medical term from the information provided.

EXAMPLE: inflammation of the sinuses
sinusitis

1. skin disease _____

2. skin inflammation _____

3. sweat gland inflammation _____

4. a fungal condition of the nail _____

5. a fungal condition of the hair _____

6. a fungal condition of the skin _____

7. yellowing of the skin _____

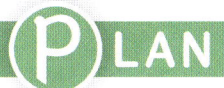
3.5 Treatments and Therapies

There is an old joke in the health community that treatment options in dermatology are very simple: If it's wet, dry it; if it's dry, wet it; and if nothing else works, use steroids. The medicines available in skin care have increased significantly, but they mostly fall in one of a few categories: anti-infection or cleansing (*antibiotics*), anti-immune (*steroids* or related), and anti-itch or allergy (*antihistamines*). In contrast to the limited number of medicines, the field of dermatology employs a variety of types of procedures in eradicating disease. They use chemicals (*chemotherapy*), vacuums (*liposuction*), cold (*cryosurgery*), lasers (*dermabrasion*), and even electricity.

One very challenging and important area of skin surgery is transplanting or grafting new skin in place of old skin. This is needed in areas where skin has been burned, scraped off, or killed. The transplanted skin can come from the patient (*autograft*), another person (*homograft*), or even another species (*heterograft*). While not all health care workers perform such in-depth procedures, most do perform skin-related procedures many times a day—specifically, injections. Inserting a needle into the skin to give medicine is a very routine part of many medical fields.

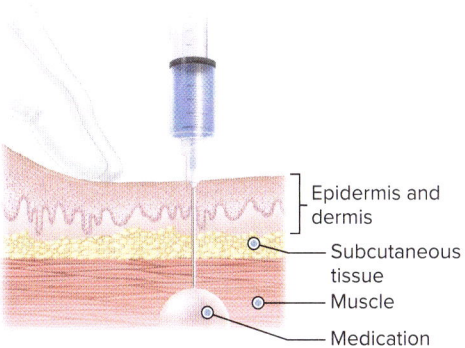

- Epidermis and dermis
- Subcutaneous tissue
- Muscle
- Medication

A wide variety of medications are administered via hypodermic needle. As the name suggests, it injects the medicine beneath (*hypo-*) the skin (*dermic*).

general terms

TERM	WORD ANALYSIS		
hypodermic hai-poh-DER-mik	hypo beneath	/ derm / skin	/ ic / pertaining to
DEFINITION pertaining to beneath the skin			
intradermal in-trah-DER-mal	intra inside	/ derm / skin	/ al / pertaining to
DEFINITION pertaining to inside the skin			
percutaneous per-kyoo-TAY-nee-us	per through	/ cutane / skin	/ ous / pertaining to
DEFINITION pertaining to through the skin			
subcutaneous sub-kyoo-TAY-nee-us	sub beneath	/ cutane / skin	/ ous / pertaining to
DEFINITION pertaining to beneath the skin			
transdermal trans-DER-mal	trans through	/ derm / skin	/ al / pertaining to
DEFINITION pertaining to through the skin			

procedures

TERM	WORD ANALYSIS		
chemotherapy KEE-moh-THEH-rah-pee	chemo chemical	/ therapy / treatment	
DEFINITION treatment using chemicals			
cryosurgery KRAI-oh-SIR-juh-ree	cryo cold	/ surgery / surgery	
DEFINITION destruction of tissue through freezing			
dermabrasion der-mah-BRAY-zhun	derm skin	/ ab / away	/ rasion / rub
DEFINITION rubbing or scraping away the outer surface of skin			

3.5 Treatments and Therapies

procedures *continued*

TERM	WORD ANALYSIS
incision and drainage (I&D) in-SIH-zhun and DRAY-nij	in / cision in / cut
DEFINITION to cut into a wound to allow trapped infected liquid to drain	
lipectomy lih-PEK-toh-mee	lip / ectomy fat / removal
DEFINITION removal of fatty tissue	
liposuction LAI-poh-SUK-shun	lipo / suction fat / vacuum
DEFINITION removal of fatty tissue using a vacuum	
onychectomy aw-nik-EK-toh-mee	onych / ectomy nail / removal
DEFINITION remove of a nail	
onychotomy aw-ni-KAW-toh-mee	onycho / tomy nail / incision
DEFINITION incision into a nail	

pharmacology

TERM	WORD ANALYSIS
anesthetic an-es-THET-ik	an / esthetic no / sensation
DEFINITION a drug that temporarily blocks sensation	
antibiotic an-tai-bai-OH-tk	anti / biotic against / life
DEFINITION a drug that destroys or opposes growth of microorganisms NOTE: The life that the drug is preventing is not the life of the patient but the life of microorganisms; similarly, a drug that encourages the growth of microorganisms (especially in the digestive system) is called a probiotic.	Christopher Kerrigan/ McGraw-Hill Education
antihistamine an-tee-HIS-tah-meen	anti / histamine against / histamine
DEFINITION a drug that opposes the effects of histamine	Christopher Kerrigan/ McGraw-Hill Education
antipruritic an-tee-pruh-RIH-tik	anti / pruritic against / itching
DEFINITION a drug that prevents or relieves itching	

Learning Outcome 3.5 Exercises

TRANSLATION

EXERCISE 1 Underline and define the word parts from this chapter in the following terms.

1. dermabrasion _____

2. lipectomy _____

3. hypodermic _____

4. onychectomy _____

5. percutaneous _____

6. subcutaneous _____

EXERCISE 2 Match the term on the left with its definition on the right.

_____ 1. anesthetic

_____ 2. antibiotic

_____ 3. antihistamine

_____ 4. antipruritic

_____ 5. incision and drainage (I&D)

a. a drug that destroys or opposes growth of microorganisms

b. to cut into a wound to allow infected liquid to drain

c. a drug that opposes the effects of histamine

d. a drug that prevents or relieves itching

e. a drug that temporarily blocks sensation

EXERCISE 3 Translate the following terms as literally as possible.

> EXAMPLE: **nasopharyngoscope** _an instrument for looking at the nose and throat_

1. cryosurgery _____

2. dermabrasion _____

3. incision _____

4. liposuction _____

5. onychotomy _____

GENERATION

EXERCISE 4 Build a medical term from the information provided.

> EXAMPLE: **inflammation of the sinuses**
> _sinusitis_

1. pertaining to upon the skin _____

2. pertaining to beneath the skin (use _cutaneo_)

_____

3. pertaining to inside the skin _____

4. pertaining to through the skin (2 terms)

_____

5. pertaining to beneath the skin (use _dermo_) __

6. chemical treatment _____

7. removing fatty tissue _____

8. removing a nail _____

EXERCISE 5 Describe the purpose of the following drugs.

1. anesthetic _____

2. antibiotic _____

3. antihistamine _____

4. antipruritic _____

3.6 Electronic Health Records

Dermatology Consult Note

Dermatology Consult

CLINIC CARE
Health and Clinical Excellence

I had the pleasure of seeing your patient John Johnson in my clinic on February 14. Your office referred him to me regarding a rash on sun-exposed areas of his body. He is a 45-year-old landscape architect who spends a large part of his days outdoors. He had noticed several spots on his arms but did not seek medical care at that time. At his routine physical, his care provider noticed the rash on his arms.

Physical exam revealed a well-developed, well-nourished, fair-skinned male. His heart was regular in rate and rhythm. His lungs were clear. His mucous membranes were moist and pink. His skin exam was significant for papules of **hyperkeratosis** with surrounding **erythema.** A few of the lesions are **hyperpigmented.** He has larger patches on his scalp.

A skin biospy performed in my office confirmed the diagnosis of **actinic keratosis (AK).** After explaining the results to Mr. Johnson, I recommended **cryotherapy** for the smaller lesions on his arms and **dermabrasion** for his scalp lesions. I explained to Mr. Johnson that **AK** can lead to **squamous cell carcinoma** and taught him about the risks of sun exposure, including further AKs and **melanoma.**

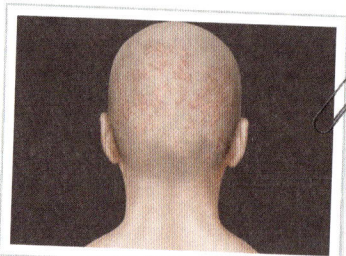

Thank you for this interesting consult.

— **James Skinner, MD**

EXERCISE 1   Match the term on the left with its definition on the right.

_____ 1. papule   a. redness

_____ 2. hyperkeratosis   b. removal of tissue in order to examine it

_____ 3. erythema   c. excessive growth of horny skin

_____ 4. hyperpigmented   d. treatment of the skin using cold

_____ 5. patch   e. a small, solid mass

_____ 6. biopsy   f. larger, flat discolored area

_____ 7. cryotherapy   g. tumor of melanin cells

_____ 8. dermabrasion   h. excessive pigment in the skin

_____ 9. melanoma   i. rubbing or scraping away the outer surface of skin

EXERCISE 2   Fill in the blanks.

1. The patient's skin exam was significant for

   _____

   (small, solid masses) of *hyperkeratosis* (excessive growth of _____ skin) with surrounding *erythema* (define:

   _____).

2. He has larger _____ (larger, flat discolored areas) on his scalp.

EXERCISE 3   Multiple-choice questions. Select the correct answer.

1. A few of Mr. Johnson's lesions are *hyperpigmented,* which means
   a. excessive pigmentation
   b. underpigmentation
   c. loss of pigmentation
   d. creation of pigmentation

2. The diagnosis of actinic keratosis was confirmed by performing
   a. biopsy   c. dermabrasion
   b. cryotherapy   d. C&S

3. Which treatment option was NOT recommended for the patient?
   a. biopsy
   b. treatment using cold
   c. rubbing or scraping away the outer surface of skin
   d. corticosteroids

4. The root word in *melanoma* means
   a. white   c. yellow
   b. black   d. red

Quick Reference

quick reference glossary of roots

ROOT	DEFINITION	ROOT	DEFINITION	ROOT	DEFINITION
adip/o	fat	kerat/o	hard, horny	steat/o	fat
alb/o	white	leuk/o	white	trich/o	hair
cutane/o	skin	lip/o	fat	ungu/o	nail
derm/o	skin	melan/o	black	xanth/o	yellow
dermat/o	skin	onych/o	nail	xer/o	dry
erythr/o	red	pil/o	hair		
hidr/o	sweat	seb/o, sebace/o	oil		

quick reference glossary of abbreviations

ABBREVIATION	DEFINITION
ABCDE	asymmetry, border, color, diameter, evolving
Bx	biopsy
C&S	culture and sensitivity
decub	decubitus ulcer
derm	dermatology
ID	intradermal
SC	subcutaneous
SQ	subcutaneous
subcut	subcutaneous
TD	transdermal
I&D	incision and drainage
UV	ultraviolet

The Musculoskeletal System—Orthopedics

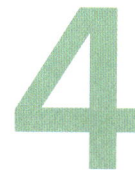

4

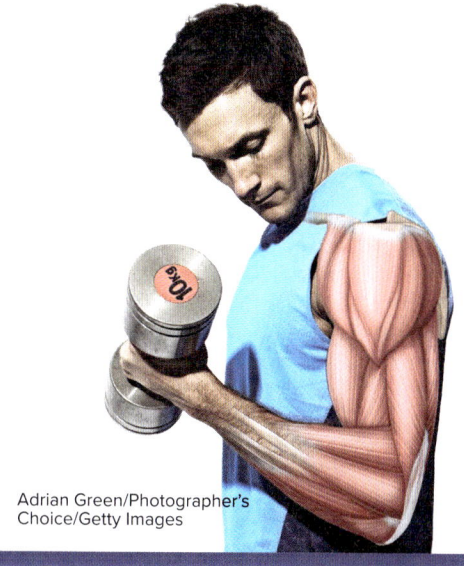

Adrian Green/Photographer's
Choice/Getty Images

Learning Outcomes

*Upon completion of this chapter,
you will be able to:*

4.1 Identify the **roots/word parts** associated with the **musculoskeletal system.**

4.2 Translate the **Subjective** terms associated with the **musculoskeletal system.**

4.3 Translate the **Objective** terms associated with the **musculoskeletal system.**

4.4 Translate the **Assessment** terms associated with the **musculoskeletal system.**

4.5 Translate the **Plan** terms associated with the **musculoskeletal system.**

4.6 Distinguish terms associated with the **musculoskeletal system** in the context of **electronic health records.**

Introduction and Overview of the Musculoskeletal System

Think of a crane at a construction site. It's an impressive piece of machinery. All the parts work together to move some very heavy objects.

Your body, specifically your musculoskeletal system, is also an amazing machine. All the parts work in just the right way to allow you to make big movements, such as lifting a heavy box, and fine movements, such as writing a note on the box.

Continuing the crane analogy, your bones are like the metal fused together to make the framework of the crane. Like the metal, your bones are strong and sturdy. They make the framework of your body. This framework supports your body and protects your internal organs. Your bones are lighter than the steel of a crane, but like steel, they are incredibly strong.

Unlike steel, however, your bones are living organs. They can grow, maintain themselves, and even self-repair.

If you look at a crane up close, you'll notice that the framework is not one solid piece. Instead, it is made up of many smaller pieces that are welded, bolted, or hinged together. Some connection points are immobile, while others allow movement. Your joints are the connection points in your body. They keep the parts together and allow for movement so the crane can actually move things.

The crane couldn't move anything without any power, though. Your muscles are the workhorses of your musculoskeletal system. They act as powerful movers and stabilizers. Some muscles, such as those in your thighs, are thick and strong, while others, such as those in your hands, are smaller and are made for delicate movements. In fact, the muscles of your eyes are at work even now as you read these words. Together, your bones, joints, and muscles move you, protect you, and give your body support.

4.1 Word Parts of the Musculoskeletal System

The Skeleton

Your bones make up the framework of your body—your skeleton. Like any good design, your skeleton has a specific layout. The bones in the middle of the skeleton are called the *axial* part of your skeleton. Your skull (*cranio*) is attached to your spine.

Your spine is made of many smaller bones (*vertebra*) that connect together. They protect your spinal cord, a very fragile and important body structure. Your spine has four sections: the neck section (*cervical*), chest/upper back section (*thoracic*), and lower back (*lumbar* and *sacral*). Your ribs (*costo*) attach to the vertebra of the thoracic section.

Your arms and legs branch off both sides of this central part of the skeleton. Your upper arm (*brachio*) leads to the two bones of your forearm (*radius* and *ulna*), then to your wrist (*carpo*), and finally to your fingers (*phalanges*). Your legs begin with your thigh bone (*femur*), work down to the two shin bones (*tibia* and *fibula*), move on to your ankle (*tarsal*), and ultimately reach your toes (*phalanges* again, just like the fingers).

---

bone

ROOT: **oste/o**

EXAMPLES: osteopathy, periosteum

NOTES: At birth, you had over 300 bones but no kneecaps. As a full-grown adult, you now have 206 bones—including two kneecaps—a net loss of at least 96 bones. A human's neck also contains the same number of bones as a giraffe's.

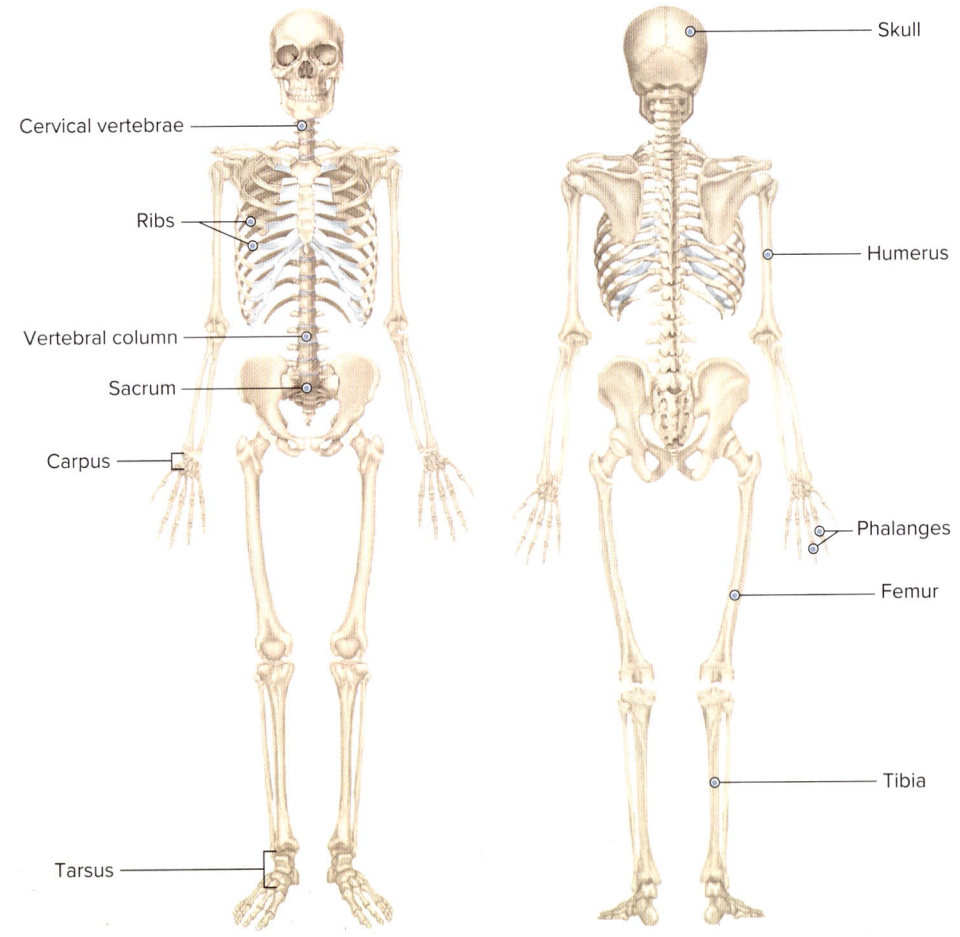

Cervical vertebrae

Ribs

Vertebral column

Sacrum

Carpus

Tarsus

Skull

Humerus

Phalanges

Femur

Tibia

head, skull

ROOT: *crani/o*

EXAMPLES: craniometer, craniomalacia

NOTES: The term *migraine* comes from the word *hemicrania,* meaning *half the head.* The term reflects the fact that most migraines are localized in half the patient's head.

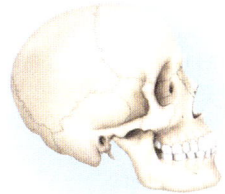

neck

ROOT: *cervic/o*

EXAMPLES: cervical spine, cervicitis

NOTES: Remember: When a *c* is followed by *a, o,* or *u,* it is pronounced hard like a *k.* When followed by *e* or *i,* it is pronounced soft like an *s.* Therefore, the two example words above are pronounced SIR-vih-kal and SIR-vih-SAI-tis.

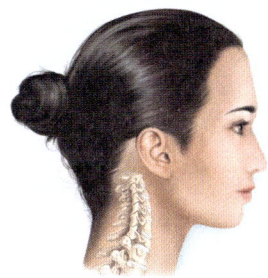

vertebra

ROOT: *spondyl/o*

EXAMPLES: spondylodynia, spondylitis

NOTES: *Vertebra* comes from Latin, for *to turn.* It is called this because the spine was once thought of as the hinge or center around which all other bones turned.

loin, lower back

ROOT: *lumb/o*

EXAMPLES: lumbar, lumbodynia

NOTES: The root *lumbo* comes from the Latin *lumbo,* for *loin.* It refers to the region between the rib cage and the pelvis, but frankly, it makes us think about steak.

finger

ROOT: *dactyl/o*

EXAMPLES: adactyly, dactylalgia

NOTES: The flying dinosaur called the pterodactlyl gets its name from *ptero* (winged) + *dactly* (fingers), which literally means *winged fingers.*

wrist

ROOT: *carp/o*

EXAMPLES: carpectomy, metacarpal

NOTES: The *carpal tunnel* is the area in the wrist where the nerves enter the hand. Repetitive motions using the wrist can cause the nerve to swell, press against the walls of the carpal tunnel, and result in numbness in the hand; this condition is called *carpal tunnel syndrome.*

rib

ROOT: *cost/o*

EXAMPLES: costectomy, intercostal

NOTES: The English word *coast* comes from this word. Think of a country's coasts as its ribs or sides. Also, the word *accost,* which means *to come alongside someone,* comes from this word.

femur (thighbone)

ROOT: *femor/o*

EXAMPLES: femoral artery

NOTES: The femur is the strongest bone in the human body (nonetheless, a hyena can bite right through it—*ouch*). The femur makes up about a fourth of a person's overall height.

tibia (shinbone)

ROOT: *tibi/o*

EXAMPLES: tibiaglia

NOTES: The term *tibia* originally meant *pipe* or *flute*. Evidently, the person who named this bone thought the shinbone bore a resemblance to this instrument.

Joints

"The toe bone's connected to the heel bone. The heel bone's connected to the foot bone . . ." and so it goes. While it doesn't exactly reflect the way anatomy is taught in medical school, the old children's song has the right idea. Every bone in the body, except the hyoid bone, is connected to another, and these connection points are known as *joints.*

Not all joints allow movement. For example, the bones in your skull are bound tightly together. Usually when we think of joints, we picture the moving ones because after all, these are the ones that we hurt when participating in sports or that cause problems in older age.

Moving joints allow motions such as bending and rotating. When a joint bends, it's called *flexion.* When it straightens, it's called *extension. Abduction* is the widening of a joint to move parts away from the body. The term *adduction* means just the opposite—during adduction, the joint narrows to bring parts back toward the body.

Moving joints often have surrounding support tissues to absorb shock, keep the bones aligned, and keep the bones moving smoothly. *Tendons* hold muscle to bone. *Ligaments* hold bone to bone. *Cartilage* surrounds bones at the joints and allows smooth movement among them. Under many tendons lie sacs of fluid, known as *bursae,* that help keep muscles and bones moving smoothly as well.

cartilage

ROOT: *chondr/o*

EXAMPLES: chondritis, chondrodynia

NOTES: People who always think they are sick are called *hypochondriacs.* This term comes from *hypo-* (beneath) + *chondro*

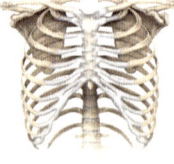

(cartilage—here specifically referring to the ribs) and reflected an ancient belief that such thoughts came from deep within the rib cage.

joint

ROOT: *arthr/o*

EXAMPLES: arthritis, arthroscopic surgery

NOTES: Insects, spiders, scorpions, and shellfish belong to the animal family known as *arthropods.* This term comes from *arthro* (joint) + *pod* (feet) and refers to their segmented limbs. If you have ever eaten crab legs, you know exactly what I mean.

bursa

ROOT: *burs/o*

EXAMPLES: bursitis, bursectomy

NOTES: A *bursa* is a small fluid-filled sac found near the body's joint. Bursae reduce friction and act as cushions. The word comes from the Greek word meaning *purse* or *bag.* In some places, the treasurer of an organization is called a *bursar* because he or she handles the purse. Also, to be *rei**burs**ed* means to have money *put back in your purse.*

Muscles

Think of a thick rope. Unlike a piece of string, it is not one strand but numerous strands bundled together. This design makes the rope much stronger. Your skeletal muscles are similar, as they are a collection of thousands of muscle fibers bundled together. The bundles are grouped together to form a muscle.

Under a microscope, these bundles appear as lines called striations. For this reason, skeletal muscle is also known as striated muscle. While cardiac muscle also has striations, it is slightly different in its packagings and is found only in the heart. Both cardiac and skeletal muscle differ from smooth muscle, which has no specific bundles or striations. Smooth muscle lines hollow organs such as blood vessels and airways. Cardiac and smooth muscle move involuntarily and are not actually part of the musculoskeletal system.

Skeletal muscle is encased in a thick membrane called *fascia.* The fascia helps keep the muscle together. Muscles attach to bones. If they didn't, they wouldn't be very useful. Their job is to move the bones, after all. Muscles attach to bones via *tendons,* which are thick bands of connective tissue.

tendon (connective tissue attaching muscle to bone)

ROOTS: *ten/o, tend/o, tendin/o*

EXAMPLES: tenodynia, tendolysis, tendinitis

NOTES: From Latin, for *to stretch*. This root is also found in the English word *attend,* which means *to stretch toward.*

muscle

ROOTS: *muscul/o, my/o, myos/o*

EXAMPLES: musculoskeletal, myopathy, myositis

NOTES: The term *muscle* comes from Latin, for *little mouse.* It was once thought that the movement of certain muscles looked like mice running underneath the skin. Personally, we don't see the connection, but linking muscle and mouse must have been commonplace, as Greek, German, and Arabic all have similar words for *muscle* and *mouse.*

Motion

Usually when you think about your muscles, you think of movement (*kinesio*). While this is a very important part of what they do, they're also hard at work when they're not moving. Your muscles not only move you, but they also support you.

This constant holding together—the built-in strength of your muscles—is your muscles' tone (*tono*). Without any muscle tone, your body would be completely limp. Your muscles require input from your nervous system to move and coordinate (*taxo*).

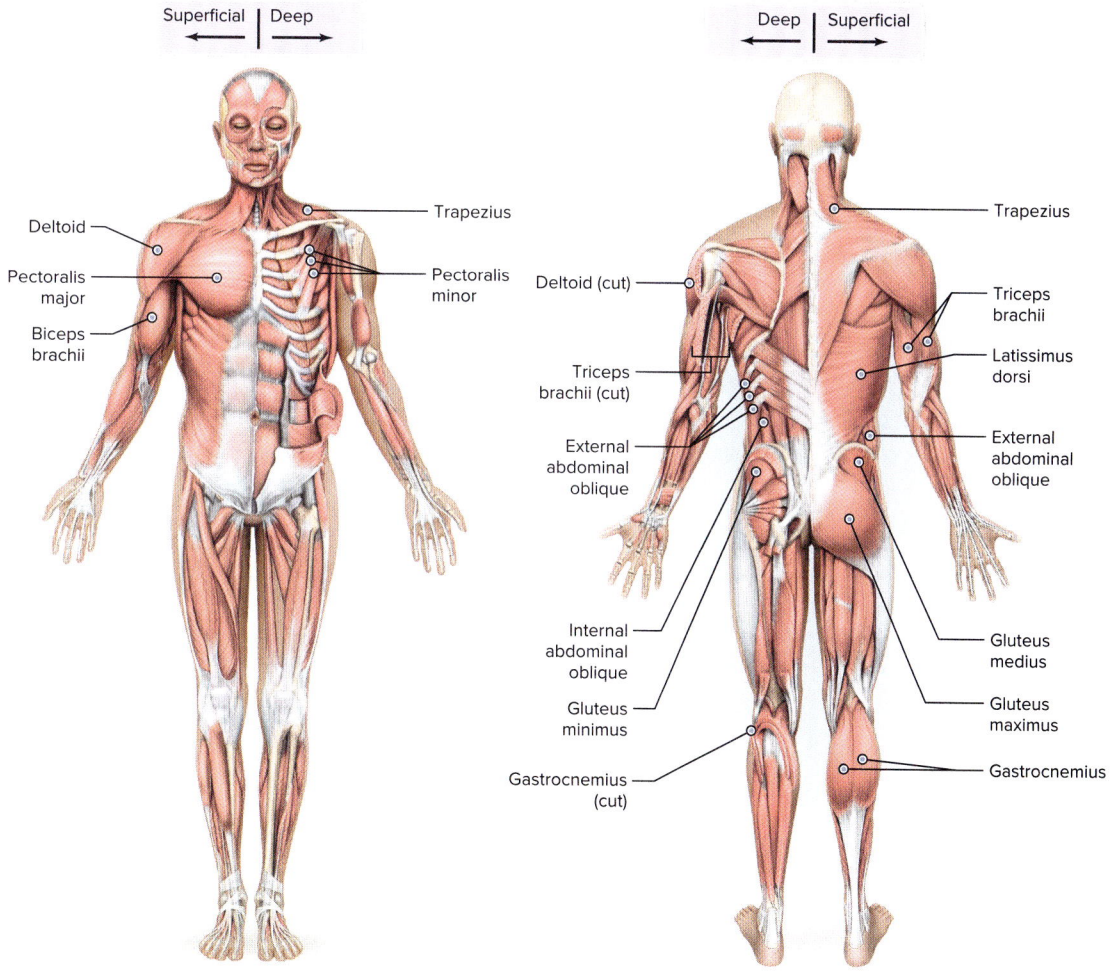

Superficial | Deep

Deltoid
Pectoralis major
Biceps brachii

Trapezius
Pectoralis minor

Deep | Superficial

Deltoid (cut)

Triceps brachii (cut)

External abdominal oblique

Internal abdominal oblique

Gluteus minimus

Gastrocnemius (cut)

Trapezius

Triceps brachii

Latissimus dorsi

External abdominal oblique

Gluteus medius

Gluteus maximus

Gastrocnemius

If you have problems transferring this input from the nervous system, you may suffer from partial paralysis (*paresis*) or complete paralysis (*plegia*).

tone, tension

ROOT: *ton/o*

EXAMPLES: dystonia, tonograph

NOTES: *Tonic* is a word for a medicinal drink. This term was used because medicinal drinks were once thought to restore a person's good muscle tone. Today, tonic water still has medicinal value. Although some people think tonic water is simply another name for carbonated soda water, tonic is actually a form of carbonated soda water in which quinine, a drug used to treat malaria, has been dissolved. Tonic water was developed to treat people who lived in tropical areas, where malaria is often prevalent.

movement, motion

ROOTS: *kinesi/o* (also sometimes *kinet/o*)

EXAMPLES: kinesiology, hyperkinesia, kinetic energy

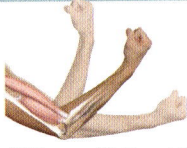
JW Ramsey/McGraw-Hill Education

NOTES: *Akinetopsia* (pronounced ah-KEE-no-TOP-see-ah) comes from the roots *a* (no) + *kinet* (movement) + *opsia* (vision) and refers to a condition where a patient can see an object if it is still but is unable to see it if it is moving.

arrangement, order, coordination

ROOT: *tax/o*

EXAMPLES: ataxia, hypotaxia

NOTES: *Syntax* is an English grammar term made up of the roots *syn* (together) + *tax* (arrangement) and refers to the study of the way words are arranged in a sentence.

Taxidermy, which comes from *taxo* (arrange) + *dermy* (skin), refers to the practice of removing and displaying the head and skin of an animal. The arrangement of military forces before a battle is called *tactics*.

Learning Outcome 4.1 Exercises

TRANSLATION

EXERCISE 1   Match the word part on the left with its definition on the right.

_____ 1. crani/o   a. bone

_____ 2. oste/o   b. head, skull

_____ 3. lumb/o   c. loin, lower back

_____ 4. femor/o   d. neck

_____ 5. cervic/o   e. rib

_____ 6. cost/o   f. thighbone

_____ 7. carp/o   g. vertebra

_____ 8. spondyl/o   h. wrist

EXERCISE 2   Translate the following word parts.

1. femor/o _____

2. crani/o _____

3. oste/o _____

4. cervic/o _____

5. lumb/o _____

6. cost/o _____

7. carp/o _____

8. spondyl/o _____

EXERCISE 3 Match the word part on the left with its definition on the right. Some definitions will be used more than once.

_____ 1. burs/o   a. arrangement, order, coordination

_____ 2. muscul/o   b. bursa

_____ 3. arthr/o   c. cartilage

_____ 4. ten/o, tend/o, d. joint
          tendin/o

_____ 5. ton/o   e. movement, motion

_____ 6. my/o, myos/o f. muscle

_____ 7. kinesi/o   g. tendon

_____ 8. chondr/o   h. tone, tension

_____ 9. tax/o

EXERCISE 4 Translate the following word parts.

1. arthr/o _____

2. burs/o _____

3. chondr/o _____

4. kinesi/o _____

5. muscul/o _____

6. my/o, myos/o _____

7. tax/o _____

8. ten/o, tend/o, tendin/o _____

9. ton/o _____

GENERATION

EXERCISE 5 Identify the word parts for the following definitions.

1. tibia _____

2. tone, tension _____

3. thighbone _____

4. cartilage _____

5. head, skull _____

6. loin, lower back _____

7. neck _____

8. finger _____

9. rib _____

EXERCISE 6 Identify the word parts for the following definitions.

1. tendon (3 roots) _____

2. bursa _____

3. tone, tension _____

4. joint _____

5. movement, motion _____

6. muscle (3 roots) _____

7. arrangement, order, coordination _____

8. cartilage _____

EXERCISE 7 Build a medical term from the information provided.

1. inflammation of the tendon _____

2. inflammation of the bursa _____

3. joint inflammation _____

4. decrease in muscle tone or tightness _____

5. decrease in muscle movement or activity _____

6. softening of a muscle _____

7. abnormal softening of the cartilage _____

4.2 Patient History, Problems, Complaints

Pain is the most common musculoskeletal medical complaint. A patient could have pain in a bone (*ostealgia*), joint (*arthralgia/arthrodynia*), tendon (*tenalgia*), or muscle (*myalgia/myodynia*). A patient may also notice a change in a muscle's appearance—a muscle may be wasting away (*atrophy*) or abnormally large (*hypertrophy*). Most of the other problems people experience relate to a change in how their muscles or joints are working.

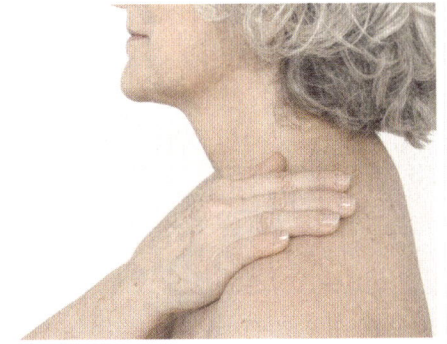

Feliz Aggelos/Getty Images

Pain is the most common musculoskeletal medical complaint.

joints

TERM	WORD ANALYSIS
arthralgia ar-THRAL-jah	arthr / algia joint / pain
DEFINITION joint pain	
arthrodynia ar-throh-DAI-nee-ah	arthro / dynia joint / pain
DEFINITION joint pain	
cervicodynia sir-vih-koh-DAI-nee-ah	cervico / dynia neck / pain
DEFINITION neck pain	

bones

TERM	WORD ANALYSIS
costalgia kaws-TAL-jah	cost / algia rib / pain
DEFINITION rib pain	
ostealgia aw-stee-AL-jah	oste / algia bone / pain
DEFINITION bone pain	
osteodynia aw-stee-oh-DAI-nee-ah	osteo / dynia bone / pain
DEFINITION bone pain	
spondylodynia spawn-dih-loh-DAI-nee-ah	spondylo / dynia vertebra / pain
DEFINITION vertebra pain	
tibialgia tih-bee-AL-ja	tibi / algia tibia / pain
DEFINITION tibia (shin) pain	

muscles

TERM	WORD ANALYSIS
bradykinesia bray-dih-kih-NEE-zhah	brady / kinesia slow / movement
DEFINITION slow movement	
dyskinesia dis-kih-NEE-zhah	dys / kinesia bad / movement
DEFINITION inability to control movement	
dystaxia dis-TAK-see-ah	dys / taxia bad / coordination
DEFINITION poor coordination	
dystonia dis-TOH-nee-ah	dys / tonia bad / muscle tone
DEFINITION poor muscle tone	
hyperkinesia hai-per-kih-NEE-zhah	hyper / kinesia over / movement
DEFINITION increase in muscle movement or activity	
hypotonia hai-poh-TOH-nee-yah	hypo / tonia under / muscle tone
DEFINITION decrease in muscle tone or tigtness	

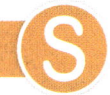

muscles _continued_	
TERM	**WORD ANALYSIS**
myalgia mai-AL-jah	**my** / algia muscle / pain
DEFINITION muscle pain	
myasthenia mai-as-THEH-nee-ah	**my** / asthenia muscle / weakness
DEFINITION muscle weakness	

muscles _continued_	
TERM	**WORD ANALYSIS**
tenalgia ten-AL-jah	**ten** / algia tendon / pain
DEFINITION tendon pain	

Learning Outcome 4.2 Exercises

TRANSLATION

EXERCISE 1   Underline and define the word parts from this chapter in the following terms.

1. tenalgia _____
2. tibialgia _____
3. costalgia _____
4. spondylodynia _____
5. cervicodynia _____
6. dyskinesia _____
7. dystaxia _____
8. dystonia _____

EXERCISE 2   Translate the following terms as literally as possible.

EXAMPLE: **nasopharyngoscope**   _an instrument for looking at the nose and throat_

1. dystonia _____
2. dyskinesia _____
3. hyperkinesia _____
4. myasthenia _____

GENERATION

EXERCISE 3   Build a medical term from the information provided.

EXAMPLE: inflammation of the sinuses
sinusitis

1. tendon pain _____
2. tibia (shin) pain _____
3. rib pain _____
4. vertebra pain _____
5. neck pain _____
6. decrease in muscle tone _____
7. slow movement _____
8. poor coordination _____

EXERCISE 4 Multiple-choice questions. Select the correct answer(s).

1. Select the term that means *bone pain.*
   a. arthralgia
   b. myalgia
   c. ostealgia
   d. arthrodynia
   e. osteodynia

2. Select the term that means *joint pain.*
   a. arthralgia
   b. myalgia
   c. ostealgia
   d. arthrodynia
   e. osteodynia

3. Select the term that means *muscle pain.*
   a. arthralgia
   b. myalgia
   c. ostealgia
   d. arthrodynia
   e. osteodynia

OBJECTIVE

4.3 Observation and Discovery

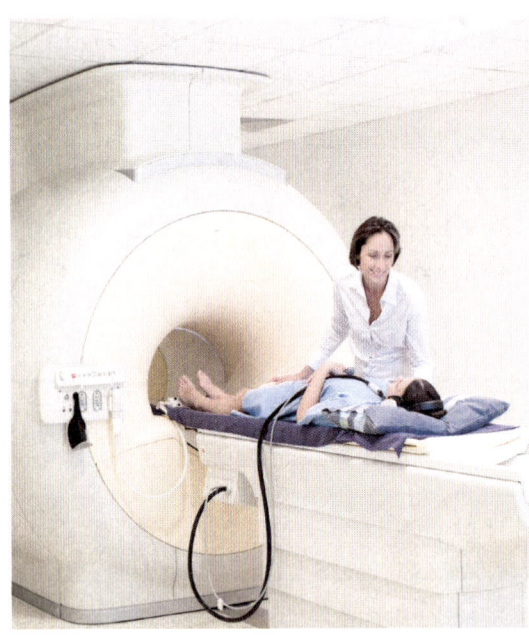

Martin Barraud/Getty Images
Evaluation of bone issues is commonly performed with imaging, including MRI.

When a patient with musculoskeletal problems is evaluated, the physical exam is very important. The exam of the muscles and bones focuses mainly on typical signs of inflammation: redness, swelling, heat, and pain. Any of these symptoms can indicate that an infection or inflammation is present.

There are not many skills that are specific to evaluating bones. Patients with fractured bones may present with a limp or pain upon touching or pressure.

Much evaluation of bone issues is performed with imaging. The bread-and-butter imaging method for bones is the simple x-ray. An x-ray can reveal fractures, bone destruction (*osteolysis*), and even extra bone growth (*exostosis*). More involved imaging methods include computed tomography (CT), computed axial tomography (CAT), or magnetic resonance imaging (MRI).

Examining a patient's joint is usually more involved. While the health care provider also checks for the same signs of inflammation, the joint's ability to move also needs to be checked. This is called the joint's range of motion (ROM). The provider also checks to make sure the joint is not moving in a direction that it's not supposed to move in. This extra movement is called *joint laxity*. The provider also checks for fluid around the joint (*effusion*). There are several diagnostic procedures specific to the joints. To get a better view, the health care provider can inject dye into the joint and perform an MRI. Other means

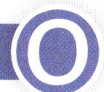

of investigating a joint include injecting a needle and collecting fluid to send to the lab (*arthrocentesis*) or even using a camera-like device to look inside the joint (*arthroscope*).

Examining muscles often means checking how they work. The function of muscles can be evaluated by checking their tone (*myotonia*) or strength. A more involved way to check this is electromyography. In this procedure, two needles are inserted into a muscle to measure the muscle activity.

diagnostic procedures

TERM	WORD ANALYSIS
arthrocentesis ar-throh-sin-TEE-sis	arthro / centesis joint / puncture
DEFINITION puncture of a joint	
arthroscope AR-throh-skohp	arthro / scope joint / instrument for looking
DEFINITION instrument for looking into a joint	
arthroscopy ar-THRAW-skoh-pee	arthro / scopy joint / looking procedure
DEFINITION procedure of looking into a joint	

radiology

TERM	WORD ANALYSIS
arthrogram AR-throh-gram	arthro / gram joint / record
DEFINITION visual record of a joint	
computed axial tomography (CAT) kom-PYOO-ted AK-see-al taw-MAW-grah-fee	axi / al axis / pertaining to tomo / graphy cut / recording procedure
DEFINITION imaging procedure using a computer to produce cross sections along an axis	

spinal curvatures

TERM	WORD ANALYSIS
kyphosis kai-FOH-sis	kyph / osis bent / condition
DEFINITION humped back; abnormal forward curvature of the upper spine	
lordosis lor-DOH-sis	lord / osis bent backward / condition
DEFINITION sway back; abnormal forward curvature of the lower spine	
scoliosis SKOH-lee-OH-sis	scoli / osis crooked / condition
DEFINITION crooked back; abnormal lateral curvature of the spine	

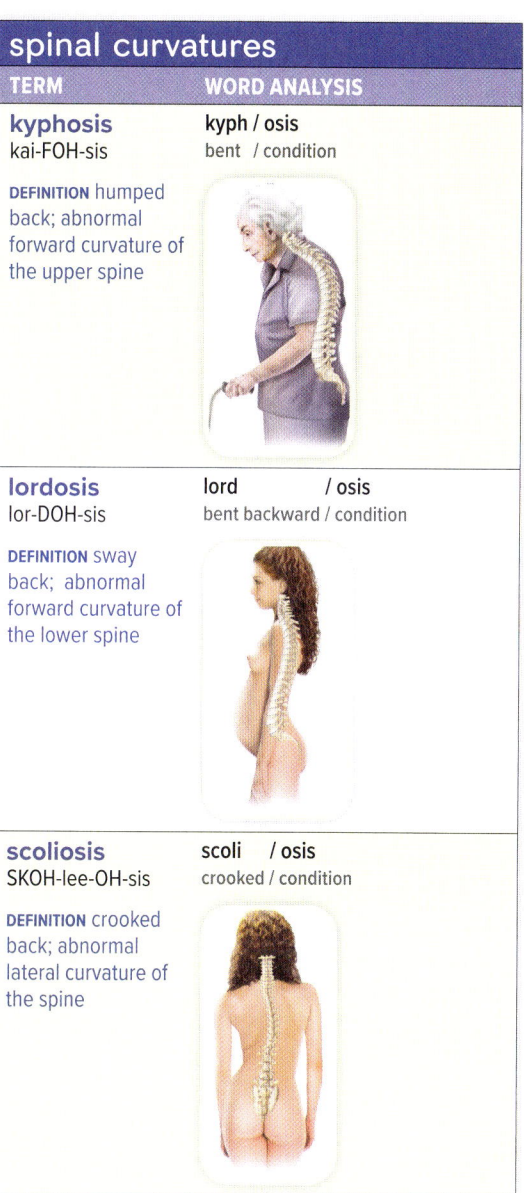

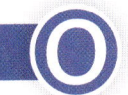

bones

TERM	WORD ANALYSIS
fracture FRAK-shur **DEFINITION** a bone break	**from Latin, for** *break*

Transverse   Oblique   Spiral   Angulated   Displaced   Angulated & displaced

TERM	WORD ANALYSIS
osteodystrophy aw-stee-oh-DIH-stroh-fee **DEFINITION** poor bone development	osteo / dys / trophy bone / bad / nourishment
spondylitis spawn-dih-LAI-tis **DEFINITION** vertebra inflammation	spondyl / itis vertebra / inflammation
spondylomalacia spawn-dih-loh-mah-LAY-shah **DEFINITION** softening of the vertebra	spondylo / malacia vertebra / softening
tarsoptosis tar-sawp-TOH-sis **DEFINITION** flat feet	tarso / ptosis ankle / drooping condition

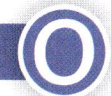

muscles

TERM	WORD ANALYSIS
atrophy A-troh-fee	a / trophy no / nourishment

DEFINITION
underdevelopment, decrease, or loss of muscle tissue

Normal

Atrophied

muscles *continued*

TERM	WORD ANALYSIS
hypertrophy hai-PER-troh-fee	hyper / trophy over / nourishment

DEFINITION overdevelopment of muscle tissue

TERM	WORD ANALYSIS
myolysis mai-AW-lih-sis	myo / lysis muscle / loss

DEFINITION loss of muscle tissue

Learning Outcome 4.3 Exercises

TRANSLATION

EXERCISE 1   Underline and define the word parts from this chapter in the following terms.

1. spondylitis _____

2. arthroscopy _____

3. tarsoptosis _____

4. osteodystophy _____

5. myotonia (2 roots) _____

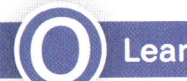

Learning Outcome 4.3 Exercises

EXERCISE 2   Match the term on the left with its definition on the right.

_____ 1. fracture

_____ 2. atrophy

_____ 3. scoliosis

_____ 4. computed axial tomography

_____ 5. hypertrophy

_____ 6. lordosis

_____ 7. kyphosis

a. imaging procedure using a computer to produce cross sections along an axis

b. humped back; abnormal forward curvature of the upper spine

c. sway back; abnormal forward curvature of the lower spine

d. crooked back; abnormal lateral curvature of the spine

e. from Latin, for _break_; a bone break

f. underdevelopment, decrease, or loss of muscle tissue

g. overdevelopment of muscle tissue

EXERCISE 3   Translate the following terms as literally as possible.

> EXAMPLE: **nasopharyngoscope**   _an instrument for looking at the nose and throat_

1. tarsoptosis _____

2. kyphosis _____

3. lordosis _____

4. scoliosis _____

GENERATION

EXERCISE 4   Build a medical term from the information provided.

> EXAMPLE: **inflammation of the sinuses**   _sinusitis_

1. vertebra inflammation _____

2. softening of the vertebra _____

3. instrument for looking into a joint _____

4. procedure of looking into a joint _____

EXERCISE 5   Multiple-choice questions. Select the correct answer(s).

1. Select the terms that pertain to bone.
   a. fracture
   b. arthrocentesis
   c. atrophy
   d. hypertrophy
   e. osteodystrophy

2. Select the terms that pertain to joints.
   a. fracture
   b. arthrocentesis
   c. atrophy
   d. hypertrophy
   e. osteodystrophy

3. Select the terms that pertain to muscle.
   a. fracture
   b. arthrocentesis
   c. atrophy
   d. hypertrophy
   e. osteodystrophy

4. What does the abbreviation _CAT_ stand for?
   a. chondro-arthrodysplasia tenotomy
   b. computed axial tomography
   c. computed arthrography telectasia
   d. chondro-axial tomography

5. Which of the following terms means _fluid build-up?_
   a. affusion
   b. effusion
   c. effision
   d. exfusure

EXERCISE 6   Briefly describe the difference between the pair of terms.

1. arthrogram, myogram _____

_____

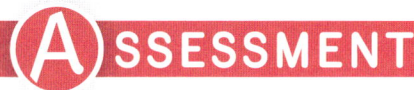

4.4 Diagnosis and Pathology

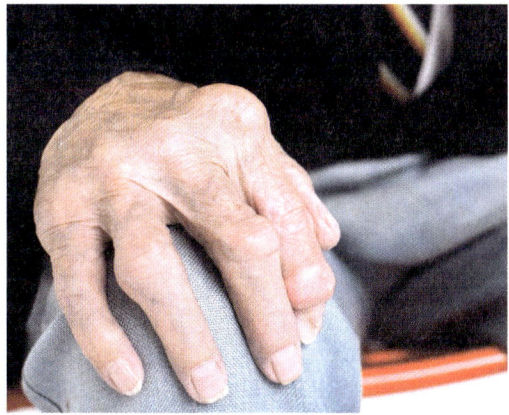

Image Source/Getty Images

As mentioned earlier, fractures are a common reason why patients see health care providers. Fractures are more common in people with weaker bones. Bone loss (*osteopenia*) can be related to age or to a diet that is deficient in calcium. Osteopenia leads to soft bones in children (*osteomalacia*) or weak, frail bones in adults (*osteoporosis*). Some patients suffer from infections of the bone (*osteomyelitis*), a serious illness that often requires hospitalization.

The vertebral column of bones is susceptible to injury. Gymnasts, football players, or weight lifters who bend their backs too far can suffer small stress fractures of their vertebra (*spondylolysis*). If the fracture is severe, the vertebrae can slip onto one another (*spondylolisthesis*). A very serious version of this condition can advance to problems with a narrowing of the space for the spinal cord (*spinal stenosis*).

You move your joints all the time. They act as shock absorbers for your body, and they take a lot of abuse. It should come as no surprise, then, that joint problems are a very common medical concern. A swollen, painful joint (*arthritis*) can have many causes—the most common being excessive wear and tear. This type is called *osteoarthritis*. As the cartilage between the bones in a joint breaks down, the bones eventually rub together and the joint becomes painful

to move. This is a very common reason for a joint replacement surgery.

Other causes of arthritis include infection (*septic arthritis*) and a disease of joint inflammation (*rheumatoid arthritis*). Other parts of the joint area that can cause problems are the bursa (*bursitis*) and tendon (*tendonitis*). These are not usually caused by an injury; instead, they are a result of normal wear and tear over time.

Unusual inflammatory conditions also affect the muscles. Muscles can become inflamed (*myositis*). Sometimes this can involve the skin as well (*dermatomyositis*). General problems with all the muscles are called *myopathies. Myasthenia gravis* and *muscular dystrophy* are two of the most common types of myopathy.

Like any system in the body, the musculoskeletal system can develop tumors. Tumors can develop in the bones (*osteosarcoma, osteocarcinoma, osteochondroma*), or they can spread to the bones from other parts of the body. Your muscles can get tumors (*myoma*) as well—one example is a *myosarcoma*.

bones	
TERM	**WORD ANALYSIS**
osteitis AW-stee-AI-tis	oste / itis bone / inflammation
DEFINITION bone inflammation	
osteochondritis AW-stee-oh-kon-DRAI-tis	osteo / chondr / itis bone / cartilage / inflammation
DEFINITION inflammation of bone and cartilage	
osteomalacia AW-stee-oh-mah-LAY-shah	osteo / malacia bone / softening
DEFINITION softening of the bone	
osteomyelitis AW-stee-oh-MAI-eh-LAI-tis	osteo / myel / itis bone / marrow / inflammation
DEFINITION inflammation of the bone and bone marrow	
osteopenia AW-stee-oh-PEE-nee-yah	osteo / penia bone / deficiency
DEFINITION reduction in bone volume	

bones *continued*

TERM	WORD ANALYSIS
osteoporosis AW-stee-oh-por-OH-sis	osteo / por / osis bone / pore / condition
DEFINITION loss of bone density	

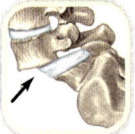

Normal

Osteoporosis

spondylolisthesis SPAWN-dih-loh-lis-THEE-sis	spondylo / listhesis vertebra / slipping
DEFINITION the slipping or dislocation of a vertebra	

spondylosis SPAWN-dih-LOH-sis	spondyl / osis vertebra / condition
DEFINITION vertebra condition	

joints

TERM	WORD ANALYSIS
arthritis ar-THRAI-tis	arthr / itis joint / inflammation
DEFINITION joint inflammation	
arthropathy ar-THRAW-pah-thee	arthro / pathy joint / disease
DEFINITION joint disease	
bursitis bur-SAI-tis	burs / itis bursa / inflammation
DEFINITION inflammation of the bursa	

joints *continued*

TERM	WORD ANALYSIS
osteoarthritis AW-stee-oh-ar-THRAI-tis	osteo / arthr / itis bone / joint / inflammation
DEFINITION inflammation of the joints, specifically those that bear weight	
rheumatoid arthritis ROO-mah-toyd ar-THRAI-tis	rheumat / oid rheumatic fever / resembling arthr / itis joint / inflammation
DEFINITION inflammation of the joints; it is called *rheumatoid* because its symptoms resemble those of rheumatic fever	

Image Source/Getty Images

muscles

TERM	WORD ANALYSIS
costochondritis KAW-stoh-kawn-DRAI-tis	costo / chondr / itis rib / cartilage / inflammation
DEFINITION inflammation of the cartilage of the rib	
muscular dystrophy MUS-kyoo-lar DIS-troh-fee	muscul / ar muscle / pertaining to dys / trophy bad / nourishment
DEFINITION disorder characterized by poor muscle development	

Realistic Reflections

myopathy mai-AW-pah-thee	myo / pathy muscle / disease
DEFINITION muscle disease	
myositis MAI-oh-SAI-tis	myos / itis muscle / inflammation
DEFINITION muscle inflammation	
tendinitis TEN-dih-NAI-tis	tendin / itis tendon / inflammation
tendonitis TEN-dah-NAI-tis	tendon / itis tendon / inflammation
DEFINITION tendon inflammation	

NOTE: These words are both accepted spellings for the same condition.

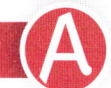

4.4 Diagnosis and Pathology

Oncology	
TERM	**WORD ANALYSIS**
osteochondroma AW-stee-oh-kon-DROH-mah	osteo / chondr / oma bone / cartilage / tumor
DEFINITION a tumor made up of bone and cartilage, also known as an exostosis made up of cartilage	
chondroma kawn-DROH-mah	chondr / oma cartilage / tumor
DEFINITION a tumor-like growth of cartilage tissue	

Oncology *continued*	
TERM	**WORD ANALYSIS**
myoma mai-OH-mah	my / oma muscle / tumor
DEFINITION a muscle tumor	
myosarcoma MAI-oh-sar-KOH-mah	myo / sarc / oma muscle / flesh / tumor
DEFINITION a cancerous muscle tumor	

A Learning Outcome 4.4 Exercises

TRANSLATION

EXERCISE 1   Underline and define the word parts from this chapter in the following terms.

1. osteitis _____

2. tendinitis _____

3. tendonitis _____

4. myositis _____

5. rheumatoid arthritis _____

6. myoma _____

7. muscular dystrophy _____

8. osteomalacia _____

9. osteopenia _____

10. osteochondroma (2 roots) _____

11. spondylolisthesis _____

12. costochondritis (2 roots) _____

EXERCISE 2   Match the term on the left with its definition on the right.

_____ 1. myosarcoma

_____ 2. osteoporosis

_____ 3. spondylosis

_____ 4. rheumatoid arthritis

_____ 5. myoma

_____ 6. chondroma

_____ 7. osteochondroma

a. loss of bone density

b. vertebra condition

c. a cancerous muscle tumor

d. a tumor made up of bone and cartilage

e. inflammation of the joints, the symptoms of which resemble rheumatic fever

f. muscle tumor

g. a tumor-like growth of cartilage tissue

EXERCISE 3 Translate the following terms as literally as possible.

> EXAMPLE: nasopharyngoscope *an instrument for looking at the nose and throat*

1. tendinitis _____

2. tendonitis _____

3. arthropathy _____

4. osteomyelitis _____

5. osteoporosis _____

6. spondylolisthesis _____

GENERATION

EXERCISE 4 Build a medical term from the information provided.

> EXAMPLE: inflammation of the sinuses
> *sinusitis*

1. inflammation of the bursa _____

2. inflammation of the cartilage and rib

   _____

3. overdevelopment (*trophic*) vertebrae inflammation _____

4. bone deficiency _____

EXERCISE 5 Multiple-choice questions. Select the correct answer(s).

1. Select the term(s) that has (have) the root meaning *muscle.*
   a. osteitis
   b. arthritis
   c. myositis
   d. osteoarthritis
   e. osteochondritis

2. Select the term(s) that has (have) the root meaning *joint.*
   a. osteitis
   b. arthritis
   c. myositis
   d. osteoarthritis
   e. osteochondritis

3. Select the term(s) that has (have) the root meaning *cartilage.*
   a. osteitis
   b. arthritis
   c. myositis
   d. osteoarthritis
   e. osteochondritis

4. Select the term(s) that has (have) the root meaning *bone.*
   a. osteitis
   b. arthritis
   c. myositis
   d. osteoarthritis
   e. osteochondritis

5. A disorder characterized by poor muscle development is known as
   a. myositis
   b. myosarcoma
   c. myopathy
   d. muscular dystrophy

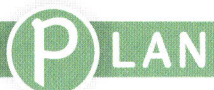

4.5 Treatments and Therapies

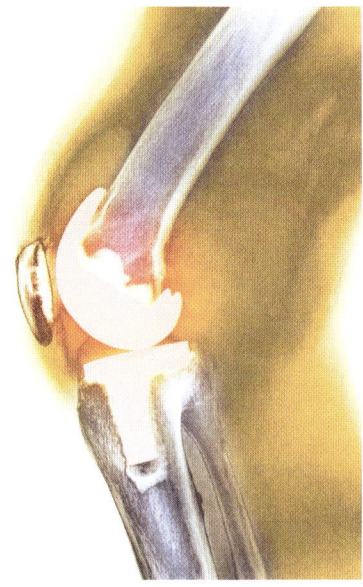

Dr. P. Marazzi/Science Photo Library/Getty Images

Common procedures for the musculoskeletal system include knee and hip replacements.

The medicines used to treat musculoskeletal problems are designed to decrease pain (*analgesic*) or inflammation (*anti-inflammatory*). The most commonly used medicines for both are known as *nonsteroidal anti-inflammatory drugs* (NSAIDs). Ibuprofen is a common example of this type of medicine. Other nonsurgical treatments include *physical therapy,* in which patients exercise and stretch in order to heal injuries, or wearing a device used to relieve tension on a joint (*orthotics*). Shoe inserts are a very common type of orthotic.

When nonsurgical treatment fails, surgery may be necessary. *Orthopedic* surgery deals with joints and bones. Many of the tools used in orthopedic surgery look like they came from a home improvement store—including drills, saws, and hammers. These tools are used to cut into bone (*osteotomy*), joints (*arthrotomy*), or muscle (*myotomy*). Sometimes they remove part or all of these structures (*osteectomy, arthrectomy, myectomy*).

When defective areas or cancer are present in a bone, the diseased area of bone must be removed before new bone (*graft*) or artificial hardware (*prosthesis*) can be installed. This reconstruction of bone procedure is called *osteoplasty.*

Similar procedures exist for joints. Sometimes, removal of a diseased joint (*arthrectomy*) is necessary, followed by a reconstruction of the joint with a prosthesis (*arthroplasty*). These are common treatments for diseased knees and hips. A less aggressive surgery for fixing diseased joints, *chondroplasty,* involves fixing the bad cartilage of a joint. It is very common in athletes and older patients with chronic osteoarthritis.

Not all orthopedic surgery involves complete reconstruction of a bone or joint. Sometimes something that has snapped must be repaired, as in a tendon repair (*tenorrhaphy*) or a muscle repair (*myorrhaphy*). Other times, new attachments must be made. This can involve attaching leftover muscle to bone (*myodesis*) after an amputation or fixing two bones surrounding a joint (*arthrodesis*). While the latter procedure results in immobility of the joint, it may be necessary to relieve pain.

pharmacology

TERM	WORD ANALYSIS
analgesic A-nal-JEE-zik	an / alge / sic no / pain / agent
DEFINITION a drug that relieves pain	

Burazin/Getty Images

TERM	WORD ANALYSIS
antiarthritic AN-tee-ar-THRIH-tik	anti / arthri / tic against / joint (pain) / agent
DEFINITION a drug that opposes joint inflammation	
anti-inflammatory AN-tee-in-FLA-mah-TOR-ee	anti / inflammatory against / inflammation
DEFINITION a drug that opposes inflammation	

4.5 Treatments and Therapies

bones

TERM	WORD ANALYSIS
carpectomy kar-PEK-toh-mee	carp / ectomy wrist / removal
DEFINITION removal of all or part of the wrist	
costectomy kaws-TEK-toh-mee	cost / ectomy rib / removal
DEFINITION removal of a rib	
craniectomy KRAY-nee-EK-toh-mee	crani / ectomy skull / removal
DEFINITION removal of a portion of the skull	
craniotomy KRAY-nee-AW-toh-mee	cranio / tomy skull / incision
DEFINITION removal of a portion of the skull NOTE: The difference between a craniectomy and a craniotomy is whether or not the piece of bone is replaced. After a craniotomy, the piece of bone that was removed to allow surgical access to the brain is replaced. In a craniectomy, the piece of bone is not replaced.	

joints

TERM	WORD ANALYSIS
arthroplasty AR-throh-PLAS-tee	arthro / plasty joint / reconstruction
DEFINITION reconstruction of a joint	
arthrotomy ar-THRAW-toh-mee	arthro / tomy joint / incision
DEFINITION incision into a joint	
chondrectomy kawn-DREK-toh-mee	chondr / ectomy cartilage / removal
DEFINITION removal of cartilage	

muscles

TERM	WORD ANALYSIS
myectomy mai-EK-toh-mee	my / ectomy muscle / removal
DEFINITION removal of muscle	
myomectomy MAI-oh-MEK-toh-mee	my / om / ectomy muscle / tumor / removal
DEFINITION removal of a muscle tumor NOTE: It is easy to miss the *oma* root in this word because the *o* looks like it belongs with *myo* and the *a* gets swallowed up by *ectomy*. The *m* is your clue. Don't just read over it—it needs to be explained.	
myoplasty MAI-oh-PLAS-tee	myo / plasty muscle / reconstruction
DEFINITION muscle reconstruction	
myorrhaphy mai-OR-ah-fee	myo / rrhaphy muscle / suture
DEFINITION muscle suture	
myotomy mai-AW-toh-mee	myo / tomy muscle / incision
DEFINITION incision into muscle	
tenorrhaphy ten-OR-ah-fee	teno / rrhaphy tendon / suture
DEFINITION suture of a tendon	

Learning Outcome 4.5 Exercises

TRANSLATION

EXERCISE 1 Underline and define the word parts from this chapter in the following terms.

1. myodesis _____

2. arthroplasty _____

3. costectomy _____

4. craniectomy _____

5. myomectomy _____

EXERCISE 2 Match the term on the left with its definition on the right.

_____ 1. arthrotomy   a. incision into a joint

_____ 2. carpectomy   b. incision into a muscle

_____ 3. chondrectomy   c. incision into the skull

_____ 4. craniotomy   d. removal of all or part of the wrist

_____ 5. myectomy   e. removal of cartilage

_____ 6. myotomy   f. removal of muscle

EXERCISE 3 Translate the following terms as literally as possible.

> EXAMPLE: nasopharyngoscope *an instrument for looking at the nose and throat*

1. myotomy _____

2. analgesic _____

3. antiarthritic _____

4. anti-inflammatory _____

GENERATION

EXERCISE 4 Build a medical term from the information provided.

> EXAMPLE: inflammation of the sinuses
> *sinusitis*

1. reconstruction of a joint _____

2. reconstruction of a muscle _____

3. removal of a rib _____

4. removal of all or part of the wrist _____

5. removal of cartilage _____

6. muscle reconstruction _____

7. suture of a muscle _____

8. suture of a tendon _____

EXERCISE 5 Briefly describe the difference between each pair of terms.

1. myectomy, myomectomy _____

2. craniectomy, craniotomy _____

4.6 Electronic Health Records

Orthopedic Clinic Note

 Subjective

History of Present Illness:
Mrs. Maureen Goldman presented to the orthopedic clinic with a chronic history of **arthralgia.** She was previously diagnosed with **osteoarthritis.** She was initially treated with **NSAIDs** and an **orthotic** that helped for a time; however, Mrs. Goldman's condition worsened and was eventually treated with an intraarticular steroid injection. She reported improved pain and range of motion. The knee pain returned last year, however, and she was treated in our clinic with **arthroscopic** surgery. While it helped some, she reports it didn't completely get rid of her symptoms, and she returns today for evaluation.
PMHx: **Septic arthritis** requiring hospitalization and **IV** antibiotics 4 years ago.

 Objective

Physical Exam:
RR: 16; HR: 70; Temp: 98.6; BP: 110/60
Gen: Alert, oriented.
CV: RRR, no murmurs.
Resp: CTA.
Musculoskeletal: **Crepitation** in right knee, decreased **ROM. Mild effusion.** Mild muscular **atrophy** of right quadriceps muscle compared to left.
Labs: **ESR** normal, joint **aspiration** normal.
X-ray: **Subchondral cysts, subchondral sclerosis,** joint space narrowing.

 Assessment

DDx: Includes **osteoarthritis, rheumatoid arthritis,** and bursitis. Given her history of osteoarthritis on exam and the results of the x-ray and joint aspiration, I believe Mrs. Goldman has **OA** that has failed to respond to previous treatments.

 Plan

I have discussed treatment options, and the patient prefers surgery. I have explained the risks and benefits of a **total knee replacement arthroplasty,** and she understands. I have scheduled her for surgery next month.
—Electronically signed by Ricchelle Mitchell, MD 01/26/2015 11:22 AM

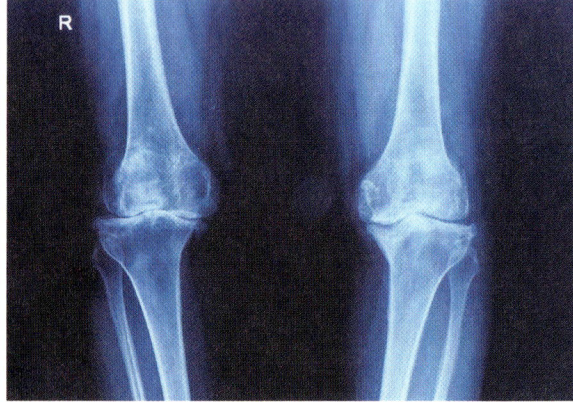

Yok_onepiece/Shutterstock

EXERCISE 1 Match the term on the left with its definition on the right.

_____ 1. ROM   a. underdevelopment, decrease, or loss of muscle tissue

_____ 2. atrophy   b. procedure of looking into a joint

_____ 3. osteoarthritis   c. beneath the cartilage

_____ 4. arthroplasty   d. reconstruction of a joint

_____ 5. arthroscopy   e. range of motion

_____ 6. subchondral   f. inflammation of the joints, specifically those that bear weight

EXERCISE 2 Fill in the blanks.

1. Mrs. Goldman was previously diagnosed with _____ (abbreviation for inflammation of the joints, specifically those that bear weight).

2. Along with _____ (nonsteroidal anti-inflammatory drugs), she was given an _orthotic_ (give definition: _____ _____).

EXERCISE 3 True or false questions. Indicate true answers with a T and false answers with an F.

1. Mrs. Goldman has a chronic history of bone pain. _____

2. Mrs. Goldman was initially treated with nonsteroidal anti-inflammatory drugs. _____

3. After the intraarticular steroid injection, Mrs. Goldman reported improved arthralgia and ROM. _____

4. Mrs. Goldman was previously hospitalized for joint inflammation caused by infection. _____

5. Mrs. Goldman's right quadricep muscle had an unusual new growth. _____

6. Mrs. Goldman's x-ray revealed hardening of the cartilage. _____

7. After understanding the risks involved, Mrs. Goldman has agreed to a TKR joint reconstruction. _____

EXERCISE 4 Multiple-choice questions. Select the correct answer.

1. _Arthroscopic surgery_ is
   a. closed reduction   c. surgery on a bone
   b. external fixation   d. surgery on a joint

2. _Septic arthritis_ requires which of the following forms of treatment?
   a. antibiotics   c. osteectomy
   b. prosthesis   d. myomectomy

3. The term _subchondral_ means
   a. beneath the cartilage c. beneath the joint
   b. beneath the knee   d. beneath the muscle

4. The term _arthrostenosis_ means
   a. joint narrowing   c. joint hardening
   b. muscle narrowing   d. muscle hardening

Additional exercises available in

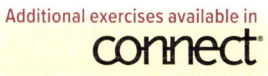

Chapter Review exercises, along with additional practice items, are available in Connect!

Quick Reference

quick reference glossary of roots

ROOT	DEFINITION	ROOT	DEFINITION
arthr/o	joint	kinesi/o	movement, motion
burs/o	bursa	lumb/o	loin, lower back
carp/o	wrist	muscul/o	muscle
cervic/o	neck	my/o, myos/o	muscle
chondr/o	cartilage	oste/o	bone
cost/o	rib	spondyl/o	vertebra
crani/o	head, skull	tax/o	arrangement, order, coordination
dactyl/o	finger	ten/o, tend/o, tendin/o	tendon
femor/o	femur	tibi/o	tibia
		ton/o	tone, tension

musculoskeletal system abbreviations

ABBREVIATION	DEFINITION
Fx	fracture
ACL	anterior cruciate ligament
MCL	medial collateral ligament
LCL	lateral collateral ligament
PCL	posterior cruciate ligament
C1–C7	cervical (of the neck) vertebrae
T1–T12	thoracic (of the chest) vertebrae
L1–L5	lumbar (of the loin) vertebrae
S1–S5	sacral vertebrae
CAT	computed axial tomography
CT	computed tomography
CTS	carpal tunnel syndrome
EMG	electromyogram
FROM	full range of motion
MD	muscular dystrophy
NSAID	nonsteroidal anti-inflammatory drug
OA	osteoarthritis
PT	physical therapy
RA	rheumatoid arthritis
ROM	range of motion
TKR	total knee replacement

The Nervous System–Neurology and Psychiatry

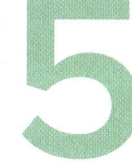

5

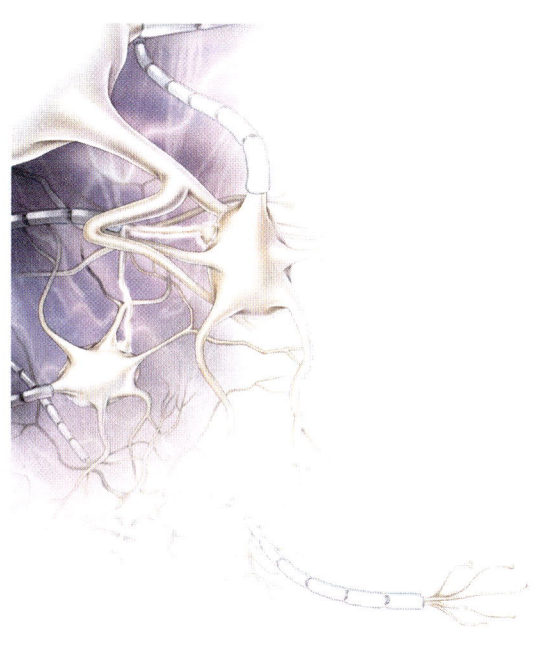

Introduction and Overview of the Nervous System

One of our defining characteristics is our ability to think. Aristotle distinguished humans as "rational animals." French philosopher René Descartes famously remarked, "I think, therefore I am." Thinking is one of the most important parts of what makes us who we are. Our knowledge, perception, and response to the world around us are due to the center of thought in our body: the nervous system. More than just the center of conscious thought, the nervous system is always at work gathering information from the world around us, deciding what to do about it, and telling the rest of the body how to respond. It functions as the body's command center for data processing, thought, and action for the conglomerate of many cells, organs, and systems that make up the human body. Thanks to the

---

Learning Outcomes

Upon completion of this chapter, you will be able to:

5.1 Identify the **roots/word parts** associated with the **nervous system**.

(S) **5.2** Translate the **Subjective** terms associated with the **nervous system**.

(O) **5.3** Translate the **Objective** terms associated with the **nervous system**.

(A) **5.4** Translate the **Assessment** terms associated with the **nervous system**.

(P) **5.5** Translate the **Plan** terms associated with the **nervous system**.

5.6 Distinguish terms associated with the **nervous system** in the context of **electronic health records**.

nervous system, the body acts as a coordinated team reacting to its surroundings with alacrity and precision. The nervous system serves as the body's communications network, coordinating data reception with appropriate reaction.

This network comprises two parts: the peripheral nervous system and central nervous system. The peripheral nervous system collects data. It receives information such as temperature, pain, light, and pressure from its surroundings. As quickly as it receives input, it transmits it to an analytic center via special conduits known as nerves. The unified collection of cells in the brain and spine is known as the central nervous system. The central nervous system processes the details and formulates a response. Commands are directed back to the appropriate body parts via nerves. This constant progression of receiving, reasoning, and reacting repeats itself continuously as we go about our daily lives.

The nervous system handles both voluntary and involuntary action of the body. In addition, we associate the brain and nervous system with conscious thought and actions. The voluntary command of the body's actions is known as the somatic nervous system. Most often, this voluntary system involves the relationship of the nervous system with the skeletal muscular system. Nerves detect input from the surroundings and send this specific information to the central nervous system for processing. These incoming nerves are called afferent neurons or nerves. The person chooses how to respond, and the central nervous system directs the body how to respond through signals sent by efferent neurons. Often these are commands sent to muscles. The signal travels down the nerve through an electric current and connects to the muscle at a special connection point (the neuromuscular junction). This voluntary observation and response represents a small part of the work of the nervous system. The central nervous system also directs the involuntary actions of the body, things that our body does without our conscious choice or awareness. This background control is called the autonomic nervous system and encompasses everything from the beating of our heart, to sweating, to digesting food.

The central nervous system also possesses supporting structures to protect and maintain itself. The skull serves as a dense external layer to protect the brain from common injury. The body also produces cerebrospinal fluid, which surrounds the brain and spinal cord and acts as a shock absorber cushioning them from injury. The brain consumes 20 to 25 percent of the body's oxygen. This huge need for oxygen necessitates a rich blood supply. Nearly 20 percent of the blood pumped from the heart is sent to the brain. This demand is met through an extensive network of blood vessels.

But the brain is more than the neurological controller of the human body's physical processes. What we see, hear, and feel affects our general perception of the world around us. We don't just move and react. We behave. We are more than just digestion, heartbeats, and breathing. We have emotions, opinions, and beliefs. We have more than brains. We have minds we call psyche (Greek for *mind*). These more complex functions fit under the umbrella of psychiatry and psychology, both of whose roots come from the Greek word *psyche,* which means *mind* or *soul.* These fields deal with problems in our perceptions, emotions, and behavior.

5.1 Word Parts of the Nervous System

Word Parts Associated with the Structure of the Nervous System

Your sensory system—specifically your eyes, ears, nose, and skin—collects data from your surroundings and sends the information to your brain (*encephalo*) by wires known as nerves (*neuro*). Your brain then makes sense of the data and determines the appropriate action. Then it sends out the action plan to the rest of the body via a web of nerves.

Together, your brain and the collecting/acting nerves make up your nervous system. The nerves that send and receive signals from the brain are collectively known as the peripheral nervous system.

Your brain and spinal cord (*myelo*) are called the central nervous system. The brain has several sections (*lobes*) and is divided in two halves (*hemispheres*). The largest portion of your brain is the cerebrum. Under the cerebrum is the *cerebellum,* which controls such things as coordination of movements. Your central nervous system is fragile and needs a protective membrane (*meninges*). The tough outer layer is known as the *dura*.

brain

ROOTS: *cerebr/o, encephal/o*

EXAMPLES: cerebropathy, cerebrospinal, encephalitis, encephalogram

NOTES: The encephalo root comes from *en* (inside) and *cephalus* (head) and literally means *the stuff inside your head*.

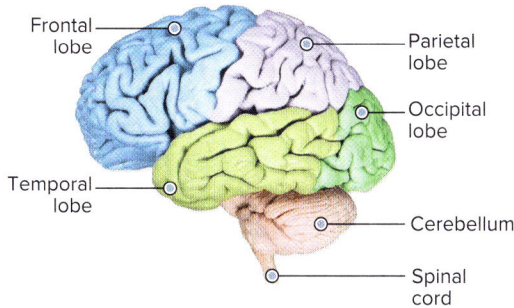

Frontal lobe · Parietal lobe · Occipital lobe · Temporal lobe · Cerebellum · Spinal cord

Christine Eckel/McGraw-Hill Education

cerebellum

ROOT: *cerebell/o*

EXAMPLES: cerebellar, cerebellitis

NOTES: This word is just the word *cerebrum* (brain) plus a diminutive suffix. It means *the little brain*. It refers to the region of the brain that controls voluntary movements and looks somewhat like a little version of the whole brain.

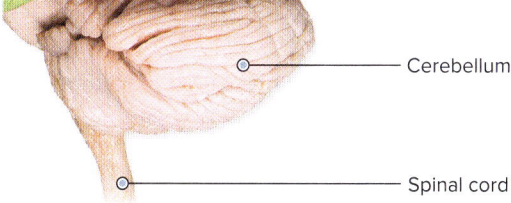

Cerebellum · Spinal cord

Christine Eckel/McGraw-Hill Education

head

ROOT: *cephal/o*

EXAMPLES: microcephaly, macrocephaly

NOTES: The scientific term for octopus, squid, and other sea creatures that are made up of a head and tentacles is *cephalopod*—literally head (*cephalo*) + feet (*pod*).

head, skull

ROOT: *crani/o*

EXAMPLES: craniometer, craniomalacia

NOTES: The term *migraine* comes from the word *hemicranias,* meaning *half the head*. It reflects the fact most migraines are localized on half the patient's head.

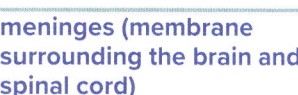

Ned Frisk/Getty Images

meninges (membrane surrounding the brain and spinal cord)

ROOTS: *mening/o, meningi/o*

EXAMPLES: meningitis, meningopathy

NOTES: When the letter *g* is followed by an *e* or an *i,* it is pronounced soft (like *j* in *jar*): men-in-JAI-tis. When the letter *g* is followed by an *a, o,* or *u,* it is pronounced hard (like *g* in *gas*): men-in-GOH-pah-thee

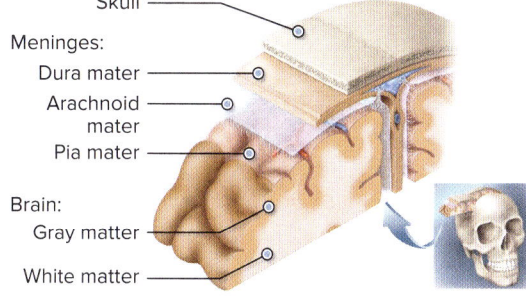

Skull · Meninges: Dura mater · Arachnoid mater · Pia mater · Brain: Gray matter · White matter

dura (tough outer membrane surrounding the brain and spinal cord)

ROOT: *dur/o*

EXAMPLES: epidural, subdural hematoma

NOTES: This root literally means *hard*. The full name of the membrane it refers to is *dura mater cerebri,* which translates to *the tough mother of the brain*. Words such as *endurance* and *durable* come from the same word.

nerve

ROOT: *neur/o*

EXAMPLES: neuralgia, neuropathy

NOTES: *Neuron* comes from a Greek word meaning *tendon* or *string*. In ancient times, when people first began examining brains, they thought neurons looked like string.

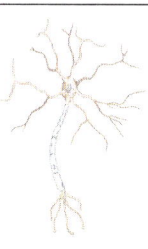

spinal cord, bone marrow

ROOT: *myel/o*

EXAMPLES: myelitis, myelodysplasia

NOTES: This root comes from a Greek word meaning *the innermost part* and is used in medicine to refer to two different things—bone marrow and the spinal cord. But if you think about it, it makes sense, as both are in the innermost part of something else. Bone marrow is in the center of bones. The spinal cord is in the center of the spine.

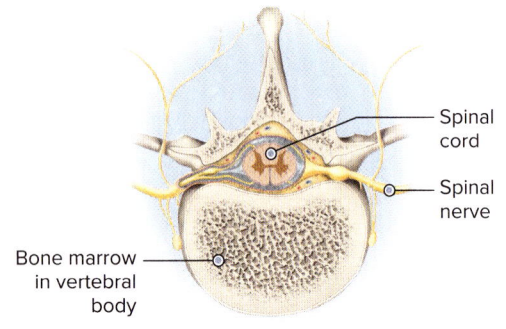

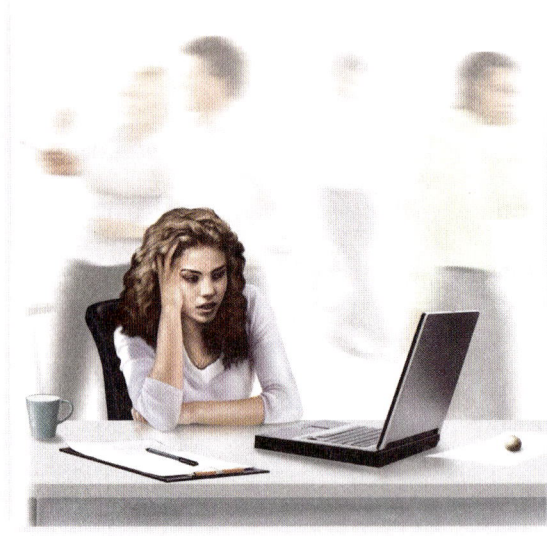

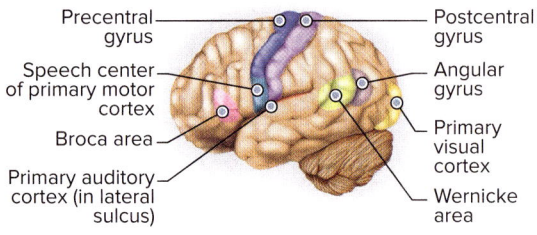

Word Parts Associated with the Function of the Nervous System

While your brain is constantly responding to the world around you, there is more to your mind than just collecting and responding to information. This is where the example of the detective show can go only so far. On those shows, the end result is generally the same—arresting a criminal.

Not all of the data that go to your brain lead to a specific action, though. Much of what you see, hear, and feel affects your general perception of the world around you. It affects your emotions, opinions, or beliefs.

Neurology focuses on actions. The more complex functions often fit under the umbrella of what we call *psyche* (from Greek, for *mind*). We don't just move and react. We *behave*. This is the realm of psychiatry and psychology. These fields of study deal with problems in human perceptions, emotions, and behavior.

feeling, sensation

ROOT: *esthesi/o*

EXAMPLES: anesthesia, hyperesthesia

NOTES: *Esthetics* (also sometimes spelled *aesthetics*) is the study of art and philosophy as it pertains to beauty. What makes something beautiful? Can you measure beauty? Is beauty really in the eye of the beholder?

speech

ROOT: *phas/o*

EXAMPLE: aphasia

NOTES: If a friend is talking too fast, perhaps he or she is stricken with the disease *tachyphasia*.

mind

ROOTS: *phren/o, psych/o*

EXAMPLES: phrenetic, psychology

NOTES: In addition to the mind, *phren/o* can also refer to the diaphragm (as in the term *phrenospasm,* a fancy medical term for a hiccup). The reason comes from the ancient Greek view of the mind. Early on, the Greeks thought of the chest as the seat of emotion and reason. As that view changed and the location of the mind moved from the chest to the brain, this term for *mind* began to be applied to both areas of the body.

"You don't know what you've got until it's gone." It's a catchy phrase used in a pop song and fortune cookies, and it also applies to the brain. Much of neurology and psychiatry deals with loss of function. A break from reality (*schizo*), a loss of speaking (*phaso*), the inability to feel (*esthesio*)—thinking about each of these conditions helps you appreciate the functions of your brain. When your mind can't keep your fears (*phobo*) or passions (*mania*) at a healthy level, they can cause problems as well. Even fears and obsessions provide a glimpse of the subtler jobs your brain performs.

know

ROOT: *gnosi/o*

EXAMPLES: agnosia, diagnosis, prognosis

NOTES: Frequently, people who have had a limb amputated report feeling or sensing the missing limb. Such an experience is called *autosomatognosis,* from *auto* (self) + *somato* (body) + *gnosis* (know).

excessive desire

SUFFIX: *-mania*

EXAMPLES: pyromania, kleptomania

NOTES: Because of the commonly used psychological term *manic-depressive,* some people mistakenly assume that *manic* refers to a type of depression. "He doesn't just have depression, he has *manic* depression." On the contrary—it actually refers to the exact opposite state.

Manic-depression is characterized by intense swings of emotion. At times, sufferers are extremely energetic (the *manic* state), and at other times, they are extremely sad (the *depressed* state). Because of these swings in mood, people with this condition are sometimes referred to as being *bipolar,* as their personality is always swinging from one extreme (pole) to the other.

excessive fear or sensitivity

SUFFIX: *-phobia*

EXAMPLES: photophobia, hydrophobia

NOTES: Phobias can refer to actual symptoms or anxieties. For example, hydrophobia is a main symptom of rabies. *Agoraphobia,* which is the fear of being outdoors or in public spaces and comes from the Greek word *agora,* meaning *marketplace,* is common in people who have experienced major traumatic accidents.

Consider these interesting phobias:
- ablutophobia—the fear of taking a bath
- acrophobia—the fear of heights
- alektorophobia—the fear of chickens
- arachnophobia—the fear of spiders
- cynophobia—the fear of dogs
- dendrophobia—the fear of trees
- gynophobia—the fear of women
- ichthyphobia—the fear of fish
- nyctophobia—the fear of night
- phobophobia—the fear of being afraid
- triskaidekaphobia—the fear of the number 13

slight or partial paralysis

SUFFIX: *-paresis*

EXAMPLE: hemiparesis

NOTES: *Paresis* comes from Greek, for *to let go,* or *to slacken;* it is used in health care to refer not to complete loss of sensation or control but instead to a partial or isolated form of paralysis.

paralysis

SUFFIX: *-plegia*

EXAMPLE: quadriplegia

NOTES: *Plegia* is from Greek, for *to strike.* So a word such as *thermoplegia* doesn't mean *heat paralysis;* instead, it means *heat stroke.*

TRANSLATION

EXERCISE 1   Match the word part on the left with its definition on the right. Some definitions will be used more than once.

_____ 1. mening/o   a. head

_____ 2. cerebell/o   b. cerebellum

_____ 3. neur/o   c. brain

_____ 4. crani/o   d. head, skull

_____ 5. cerebr/o   e. tough outer membrane surrounding the brain and spinal cord

_____ 6. encephal/o   f. meninges; membrane surrounding the brain and spinal cord

_____ 7. cephal/o   g. nerve

_____ 8. myel/o   h. spinal cord

_____ 9. dur/o

EXERCISE 2   Translate the following word parts.

1. crani/o _____

2. cerebr/o _____

3. cerebell/o _____

4. cephal/o _____

5. encephal/o _____

6. mening/o, meningi/o _____

7. neur/o _____

8. dur/o _____

9. myel/o _____

EXERCISE 3   Break down the word into its component parts and translate.

> EXAMPLE: **sinusitis**   _sinus | itis_
> _inflammation of the sinuses_

1. cerebral _____

2. epidural _____

3. meningitis _____

4. myelitis _____

5. cerebellitis _____

6. cephalalgia _____

7. neuralgia _____

8. craniotomy _____

9. encephalopathy _____

EXERCISE 4   Match the word part on the left with its definition on the right. Some definitions will be used more than once.

_____ 1. psych/o   a. feeling, sensation

_____ 2. -phobia   b. know

_____ 3. -mania   c. excessive desire

_____ 4. -plegia   d. slight or partial paralysis

_____ 5. -paresis   e. speech

_____ 6. esthesi/o   f. excessive fear or sensitivity

_____ 7. gnosi/o   g. mind

_____ 8. phas/o   h. paralysis

_____ 9. phren/o

EXERCISE 5   Translate the following word parts.

1. -phobia _____

2. -mania _____

3. -paresis _____

4. phren/o _____

EXERCISE 6   Break down the following words into their component parts and translate.

> EXAMPLE: **sinusitis**   _sinus | itis_
> _inflammation of the sinuses_

1. psychology _____

2. aphasia _____

3. monoplegia _____

GENERATION

EXERCISE 7 Underline and define the word parts from this chapter in the following terms.

1. cerebral thrombosis _____
2. subdural hematoma _____
3. craniosclerosis _____
4. encephalocele _____
5. meningioma _____
6. cephalodynia _____
7. myelodysplasia _____
8. neuropharmacology _____

EXERCISE 8 For the following words, identify and translate the word parts from this chapter.

1. pyromania _____
2. hydrophobia _____
3. schizophrenia _____
4. psychosomatic _____
5. hemiparesis _____

EXERCISE 9 Build a medical term from the information provided.

1. incision into the brain (use *cerebral*) _____
2. incision into the skull _____
3. incision into a nerve _____
4. inflammation of the dura _____
5. inflammation of the cerebellum _____
6. hernia of the meninges _____
7. hernia of the spinal cord _____
8. hernia of the brain (use *encephalo*) _____
9. large head (use *cephalo*) _____

EXERCISE 10 Build a medical term from the information provided.

1. half paralysis (use *-plegia*) _____
2. no feeling _____
3. bad speaking condition _____

$\textstyle\bigcirc$UBJECTIVE

5.2 Patient History, Problems, Complaints

When someone comes to a health care professional with neurological complaints, the complaint will usually fall into problems with either the peripheral or central nervous system. Some patients with peripheral nervous system complaints have problems with the signals being sent to the brain. Their brains may be sending painful signals, or their brains could have problems receiving sensations. Other problems with the peripheral nervous system relate to interruptions in receiving signals from the brain or spinal cord, which could lead to partial or complete paralysis. Central nervous system problems can affect the entire body, as with fainting (*syncope*). Other problems can be more focused, such as problems with speaking (*aphasia, dysphasia*).

The most common psychiatric complaints health care professionals see deal with emotions, such as depression and anxiety. Other common complaints may include concerns over erratic behaviors, abnormal fears *(phobias),* or unhealthy obsessions *(manias).* When a patient enters a sudden state of confusion or abrupt loss of awareness of his or her surroundings, it is *delirium.* When it is a more permanent loss in orientation and thinking ability, it is *dementia.*

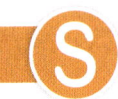

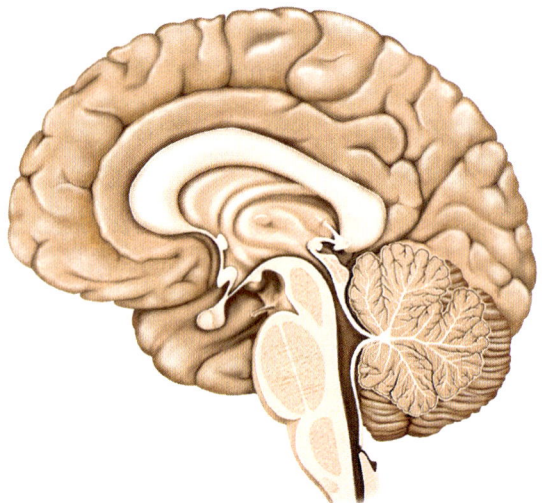

A sagittal cross section of the brain showing the cerebrum, cerebellum, brain stem, and other supporting structures.

pain

TERM	WORD ANALYSIS
cephalalgia SEH-ful-AL-jah	cephal / algia head / pain
DEFINITION head pain	
neuralgia nur-AL-jah	neur / algia nerve / pain
DEFINITION nerve pain	

paralysis

TERM	WORD ANALYSIS
paralysis puh-RAH-lu-sis	from Greek, for *to disable*
DEFINITION complete loss of sensation and motor function	
paresis puh-REE-sis	from Greek, for *to let go*
DEFINITION partial paralysis characterized by varying degrees of sensation and motor function	

impairments

TERM	WORD ANALYSIS
aphasia ah-FAY-zhah	a / phas / ia not / speaking / condition
DEFINITION inability to speak	
dementia da-MEN-chah	de / ment / ia down / mind / condition
DEFINITION loss/decline in mental function	
dysphasia dis-FAY-zhah	dys / phas / ia bad / speaking / condition
DEFINITION difficulty speaking	
neurasthenia NUR-as-THEN-ee-ah	neur / asthenia nerve / weakness
DEFINITION nerve weakness	
syncope SIN-koh-pee	from Greek, for *contraction* or *cut off*
DEFINITION fainting; losing consciousness due to temporary loss of blood flow to brain	

phobia/mania

TERM	WORD ANALYSIS
acrophobia AK-roh-FOH-bee-ah	acro / phobia heights / excessive fear
DEFINITION fear of heights	
agoraphobia ah-GOR-ah-FOH-bee-ah	agora / phobia marketplace / excessive fear
DEFINITION fear of outdoor spaces NOTE: *Agora* is Greek for *marketplace*; similar to the Roman *forum*.	
hydrophobia HAI-droh-FOH-bee-ah	hydro / phobia water / excessive fear
DEFINITION fear of water	
kleptomania KLEP-toh-MAY-nee-ah	klepto / mania theft / excessive desire
DEFINITION desire to steal	
pyromania PAI-roh-MAY-nee-ah	pyro / mania fire / excessive desire
DEFINITION desire to set fire	

PRONUNCIATION

EXERCISE 1 Indicate which syllable(s) is emphasized when pronounced.

EXAMPLE: bronchitis bron<u>chi</u>tis

1. paresis _____

2. neuralgia _____

3. aphasia _____

4. paralysis _____

5. dysphasia _____

TRANSLATION

EXERCISE 2 Break down the following words into their component parts.

EXAMPLE: nasopharyngoscope
naso | pharyngo | scope

1. dementia _____

2. pyromania _____

3. hydrophobia _____

4. dysphasia _____

5. neuralgia _____

EXERCISE 3 Underline and define the word parts from this chapter in the following terms.

1. neurasthenia _____

2. cephalalgia _____

3. kleptomania _____

4. agoraphobia _____

5 aphasia _____

6. dementia _____

7. dysphasia _____

EXERCISE 4 Match the term on the left with its definition on the right.

_____ 1. paralysis

_____ 2. acrophobia

_____ 3. syncope

_____ 4. paresis

a. fear of heights

b. fainting; losing consciousness due to temporary loss of blood flow to the brain

c. from Greek, for *to disable;* complete loss of sensation and motor function

d. from Greek, for *to let go;* partial paralysis characterized by varying degrees of sensation and motor function

EXERCISE 5 Translate the following terms as literally as possible.

EXAMPLE: nasopharyngoscope *an instrument for looking at the nose and throat*

1. aphasia _____

2. neuralgia _____

3. hydrophobia _____

4. pyromania _____

GENERATION

EXERCISE 6 Multiple-choice questions. Select the correct answer(s).

1. The main categories for nerve complaints are
   a. peripheral and central nervous system problems
   b. central nervous system and psychiatric problems
   c. peripheral and psychiatric problems
   d. autonomic and pyramidal problems

2. Select the terms that pertain to peripheral nerve problems.
   a. sending painful signals to the brain (*algia*)
   b. excessive desire (*mania*)
   c. problems speaking (*phaso*)
   d. abnormal fear (*phobia*)
   e. paralysis (*plegia*)

3. Select the terms that pertain to central nervous system problems.
   a. sending painful signals to the brain (*algia*)
   b. excessive desire (*mania*)
   c. problems speaking (*phaso*)
   d. abnormal fear (*phobia*)
   e. paralysis (*plegia*)

4. Select the terms that pertain to psychiatric problems.
   a. sending painful signals to the brain (*algia*)
   b. excessive desire (*mania*)
   c. problems speaking (*phaso*)
   d. abnormal fear (*phobia*)
   e. paralysis (*plegia*)

5. Which of the following means *fear of heights?*
   a. hydrophobia   c. acrophobia
   b. agoraphobia   d. photophobia

EXERCISE 7 Build a medical term from the information provided.

> **EXAMPLE:**   inflammation of the sinuses
> *sinusitis*

1. bad speaking condition _____
2. nerve weakness _____
3. fear of outdoor spaces _____
4. excessive sensitivity to light _____
5. desire to steal _____

EXERCISE 8 Briefly describe the difference between each pair of terms.

1. paralysis, paresis _____
2. neuralgia, cephalalgia _____

OBJECTIVE

5.3 Observation and Discovery

When a health care professional sees a patient with a neurologic or psychiatric problem, the exam is often quite involved. The neurologic exam involves checking the patient's muscle strength and coordination, sensation, and reflexes. A reflex is a muscle contraction that bypasses the brain. When certain tendons are tapped, an impulse flows directly to the spinal cord, which sends a quick command to the nearby muscle to contract. Checking sensation involves studying afferent nerve paths, which are

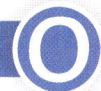

the paths that lead from the peripheral to the central nervous system. Checking strength and coordination involves studying efferent nerve paths, which are paths that lead from the brain to the peripheral nervous system. Psychiatric evaluation is very involved because it depends on extensive questions and history to help discover the root of the patient's problem.

The most common lab work done in the evaluation of the neurologic system focuses on testing a patient's cerebrospinal fluid, which is obtained via lumbar puncture. This is a procedure in which a needle is gently inserted between the vertebrae of the lower spine, and a small amount of fluid is drawn and evaluated for signs of infection and other types of inflammation.

Imaging the brain is commonly performed to evaluate for bleeding after an injury, to determine the presence of diseased brain tissue, and to look for brain tumors. The most common imaging technique is the computed tomography (CT) scan, which is a complex type of x-ray. The benefit of a CT is its speed. When a more detailed view is needed or when the cerebellum is of special importance, a magnetic resonance image (MRI) is beneficial. Ultrasounds can be used to assess blood circulation to the brain and monitor the speed of the blood passing through the vessels, which is helpful in detecting both blockages and bleeding. Another type of image utilizing dye is a myelogram, in which an x-ray of the spine is completed after dye is injected into the vertebrae. Another very common procedure for analyzing the electric function of the brain is an electroencephalogram (EEG). An EEG is not exactly an image of the brain; electrodes are placed around the skull and the brain's electric currents are monitored. This is the most effective means to detect seizure activity in the brain.

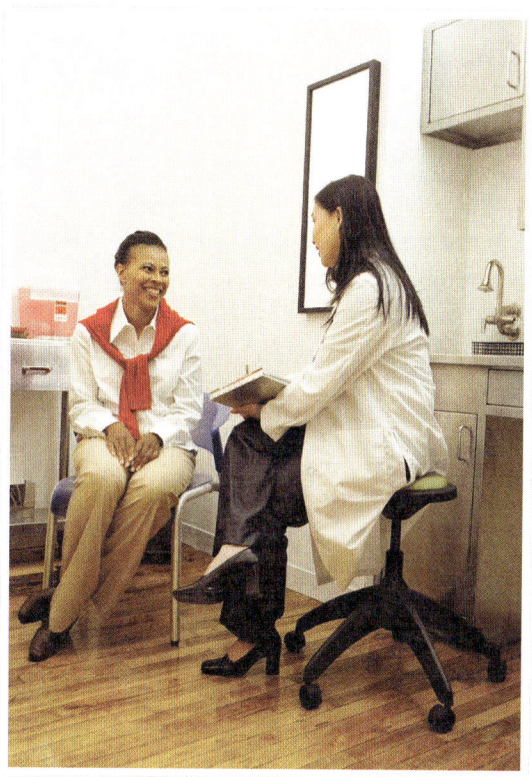

Photomondo/Getty Images

Two of the most common ways of obtaining data to be used in diagnosing neurological or psychiatric disorders involve interviewing the patient and imaging.

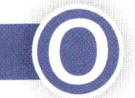

diagnostic procedures

TERM	WORD ANALYSIS
electroencephalog-raphy (EEG) eh-LEK-troh-en-SEH-fah-LAW-grah-fee	electro / encephalo / electricity / brain / **graphy** writing procedure

DEFINITION procedure used to examine the electrical activity of the brain

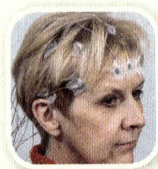

Bob Coyle/McGraw-Hill Education

TERM	WORD ANALYSIS
lumbar puncture (LP) LUM-bar PUNK-chir	lumb / ar puncture lower back / pertaining to

DEFINITION inserting a needle into the lumbar region of the spine in order to collect spinal fluid, commonly called a "spinal tap"

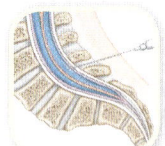

radiology

TERM	WORD ANALYSIS
cerebral angiography sih-REE-bral AN-jee-AW-grah-fee	cerebr / al brain / pertaining to **angio** / **graphy** vessel / writing procedure

DEFINITION procedure used to examine blood vessels in the brain

TERM	WORD ANALYSIS
myelogram MAI-el-oh-gram	myelo / gram spinal cord / record

DEFINITION image of the spinal cord, usually done using x-ray

TERM	WORD ANALYSIS
positron emission tomography (PET) scan PAWZ-ih-trawn ee-MISH-un taw-MAW-gra-fee	e / mission out / send **tomo** / **graphy** cut / writing procedure

DEFINITION an imaging procedure that uses radiation (positrons) to produce cross sections of the brain

structure

TERM	WORD ANALYSIS
encephalocele en-SEF-ah-loh-SEEL	encephalo / cele brain / hernia

DEFINITION hernia of the brain (normally through a defect in the skull)

TERM	WORD ANALYSIS
hematoma HEE-mah-TOH-mah	hemat / oma blood / tumor

DEFINITION a tumor-like mass made up of blood

TERM	WORD ANALYSIS
epidural hematoma EH-pi-DIR-al HEE-mah-TOH-mah	epi / dur / al upon / dura / pertaining to **hemat** / **oma** blood / tumor

DEFINITION a hematoma located on top of the dura

TERM	WORD ANALYSIS
intracerebral hematoma IN-trah-se-REE-bral HEE-mah-TOH-mah	intra / cerebr / al inside / brain / pertaining to **hemat** / **oma** blood / tumor

DEFINITION a hematoma located inside the brain

TERM	WORD ANALYSIS
subdural hematoma sub-DIR-al HEE-mah-TOH-mah	sub / dur / al beneath / dura / pertaining to **hemat** / **oma** blood / tumor

DEFINITION a hematoma located beneath the dura

Medical Body Scans/Getty Images

TERM	WORD ANALYSIS
meningocele meh-NIN-goh-seel	meningo / cele meninges / hernia

DEFINITION a hernia of the meninges

TERM	WORD ANALYSIS
neuritis nir-AI-tis	neur / itis nerve / inflammation

DEFINITION nerve inflammation

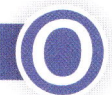

5.3 Observation and Discovery

professional terms

TERM	WORD ANALYSIS
afferent nerve A-fir-ent nirv	af / ferent nerve toward / carry

DEFINITION a nerve that carries impulses toward the central nervous system
NOTE: The prefix *af-* is actually *ad-* (toward), as in *admit* or *address*. When *ad-* is added to *-ferent,* the word *adferent* changes to *afferent*—it's just easier to easier to say.

TERM	WORD ANALYSIS
efferent nerve EH-fir-ent nirv	ef / ferent nerve away / carry

DEFINITION a nerve that carries impulses away from the central nervous system
NOTE: The prefix *ef-* is actually *ex- (out or away),* as in *exit.* When added to *-ferent,* it changes for the same reasons as described for *afferent.*

TERM	WORD ANALYSIS
psychiatrist sai-KAI-ah-trist	psych / iatrist mind / treatment specialist

DEFINITION doctor who specializes in treatment of the mind

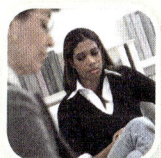

Andrea Morini/Getty Images

professional terms *continued*

TERM	WORD ANALYSIS
psychiatry sai-KAI-ah-tree	psych / iatry mind / specialty

DEFINITION branch of medicine that focuses on the treatment of the mind

TERM	WORD ANALYSIS
psychologist sai-KAW-loh-jist	psycho / logist mind / specialist

DEFINITION doctor who specializes in the study of the mind.

TERM	WORD ANALYSIS
psychology sai-KAW-loh-jee	psycho / logy mind / study of

DEFINITION branch of medicine that focuses on the study of the mind
NOTE: The chief differences between a psychologist and a psychiatrist are their training and approach; a psychologist has a PhD and normally uses psychotherapy, and a psychiatrist has an MD or a DO and can prescribe medication.

TERM	WORD ANALYSIS
psychosomatic SAI-koh-soh-MA-tik	psycho / somat / ic mind / body / pertaining to

DEFINITION pertaining to the relationship between the body and the mind

Learning Outcome 5.3 Exercises

TRANSLATION

EXERCISE 1 Break down the following words into their component parts.

> EXAMPLE: nasopharyngoscope
> *naso | pharyngo | scope*

1. neuritis _____
2. psychiatry _____
3. psychology _____
4. psychosomatic _____
5. intracerebral hematoma _____
6. subdural hematoma _____

EXERCISE 2 Underline and define the word parts from this chapter in the following terms.

1. psychologist _____
2. meningocele _____
3. encephalocele _____
4. myelogram _____
5. cerebral angiography _____
6. epidural hematoma _____
7. electroencephalography _____

EXERCISE 3 Match the term on the left with its definition on the right.

_____ 1. hematoma

_____ 2. lumbar puncture (LP)

_____ 3. positron emission tomography (PET) scan

_____ 4. afferent nerve

_____ 5. efferent nerve

a. inserting a needle into the lumbar (lower back) region of the spine in order to collect spinal fluid

b. an imaging procedure that uses radiation (positrons) to produce cross sections of the brain

c. a nerve that carries impulses toward the CNS

d. nerve that carries impulses away from the CNS

e. a tumor-like mass made up of blood

EXERCISE 4 Translate the following terms as literally as possible.

EXAMPLE: nasopharyngoscope _an instrument for looking at the nose and throat_

1. encephalocele _____

2. psychosomatic _____

3. afferent nerve _____

4. efferent nerve _____

GENERATION

EXERCISE 5 Build a medical term from the information provided.

EXAMPLE: inflammation of the sinuses _sinusitis_

1. inflammation of the nerves _____

2. inflammation of the cerebellum _____

3. pertaining to the body and mind _____

4. a hernia of the meninges _____

5. spinal cord record _____

6. branch of medicine that focuses on the treatment of the mind _____

7. branch of medicine that focuses on the study of the mind _____

EXERCISE 6 Multiple-choice questions. Select the correct answer(s).

1. Which diagnostic procedure is used to examine blood vessels in the brain?
   a. cerebral angiography
   b. lumbar puncture
   c. positron emission tomography
   d. myelogram

2. During a lumbar puncture (LP), the needle is inserted into what part of the body?
   a. arm
   b. brain
   c. heart
   d. spine

3. Which term means _a tumor-like mass made up of blood located inside the brain?_
   a. epidural hematoma
   b. intracerebral hematoma
   c. subdural hematoma
   d. encephaloma

EXERCISE 7 Briefly describe the difference between each pair of terms.

1. psychiatrist, psychologist _____

2. afferent nerve, efferent nerve _____

3. epidural hematoma, subdural hematoma _____

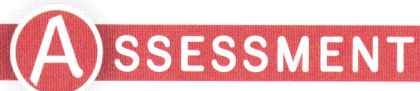
5.4 Diagnosis and Pathology

When assessing a patient with neuropsychiatric problems, it's helpful to determine whether the problem originates from the nervous system (*neurogenic*) or mind (*psychogenic*).

Neurogenic problems may arise from conditions involving the supporting structures, such as the skull or blood supply. Disorders of the skull, such as premature closure of the bones, can limit brain growth and lead to pressure on the brain. Increased pressure can also arise from too much fluid around the brain, as seen in hydrocephalus. Pressure in the brain (*intracranial pressure*) from these conditions can present as headache and vomiting. Disruption of critical blood supply to the brain presents with sudden changes in neurologic function, such as slurring of speech. It can happen from a rupture in the blood vessel (*hemorrhagic stroke*) or a blockage cutting off blood supply (*ischemic stroke*). These vascular events constitute a medical emergency.

Problems of the central nervous system may also arise from direct injury or irritation to nerves or brain cells. The symptoms depend on which part of the nervous system is affected. For example, problems involving only the spinal cord, such as myelitis or spinal injury, do not cause problems with thought but can lead to muscle weakness or even paralysis. Infections of the tissue surrounding the brain and spinal cord (*meningitis*) cause headache and a stiff neck, whereas infections of the brain matter (*encephalitis*) lead to generalized dysfunction of the brain, characterized by an altered mental state (*encephalopathy*). Other causes of encephalopathy include prolonged deprivation of oxygen, exposure to toxins, increased pressure in the brain, and chronic injuries. Not all conditions of the brain matter lead to changes in general mental state. Abnormal firing of nerves leads to involuntary changes in muscle tone (*seizure*), and a dysfunction in higher functions such as personal interaction and communication is seen in autism.

Nerves can be affected directly by injury or compression, or indirectly through diseases or toxins. Typically, injury or compression will cause a decrease or total loss of function of a single nerve or a group of nerves that exits the spinal cord in the same place.

This may lead to pain (*neuralgia*) and/or loss of function (*paresis* or *paralysis*). Diseases such as diabetes and medicines such as chemotherapy drugs can be toxic to nerves. Often, this has a greater effect on the nerves that are farther from the brain and spinal cord (*peripheral neuropathy*).

Common psychogenic problems include depression and anxiety. Some people have an inability to control their urges for periods of time, which is known as mania. Most often, these manic phases alternate with bouts of depression, producing a condition known as bipolar disorder or manic-depressive disorder. Some patients have an altered perception of reality known as a psychosis. One of the more common psychotic conditions is schizophrenia. Patients often struggle with distorted perceptions of reality (*delusions*) and may even hear or see things that are not there (*hallucinations*). Furthermore, their thinking patterns are disorganized and emotions are erratic. Another condition characterized by a patient's distorted view of reality occurs in eating disorders. Rather than misunderstanding the world around them, patients with eating disorders such as anorexia and bulimia suffer from an altered perception of their own body.

structure

TERM	WORD ANALYSIS
Cerebrovascular Accident	
cerebrovascular accident (CVA) seh-REE-broh-VAS-kyoo-lar AK-sih-dent	cerebro / vascul / ar brain / blood vessel / pertaining to
DEFINITION an accident involving the blood vessels of the brain	
stroke STROHK	*stroke*
DEFINITION loss of brain function caused by interruption of blood flow/supply to the brain	

structure *continued*

TERM	WORD ANALYSIS
transient ischemic attack (TIA) TRAN-zee-ent ih-SKEE-mik ah-TAK	trans / ient across / go isch / em / ic hold back / blood / pertaining to
DEFINITION a "mini-stroke" caused by the blockage of a blood vessel, which resolves (goes away) within 24 hours	
hydrocephaly HAI-droh-SEH-fah-lee	hydro / cephal / y water / head / condition
DEFINITION abnormal accumulation of spinal fluid in the brain	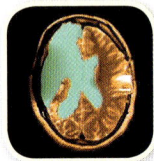 Medical Body Scans/ Getty Images

Other

TERM	WORD ANALYSIS
encephalitis en-SEF-ah-LAI-tis	encephal / itis brain / inflammation
DEFINITION inflammation of the brain	
encephalopathy en-SEF-ah-LAW-pah-thee	encephalo / pathy brain / disease
DEFINITION disease of the brain	
meningitis MEH-nin-JAI-tus	mening / itis meninges / inflammation
DEFINITION inflammation of the meninges	
myelitis MAI-el-AI-tis	myel / itis spinal cord / inflammation
DEFINITION inflammation of the spinal cord	
neuropathy nir-AW-pah-thee	neuro / pathy nerve / disease
DEFINITION disease of the nervous system	
poliomyelitis POH-lee-oh-MAI-el-AI-tis	polio / myel / itis gray / spinal cord / inflammation
DEFINITION inflammation of the gray matter of the spinal cord NOTE: This is the full name of the disease known as polio.	

function

TERM	WORD ANALYSIS
anorexia a-noh-REK-see-ah	an / orex / ia no / appetite / condition
DEFINITION an eating disorder characterized by the patient's refusal to eat	
autism AW-tiz-um	aut / ism self / condition
DEFINITION a psychiatric disorder characterized by withdrawal from communication with others; the patient is focused only on the self	
bulimia boo-LEE-mee-ah	bu / lim / ia ox / hunger / condition
DEFINITION an eating disorder characterized by overeating and usually followed by forced vomiting or other compensatory behaviors	
cerebral palsy sih-REE-bral PAL-zee	cerebr / al palsy brain / pertaining to paralysis
DEFINITION paralysis caused by damage to the area of the brain responsible for movement NOTE: *Palsy* is a less common word for paralysis.	
epilepsy eh-pih-LEP-see	epi / lepsy upon / seize
DEFINITION a disease marked by seizures	
narcolepsy NAR-coh-LEP-see	narco / lepsy sleep / seize
DEFINITION a disease characterized by sudden, uncontrolled sleepiness	
neurosis neh-ROH-sis	neur / osis nerve / condition
DEFINITION a nerve condition	
psychosis sai-KOH-sis	psych / osis mind / condition
DEFINITION a mind condition NOTE: Both neurosis and psychosis are general terms of psychiatric conditions, but a neurosis doesn't interfere with rational thought or daily functioning; a psychosis involves some sort of break with reality.	
schizophrenia SKIT-zoh-FREH-nee-ah	schizo / phren / ia divide / mind / condition
DEFINITION a mental illness characterized by delusions, hallucinations, and disordered speech NOTE: *Schizo* refers to the division in the mind between the mind itself and reality, not the division of the mind into multiple personalities.	

TRANSLATION

EXERCISE 1 Break down the following words into their component parts.

> EXAMPLE: nasopharyngoscope
> *naso | pharyngo | scope*

1. intracerebral _____
2. cerebrovascular _____
3. meningitis _____
4. encephalitis _____
5. poliomyelitis _____
6. encephalopathy _____

EXERCISE 2 Underline and define the word parts from this chapter in the following terms.

1. encephalopathy _____
2. hydrocephaly _____
3. myelitis _____
4. neuropathy _____
5. cerebral palsy _____
6. neurosis _____
7. psychosis _____
8. schizophrenia _____

EXERCISE 3 Match the term on the left with its definition on the right.

_____ 1. autism

_____ 2. bulimia

_____ 3. anorexia

_____ 4. epilepsy

_____ 5. stroke

_____ 6. transient ischemic attack (TIA)

_____ 7. narcolepsy

_____ 8. cerebrovascular accident (CVA)

a. an accident involving the blood vessels of the brain

b. loss of brain function caused by interruption of blood flow/supply to the brain

c. a mini-stroke caused by the blockage of a blood vessel that resolves (goes away) within 24 hours

d. an eating disorder characterized by overeating and usually followed by forced vomiting or other compensatory behavior

e. an eating disorder characterized by the patient's refusal to eat

f. a psychiatric disorder characterized by the withdrawal from communication with others; the patient is focused only on the self

g. a disease marked by seizures

h. a disease characterized by sudden, uncontrolled sleepiness

EXERCISE 4 Translate the following terms as literally as possible.

> EXAMPLE: nasopharyngoscope *an instrument for looking at the nose and throat*

1. meningitis _____
2. epilepsy _____
3. neuropathy _____
4. poliomyelitis _____
5. bulimia _____
6. cerebrovascular accident _____

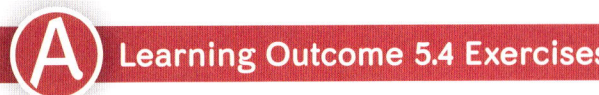

GENERATION

EXERCISE 5 Build a medical term from the information provided.

> EXAMPLE: inflammation of the sinuses
> *sinusitis*

1. inflammation of the spinal cord _____

2. inflammation of the brain (use *encephalo*) ____

3. literally, *water head condition* _____

EXERCISE 6 Multiple-choice questions. Select the correct answer.

1. Anorexia is
   a. a disease marked by seizures
   b. an eating disorder characterized by the patient's refusal to eat
   c. an eating disorder characterized by overeating and usually followed by forced vomiting or other compensatory behavior
   d. a psychiatric disorder characterized by the withdrawal from communication with others

2. Autism is
   a. a disease marked by seizures
   b. an eating disorder characterized by the patient's refusal to eat
   c. an eating disorder characterized by overeating and usually followed by forced vomiting or other compensatory behaviors
   d. a psychiatric disorder characterized by the withdrawal from communication with others

3. Epilepsy is
   a. a disease marked by seizures
   b. an eating disorder characterized by the patient's refusal to eat
   c. an eating disorder characterized by overeating and usually followed by forced vomiting or other compensatory behaviors
   d. a psychiatric disorder characterized by the withdrawal from communication with others

4. A person who is *narcoleptic* has a disease characterized by sudden, uncontrolled
   a. desire for food
   b. sleepiness
   c. desire for medication
   d. withdrawal into self

5. A person with *cerebral palsy* has paralysis caused by damage to the area of the brain responsible for
   a. emotion   c. movement
   b. hunger   d. feeling/sensation

6. A loss of brain function caused by interruption of blood flow/supply to the brain is
   a. stroke   d. neurosis
   b. hemorrhagia   e. myelitis
   c. psychosis

7. Excessive bleeding inside the brain is a(n)
   a. stroke   d. neurosis
   b. hemorrhagia   e. myelitis
   c. psychosis

8. Which of the following characteristics is *not* displayed by a schizophrenic?
   a. delusions
   b. disordered speech
   c. hallucinations
   d. multiple personalities

EXERCISE 7 Briefly describe the difference between each pair of terms.

1. neurosis, psychosis _____

2. encephalopathy, neuropathy _____

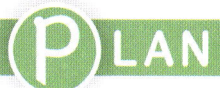

5.5 Treatments and Therapies

There are few medicines that work directly on the neurologic system. The largest class of neurologic medicine works to dull the pain reception from nerves (*anesthetics*). Anesthetics have revolutionized medicine. They may be injected into a small area (*local*), injected into a group of nerves (*epidural*), or even affect the entire body (*general*). In fact, this type of medicine is so critical, there is an entire medical specialty devoted to its use (*anesthesiology*). Another large class of neurologic medicine treats seizures (*anticonvulsants*).

Perhaps one of the fastest-growing areas in drug development has been in the field of psychiatry. There are numerous medicines to treat problems of the mind. Whether they treat depression (*antidepressants*), anxiety (*anxiolytics*), or psychosis (*antipsychotics*), these medicines all work in a similar fashion—by altering the response or availability of the chemicals that allow communication between nerves (*neurotransmitters*). Psychiatric medicines work by increasing or decreasing the activity of specific neurotransmitters that lead to an increase or decrease in activity of certain areas of the brain.

Surgical interventions to treat neurologic disorders can involve direct cutting and cleaning of a partially blocked artery, as in endarterectomy. Treating diseased blood vessels in the brain may also be carried out by less invasive techniques such as radiology guided therapy. In endovascular neurology, medicines are injected into specific areas to cause or destroy clots, depending on the need. Neurosurgery can also be used to treat problems of the nervous system's support structures. These procedures can help remedy skull problems (*cranioplasty*), or remove part of the vertebral bone (*laminectomy*) or an intervertebral disc (*discectomy*). In cases of hydrocephalus, a special drain can be inserted leading from the brain into another part of the body. Most commonly, the drain is placed in the open area surrounding the inside of the abdomen. This type of shunt is called a ventriculoperitoneal (VP) shunt. Invasive brain surgery may be necessary to remove a tumor, to place a device to monitor the pressure in the brain, to insert a device to treat seizures, or to remove part of a lobe of the brain (*lobectomy*). Nerves have traditionally posed a challenge to repair surgically, but advances are being made that allow for nerves to be reconnected (*neurorrhaphy*).

anesthesiology

TERM	WORD ANALYSIS
anesthetic an-es-THET-ik	an / esthetic not / sensation
DEFINITION a drug that causes loss of sensation	

pharmacology

TERM	WORD ANALYSIS
analgesic an-al-JEE-zik	an / alge / sic not / pain / agent
DEFINITION a drug that relieves pain	
anticonvulsant AN-tee-kon-VUL-sant	anti / convuls / ant against / convulsion / agent
DEFINITION a drug that opposes convulsions	
antipsychotic AN-tee-sai-KAW-tik	anti / psycho / tic against / psychosis / agent
DEFINITION a drug that opposes psychoses	
anxiolytic ANG-zee-oh-LIH-tik	anxio / lyt / ic anxiety / loss / agent
DEFINITION a drug that lessens anxiety	

surgical procedures and treatments

TERM	WORD ANALYSIS
craniectomy KRAY-nee-EK-toh-mee	crani / ectomy skull / removal
DEFINITION removal of a piece of the skull	
craniotomy KRAY-nee-AW-toh-mee	cranio / tomy skull / incision
DEFINITION incision into the skull	
neurectomy nir-EK-toh-mee	neur / ectomy nerve / removal
DEFINITION removal of a nerve	

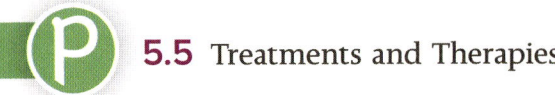

5.5 Treatments and Therapies

surgical procedures and treatments *continued*	
TERM	**WORD ANALYSIS**
neurolysis nir-AW-lih-sis	neuro / lysis nerve / loose
DEFINITION destruction of nerve tissue NOTE: You may wonder why this term is under treatment and not disease; the reason is because one common treatment for chronic nerve pain is to destroy the nerve causing it.	
neuroplasty NIR-oh-PLAS-tee	neuro / plasty nerve / reconstruction
DEFINITION reconstruction of a nerve	

surgical procedures and treatments *continued*	
TERM	**WORD ANALYSIS**
neurorrhaphy nir-OR-ah-fee	neuro / rrhaphy nerve / suture
DEFINITION suturing of a nerve (often the severed ends of a nerve)	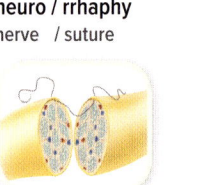

 Learning Outcome 5.5 Exercises

PRONUNCIATION

EXERCISE 1   Indicate which syllable(s) is emphasized when pronounced.

EXAMPLE: bronchitis bron<u>chi</u>tis

1. analgesic _____
2. neurectomy _____
3. craniotomy _____
4. neuroplasty _____

TRANSLATION

EXERCISE 2   Break down the following words into their component parts.

EXAMPLE: nasopharyngoscope
naso | pharyngo | scope

1. craniotomy _____
2. neurolysis _____
3. neuroplasty _____
4. antipsychotic _____

EXERCISE 3   Underline and define the word parts from this chapter in the following terms.

1. anesthetic _____
2. neurectomy _____
3. craniectomy _____
4. neurorrhaphy _____

EXERCISE 4 Match the term on the left with its definition on the right.

_____ 1. analgesic

_____ 2. anticonvulsant

_____ 3. anxiolytic

_____ 4. neurectomy

a. a drug that lessens anxiety

b. a drug that opposes convulsions

c. removal of a nerve

d. a drug that relieves pain

EXERCISE 5 Translate the following terms as literally as possible.

EXAMPLE: **nasopharyngoscope** *an instrument for looking at the nose and throat*

1. anesthetic _____

2. craniectomy _____

3. neurolysis _____

4. neurorrhaphy _____

GENERATION

EXERCISE 6 Build a medical term from the information provided.

EXAMPLE: inflammation of the sinuses
sinusitis

1. skull incision _____

2. nerve removal _____

3. nerve reconstruction _____

4. a drug (literally, *agent*) that opposes psychosis
_____

EXERCISE 7 Multiple-choice questions. Select the correct answer.

1. A medical professional may recommend which drug to relieve pain?
   a. analgesic   c. neurolysis
   b. anxiolytic   d. anticonvulsant

2. Which term means the *removal of a nerve*?
   a. neurolysis   c. neuroplasty
   b. neurectomy   d. neurorraphy

3. The root *crani* in the terms *craniectomy* and *craniotomy* means
   a. skull   c. brain
   b. nerve   d. head

5.6 Electronic Health Records

Emergency Department Visit

Patient Name: Manuel Skayken

Chief Complaint: Confusion, fever.

History of Present Illness:

Manuel Skayken is a 15-year-old boy who presents with a 2-day history of fever to 104°F. He has been more lethargic today, and his headache has worsened. He has **photophobia,** and his parents are concerned that he is acting abnormally. He is not using his right arm and leg as much as his left. He appears **ataxic** in his gait and has been **hypersomnolent** at home. His parents are concerned that he is not responding to questions normally.

Past Medical History: **Somnambulation,** otherwise noncontributory.

Medications: None.

Allergies: NKDA.

Social History: Lives at home with his parents.

Sophomore in high school. A/B student. Nonsmoker.

Surgical History: None.

Physical Exam:

RR: 30; HR: 98; Temp: 104.2; BP: 88/60

Gen: WDWN. Lethargic.

Confused and disoriented.

HEENT: PERRLA, mild **nystagmus.**

Neck: Stiff.

CV: Mildly fast heart rate. No murmurs.

Juanmonino/Getty Images

Resp: Clear.

GI: Normal.

Neuro: CN II-XII grossly intact; DTRs normal.

Hemiparesis: Strength in right arm and leg. Failed mini-mental status exam.

Emergency Department Course:

Manuel was driven to the emergency room by his parents. On arrival, he appeared very confused, though not agitated. With his encephalopathic picture, we were most worried about **psychotropic** drug abuse or infection. A normal urine drug screen and a CBC with an elevated WBC count were suspicious for infection. Because **encephalitis** and **meningitis** were the main concerns, we performed a **lumbar puncture.** The opening pressure was consistent with elevated **intracranial pressure.** The **CSF** showed an elevated WBC count. The culture is pending. Shortly after his lumbar puncture, Manuel had a tonic-clonic **seizure.** We treated him with an **anticonvulsant** and the seizure stopped. The **electroencephalogram** showed paroxysmal lateral epileptiform discharges (PLEDs), which are characteristic of herpes encephalitis. The pediatric team was called, and they admitted him to the PICU.

EXERCISE 1 Match the term on the left with its definition on the right.

_____ 1. anticonvulsant

_____ 2. encephalitis

_____ 3. meningitis

_____ 4. EEG

_____ 5. ICP

_____ 6. photophobia

a. excessive sensitivity to light

b. inflammation of the brain

c. inflammation of the meninges

d. intracranial pressure

e. electroencephalography

f. a drug that opposes convulsions

EXERCISE 2 Refer to the document on the previous page and fill in the blanks.

1. The root word in *encephalopathic* is *encephalo,* which means _____.

2. The term *intracranial* comes from combining _____ (inside) and *cranio,* which means _____.

EXERCISE 3 True or false questions. Refer to the document on the previous page and indicate true answers with a T and false answers with an F.

1. The medical professionals worried that Manuel was abusing drugs. _____

2. Because of their concern about encephalitis and meningitis, the health professionals performed an LP. _____

3. In response to his seizure, Manuel was given a thrombolytic. _____

EXERCISE 4 Multiple-choice questions. Select the correct answer.

1. The health professionals were concerned about the possibility of which two conditions?
   a. inflammation of the brain and the membrane surrounding the brain and spinal cord
   b. inflammation of the brain and spinal cord
   c. inflammation of the spinal cord and the tough outer membrane surrounding the brain and spinal cord
   d. inflammation of the spinal cord and the membrane surrounding the brain and spinal cord

2. Which procedures were used to assist in the diagnosis and treatment of the patient?
   a. LP, EEG   d. EEG, LP, ICP
   b. CSF, EEG   e. ICP, LP, CSF
   c. LP, CSF

Quick Reference

glossary of roots and suffixes

TERM	DEFINITION	TERM	DEFINITION
cephal/o	head	-mania	excessive desire
cerebell/o	cerebellum	mening/o, meningi/o	meninges; membrane surrounding the brain and spinal cord
cerebr/o	brain	myel/o	spinal cord, bone marrow
crani/o	head, skull	neur/o	nerve
dur/o	tough outer membrane surrounding the brain and spinal cord	-paresis	slight or partial paralysis
encephal/o	brain	phas/o	speech
esthesi/o	feeling, sensation	-phobia	excessive fear
gnosi/o	know	phren/o	mind
		-plegia	paralysis
		psych/o	mind

nervous system abbreviations

ABBREVIATION	DEFINITION
ADHD	attention-deficit hyperactivity disorder
ALS	Lou Gehrig's disease (amyotrophic lateral sclerosis)
CNS	central nervous system
CP	cerebral palsy
CSF	cerebrospinal fluid
CVA	cerebrovascular accident
EEG	electroencephalogram
ICP	intracranial pressure
LP	lumbar puncture
MS	multiple sclerosis
OCD	obsessive compulsive disorder
PET	positron emission tomography
PNS	peripheral nervous system
TIA	transient ischemic attack

The Sensory System— Ophthalmology and Otolaryngology

6

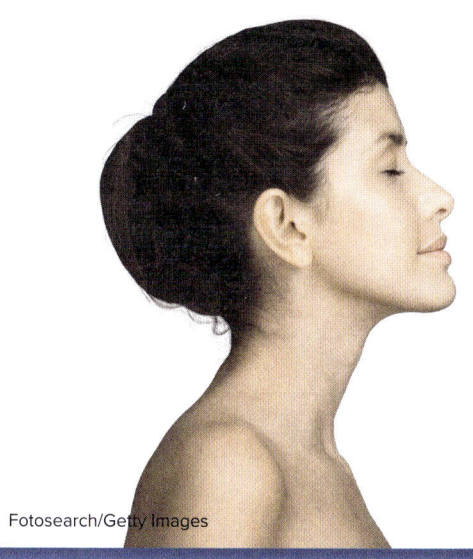

Fotosearch/Getty Images

Learning Outcomes

Upon completion of this chapter, you will be able to:

6.1 Identify the **roots/word parts** associated with the **sensory system.**

(S) **6.2** Translate the **Subjective** terms associated with the **sensory system.**

(O) **6.3** Translate the **Objective** terms associated with the **sensory system.**

(A) **6.4** Translate the **Assessment** terms associated with the **sensory system.**

(P) **6.5** Translate the **Plan** terms associated with the **sensory system.**

6.6 Distinguish terms associated with the **sensory system** in the context of **electronic health records.**

Introduction and Overview of Sensory Organs

You are standing at a music festival listening to live music. The feeling is electric and the experience is unforgettable. What makes it so memorable? The sound is fantastic, but you could download the music. The sights are great. The band is in top form and everyone around you is excited. However, you could watch and hear it all online. There are distinct smells. Many of them are unpleasant, but for some reason, as part of a whole, they are acceptable. You feel the bass. You sweat as you dance. Overall, the experience is far greater than the parts. Why is that the case? Your brain processes each component of these things and integrates them into a whole. Yet each sense is important in defining the experience. The function of the sensory system is collecting specific details about the surroundings and sending the information on to the central nervous system.

Sensory organs and cells are found throughout your entire body. As mentioned before, your skin is your largest sensory organ. It contains thousands upon thousands of cells sending information to your brain, including information about pain, pressure, and temperature. Your most complex sensory organs, however, are your eyes and ears. They provide you with a wealth of information about the world around you.

6.1 Word Parts of the Sensory System

Word Roots Associated with the Eye

OUTER STRUCTURES AND VISION

The eye (*oculo*) is a very valuable but vulnerable organ. There are many protective structures around the eye that help keep it safe and wet. The eye rests in a socket made of seven connecting bones in the skull. This socket is also known as the orbit. Just outside the eye are a set of eyelids (*blepharo*) that protect the eyes from dust and other floating particles in the air. In addition, eyelids aid in keeping the eye moist. It is extremely important for the eye to remain wet. For this reason, there are additional structures that help keep the eye moist. The lacrimal gland is a small gland that sits just above and to the side of the eye. It produces tears that stream across the eye and keep it wet. Finally, the eyes and eyelids are lined with a thin invisible membrane known as the conjunctiva.

eye

ROOTS: *ocul/o, ophthalm/o, opt/o*

EXAMPLES: oculopathy, ophthalmologists, optometrist

NOTES: It might sound nitpicky, but *ophthalmo* has two *h*s, not one. Many people think the root is *OPthalmo*, but it is actually *OPHthalmo*.
Some people think the word *antler* comes from the Latin phrase *ante ocular,* which means *in front of the eye,* because that is where the horns grow on deer and cows.

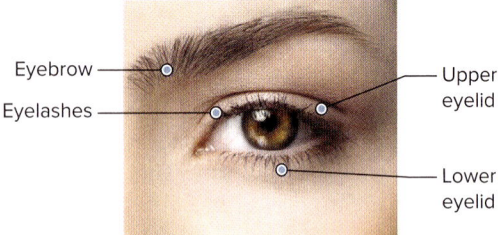

Eyebrow
Eyelashes
Upper eyelid
Lower eyelid

Frank P Wartenberg/Picture Press/Getty Images

tear

ROOTS: *lacrim/o, dacry/o*

EXAMPLES: lacrimation, dacryorrhea

NOTES: Often the term *lacrimal* is used interchangeably for the word *tear*. Keep in mind that the lacrimal gland and the tear gland refer to the same thing. Although it isn't the origin of the term, you may find it easy to remember that *dacryo* means *tear* because it has the word *cry* in the middle of it—daCRYo.

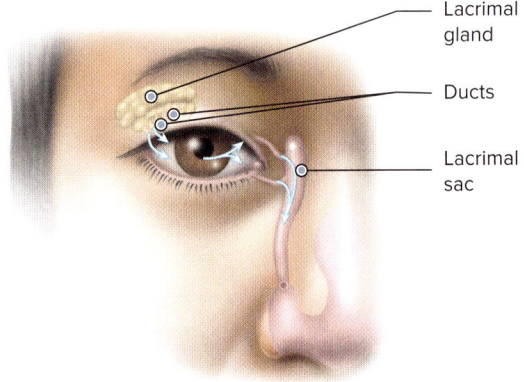

Lacrimal gland

Ducts

Lacrimal sac

McGraw-Hill Global Education Holdings, LLC

vision condition

SUFFIXES: *-opia, -opsia*

EXAMPLES: hyperopia, akinetopsia

NOTES: Akinetopsia = *a* + *kinet* + *-opsia* = no movement vision condition. It refers to a condition in which patients are unable to see objects in motion.

eyelid

ROOT: *blephar/o*

EXAMPLES: blepharedema, blepharoplasty

NOTES: Blepharoplasty = *blepharo* + *plasty* = surgical reconstruction of the eyelid. Also, remember that the *ph* is pronounced *f.* The word is ble*ph*aroplasty, *not* ble*p*aroplasty.

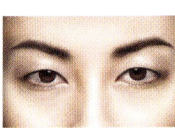
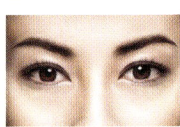

McGraw-Hill Global Education Holdings, LLC

SCLERA AND CORNEA

An eye is like a video camera with three layers. The outermost layer includes the *sclera* and the *cornea*. The *sclera* is the white part of the eye—a dense, protective layer, like the hard shell on the outside of the video camera. The *cornea* is a clear surface in the middle of the eye. Like the glass on a video camera, the cornea protects the lens and begins the work of focusing light to the back of the eye.

conjunctiva

ROOT: *conjunctiv/o*

EXAMPLE: conjunctivitis

NOTES: The *conjunctiva* is a clear membrane that covers the sclera and lines the eyelids. The root comes from two Latin words, *con* (with/together) and *junct* (join). Evidently, someone thought it joined the eye to the rest of body.

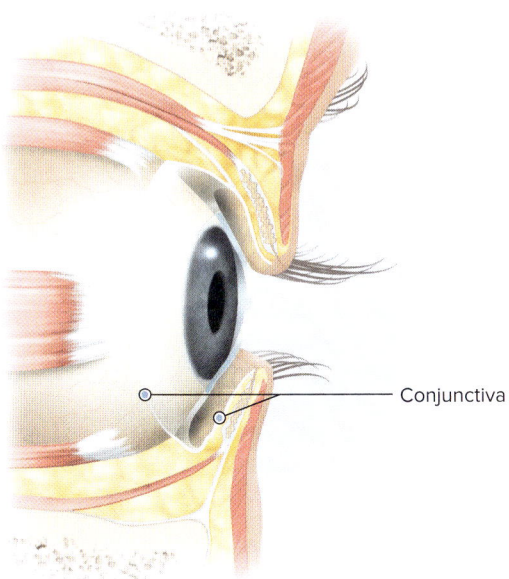

McGraw-Hill Global Education Holdings, LLC

cornea

ROOTS: *corne/o, kerat/o*

EXAMPLES: corneal transplant, keratitis

NOTES: *Kerato* is a tricky root because it has multiple meanings. In the context of the eye, *kerato* means *cornea*. In the context of the skin, *kerato* refers to a horny texture to the skin. What's the connection? *Kerato* comes from a Greek word meaning *horn* (think of a rhinoCEROS) and *corneo* comes from a

Latin word meaning *horn* (think of a CORNUcopia, a horn of plenty). Apparently someone thought the cornea of the eye looked like a horn.

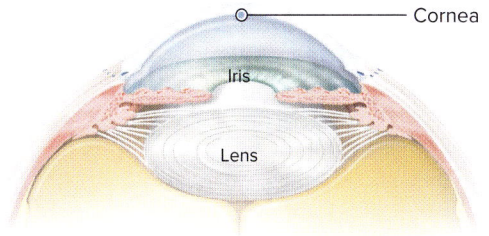

McGraw-Hill Global Education Holdings, LLC

sclera (the white of the eye)

ROOT: *scler/o*

EXAMPLE: scleritis

NOTES: Just like *kerato*, sclera has multiple meanings. In other contexts, *sclero* means *hard* and can refer to the abnormal hardening of any tissue or organ. In the eye, it refers to the white, tough, and fibrous protective covering of the eye. Words having to do with the eye use *sclero* in both ways:

phacosclerosis = *phaco* + *scler* + *osis* = an abnormal hardening of the lens

scleromalacia = *sclero* + *malacia* = an abnormal softening of the sclera

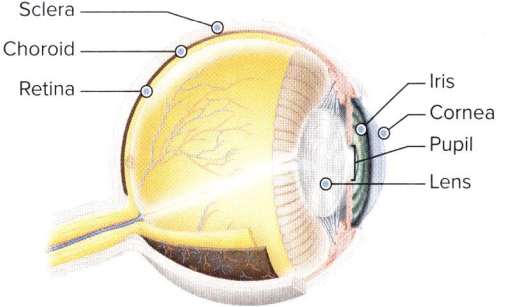

McGraw-Hill Global Education Holdings, LLC

CHOROID AND RETINA

The next layer down is the *choroid*. It includes the *lens,* which gathers light and focuses on images in the same way a lens on a camera does. The choroid also includes the *iris* and the *ciliary muscles.*

The iris is what gives eyes their color. By expanding (*dilating*) or shrinking (*constricting*) the pupil, the iris controls how much light hits the back of the eye.

The ciliary muscles adjust the shape of the eye and lens to focus on near or far objects. As light passes through the lens, it passes through liquid in the eye (*vitreous*) that bends the light and aims it to the back of the eyeball—all the way to the deepest layer, the *retina,* which is the eye's image processor. The retina helps turn visual stimuli into electric signals. The collected information is then sent to the brain by electric signals along the optic nerve.

---

retina

ROOT: **retin/o**

EXAMPLES: retinitis, retinoscope

NOTES: *Retina* comes from a word that means *net;* it refers to the netlike pattern of light-sensitive tissue on the inside surface of the eye.

---

iris

ROOTS: **ir/o, irid/o**

EXAMPLES: iritis, iridalgia

NOTES: The iris is the colored part of the eye. It is responsible for adjusting the size of the pupil to control the amount of light that enters the eye. In Greek mythology, Iris was a female messenger of the gods. She was the personification of the rainbow, which is why her name was given to the colored part of the eye.

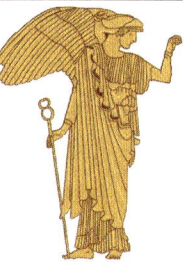
McGraw-Hill Global Education Holdings, LLC

---

lens

ROOTS: **phac/o, phak/o**

EXAMPLES: phacoscope, phakitis

NOTES: *Phaco* is a Greek word meaning *lentil,* a type of bean, which is where we get the word *lens.* Notice that *phaco* can be spelled with a *c* (*phaco*) or a *k* (*phako*). Because *c* sounds like *s* before *i* and *e,* the *k* sound is used sometimes to be sure the syllable is pronounced hard. For example, *phacitis* could be pronounced fah-SAI-tis. To avoid confusion, the word is sometimes spelled *phakitis* so it is pronounced fah-KAI-tis.

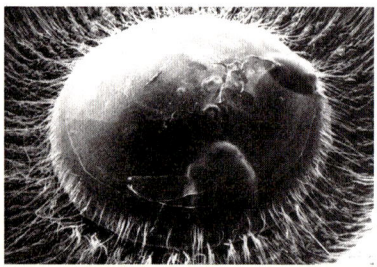

An up-close picture of the eye's lens.
Ralph C. Eagle/MD/Science Source

Word Roots Associated with the Ear

THE EAR AND HEARING

Ears work like stereo speakers in reverse. While stereo speakers turn electrical signals into sounds (*acouso, audio*), ears (*auro, oto*) turn sounds into electrical signals. First, they collect sounds. Next, they turn the energy from the sounds into movements, and then they convert them again into electrical signals. Last, they send the signals to the brain, where it all gets sorted out into meaning.

---

ear

ROOTS: **aur/o, ot/o**

EXAMPLES: aural, otoscope

NOTES: If you learn better by hearing something than by reading it, then you are an *aural learner.* It's easy to confuse *aural* with *oral.* But since *oral* means *mouth,* we guess an oral learner would be someone who learns by eating.

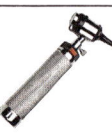
Photodisc Collection/ Getty Images

Also, the root *oto* is pronounced OH- toh, not AW-toh. An instrument a doctor uses to look in the ear is called an *otoscope,* which is pronounced OH-toh-skohp, not AW-toh-skohp.

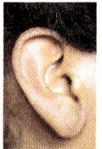
Joe DeGrandis/ McGraw-Hill Education

---

sound, hearing

ROOTS: **acous/o, audi/o**

EXAMPLES: acoustic, audiogram

NOTES: Sound travels at 768 miles per hour. That's about 12 miles per minute, or about 1 mile every 5 seconds. Light, however, travels a lot faster—186,282 miles per second, which is about 5.6 million miles per minute, or more than 335 million miles per hour. That's why you see a flash of lightning before you hear the thunder.

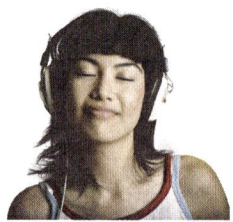
Hill Street Studios/ Photolibrary/Getty Images

---

hearing condition

SUFFIX: **-acusis**

EXAMPLES: hyperacusis, osteoacusis

NOTES: Have you ever wondered why your voice sounds different to you than it does to other people, or why you seem to sound different when you hear a recording of yourself? That's because of *osteoacusis (osteo + -acusis = bone hearing* condition). When you speak, your voice passes through the air and hits other people's eardrums. But it reaches your own ear in two very different ways—through the air, as it does for others, but also through the bones of your head, which is why you can hear yourself talk even if you plug your ears. Sound waves travel differently through bone than through air, so your voice sounds different to you than it does to other people.

OUTER/MIDDLE EAR

There are three main divisions of the ear: the outer ear, the middle ear, and the inner ear.

The outer ear includes the *pinna* and the *ear canal.* The pinna is what we first think of when we think about the ear—it's the fleshy part we pierce, tug on, and cover up in the winter. The pinna sits on the mastoid bone of the skull. Its funnel shape helps collect sounds from the air and send it down the ear canal toward the eardrum (*tympanic membrane*).

The eardrum is part of the middle ear and is a very important structure. It turns sound waves into physical energy. To keep the eardrum free from interference, the body protects it from both sides. From the outside, the ear canal produces ear wax (*cerumen*). Despite its gross appearance, ear wax is very helpful—it is a natural antibiotic and also a lubricant that keeps the ear canal moist. On the other side of the eardrum is a drainage system. The middle ear is connected to the nose and throat through a tube (*salpinx*). This tube helps drain the ear of any fluid and keeps the pressure inside the middle ear the same as outside the ear. Your eardrum is attached to three bones that make up the rest of the middle ear. These bones are the *incus, stapes,* and *malleus* (anvil, stirrup, and hammer). When the eardrum moves, these tiny bones move too. They transfer their movement to the inner ear.

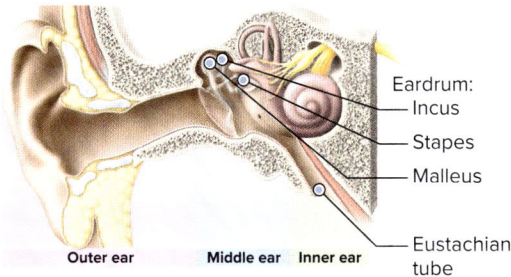

Eardrum:
— Incus
— Stapes
— Malleus
— Eustachian tube

Outer ear   Middle ear   Inner ear

McGraw-Hill Global Education Holdings, LLC

eardrum

ROOTS: *tympan/o, myring/o*

EXAMPLES: tympanostomy, myringotomy

NOTES: The root *tympano* comes from a Greek word meaning *drum.* Orchestras' big kettle drums are called *tympany,* so *eardrum* is not a bad translation. If you take a peek inside someone's ear sometime, you'll probably agree that it does resemble a drum.

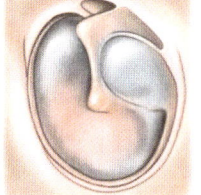

McGraw-Hill Global Education Holdings, LLC

ear wax

ROOT: *cerumin/o*

EXAMPLE: ceruminolysis

NOTES: Remember: *C* is pronounced like an *s* before *e* and *i* and like a *k* before *a, o,* and *u.* So *cerumen* is pronounced SEH-roo-men.

eustachian tube

ROOT: *salping/o*

EXAMPLE: rhinosalpingitis

NOTES: *Salpingo* is derived from the Latin word *salpinx,* which means *trumpet.* It refers to the long, straight kind used by Roman legions in battle, not the curvy kind with keys that is used today. This is important because *salpingo* is used in two body systems: in the ear, referring to the eustachian tubes, and in the female reproductive system, referring to the fallopian tubes. Both have long, tubelike shapes. And what are eustachian tubes? They connect the middle ear to the throat. Hold your nose, close your mouth, and blow. You'll make your eardrum pop by forcing air into your middle ear through the eustachian tubes. Ear infections occur when the eustachian tubes are prevented from draining fluid out of the middle ear.

INNER EAR

The bones of the middle ear are connected to the *cochlea,* a shell-shaped organ in your inner ear (*labyrinth*) filled with fluid and hair. When the *stapes* (pronounced STAY-peez) moves, it presses on the cochlea and causes the fluid to move. Just as the ocean waters move through seaweed, when the fluid moves, the hairs bend. The hairs, which are connected to the nervous system, create an electric signal carried by the *acoustic nerve* to the brain. Finally, the brain receives and processes the electric signals.

The inner ear also has another critical job: helping maintain balance. The *vestibular system* sends information to the brain about the tilt, rotation, and motion of the head. Like the cochlea, it is made up of small canals filled with fluid and hair. These hairs are moved not by sound but by movement and head angle. This helps maintain balance and also allows the brain to coordinate movement with the eyes.

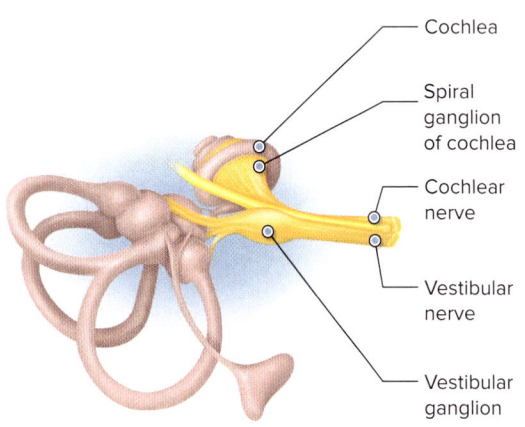

McGraw-Hill Global Education Holdings, LLC

vestibule

ROOT: *vestibul/o*

EXAMPLE: vestibulitis

NOTES: The term *vestibule* literally means the lobby of a building. Sometimes church lobbies are called vestibules. In medicine, *vestibule* refers to a small space at the beginning of a canal. In the ear, it refers to the area in front of semicircular canals (hence the name); it contains structures that help regulate balance.

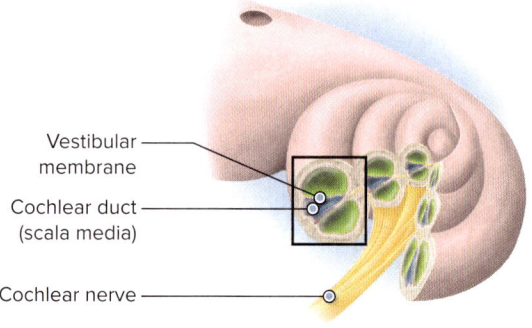

McGraw-Hill Global Education Holdings, LLC

cochlea

ROOT: *cochle/o*

EXAMPLE: cochleitis

NOTES: From Greek, for *snail shell,* the *cochlea* (pronounced KOH-klee-ah) is a spiral, snail shell–shaped tube in the inner ear that contains hearing receptors.

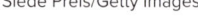

Siede Preis/Getty Images

labyrinth

ROOT: *labyrinth/o*

EXAMPLE: labyrinthitis

NOTES: The *labyrinth* is the innermost part of the ear. It contains two structures: the *cochlea,* which controls hearing, and the *vestibular system,* which controls balance.

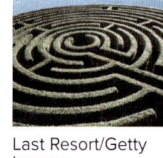

Last Resort/Getty Images

The term *labyrinth* comes from Greek mythology. It is the name of an elaborate maze built by King Minos to imprison the Minotaur, a half-man, half-bull creature.

TRANSLATION

EXERCISE 1 Match the word part on the left with its definition on the right.

_____ 1. ophthalm/o   a. eye

_____ 2. dacry/o   b. eye condition

_____ 3. -opia   c. eyelid

_____ 4. blephar/o   d. tear

EXERCISE 2 Translate the following word parts.

1. opt/o _____

2. ocul/o _____

3. -opsia _____

4. ophthalm/o _____

5. blephar/o _____

6. dacry/o _____

7. lacrim/o _____

EXERCISE 3 Break down the following words into their component parts and translate.

> EXAMPLE: **sinusitis**   _sinus | itis_
> _inflammation of the sinuses_

1. optic _____

2. oculopathy _____

3. ophthalmitis _____

4. blepharitis _____

5. hyperopia _____

6. dacryorrhea _____

EXERCISE 4 Match the word part on the left with its definition on the right.

_____ 1. retin/o   a. conjunctiva

_____ 2. corne/o   b. cornea

_____ 3. conjunctiv/o   c. iris

_____ 4. scler/o   d. lens

_____ 5. ir/o   e. retina

_____ 6. phac/o   f. sclera

EXERCISE 5 Translate the following roots.

1. corne/o _____

2. retin/o _____

3. irid/o _____

4. conjunctiv/o _____

5. ir/o _____

6. phac/o _____

7. kerat/o _____

8. phak/o _____

EXERCISE 6 Break down the following words into their component parts and translate.

> EXAMPLE: **sinusitis**   _sinus | itis_
> _inflammation of the sinuses_

1. corneal transplant _____

2. conjunctivitis _____

3. iritis _____

4. scleromalacia _____

5. retinopathy _____

6. keratopathy _____

7. phacoscope _____

8. iridalgia _____

9. scleritis _____

10. sclerokeratitis _____

EXERCISE 7 Match the word part on the left with its definition on the right. Some definitions will be used more than once.

_____ 1. audi/o   a. ear

_____ 2. -acusis   b. hearing condition

_____ 3. acous/o   c. sound

_____ 4. aur/o

_____ 5. ot/o

EXERCISE 8   Translate the following word parts.

1. -acusis _____
2. acous/o _____
3. aur/o _____
4. audi/o _____
5. ot/o _____

EXERCISE 9   Break down the following words into their component parts and translate.

EXAMPLE: **sinusitis**   *sinus | itis*
inflammation of the sinuses

1. audiologist _____
2. hyperacusis _____
3. hypoacusis _____
4. otalgia _____
5. otoscope _____
6. acoustic neuroma _____

EXERCISE 10   Match the word part on the left with its definition on the right.

_____   1. cochle/o   a. cochlea
_____   2. salping/o   b. eardrum
_____   3. labyrinth/o   c. ear wax
_____   4. vestibul/o   d. eustachian tube
_____   5. myring/o   e. labyrinth
_____   6. cerumin/o   f. vestibule

EXERCISE 11   Translate the following word parts.

1. cochle/o _____
2. vestibul/o _____
3. labyrinth/o _____
4. tympan/o _____
5. cerumin/o _____
6. myring/o _____
7. salping/o _____

EXERCISE 12   Break down the following words into their component parts and translate.

EXAMPLE: **sinusitis**   *sinus | itis*
inflammation of the sinuses

1. cochleitis _____
2. labyrinthitis _____
3. vestibulitis _____
4. myringitis _____
5. salpingoscope _____
6. tympanostomy _____
7. labyrinthectomy _____
8. myringodermatitis _____

GENERATION

EXERCISE 13   Identify the word parts from this chapter for the following terms.

1. amblyopia _____
2. ophthalmologist _____
3. blepharospasm _____
4. lacrimation _____
5. oculomycosis _____
6. optomyometer _____
7. hemianopsia _____
8. dacryohemorrhea _____
9. optokinetic _____

EXERCISE 14 Build a medical term from the information provided.

1. surgical reconstruction of the eye (use *ocul/o*)

   _____

2. surgical reconstruction of the eyelid

   _____

3. disease of the eye (use *ophthalm/o*)

   _____

4. specialist in measuring the eye (use *opt/o*)

   _____

5. over vision condition (use *-opia*)

   _____

6. excessive discharge of tears (use *dacry/o*)

   _____

EXERCISE 15 Identify the word parts from this chapter for the following terms.

1. corneal xerosis _____
2. keratomalacia _____
3. retinopexy _____
4. iridemia _____
5. phacoemulsification _____
6. aphakia _____
7. blepharoconjunctivitis _____
8. sclerokeratoiritis _____

EXERCISE 16 Build a medical term from the information provided.

1. inflammation of the lens (use *phak/o*)

   _____

2. inflammation of the conjunctiva _____

   _____

3. inflammation of the cornea (use *kerat/o*)

   _____

4. inflammation of the iris (use *ir/o*)

   _____

5. lens softening (use *phac/o*) _____

   _____

6. incision into the retina _____

7. incision into the sclera _____

EXERCISE 17 Identify the word parts from this chapter for the following terms.

1. otitis media _____
2. aural _____
3. audiogram _____
4. auditory prosthesis _____
5. pneumatic otoscopy _____
6. osteoacusis _____
7. otoneurology _____

EXERCISE 18 Build a medical term from the information provided.

1. pertaining to the ear (use *aur/o*) _____

   _____

2. pertaining to sound/hearing (use *acous/o*)

   _____

3. surgical reconstruction of the ear (use *ot/o*)

   _____

4. ear hardening condition (use *ot/o*) _____

   _____

5. procedure for looking in the ear (use *ot/o*)

   _____

6. procedure for measuring hearing (use *audi/o*)

   _____

7. instrument for measuring hearing (use *audi/o*)

   _____

EXERCISE 19 Identify the word parts from this chapter for the following terms.

1. tympanic perforation _____
2. cochlear implant _____
3. ceruminolysis _____

4. vestibular neuritis _____

5. myringomycosis _____

6. salpingopharyngeal _____

EXERCISE 20 Build a medical term from the information provided.

1. inflammation of the cochlea _____

2. ear wax condition _____

3. surgical reconstruction of the eardrum (use *myring/o*) _____

4. surgical reconstruction of the eardrum (use *tympan/o*) _____

5. incision into the vestibule _____

6. incision into the labyrinth _____

7. instrument for looking at the eustachian tubes _____

SUBJECTIVE

6.2 Patient History, Problems, Complaints

The Eye

When a patient goes to a health clinic for an eye problem, often the problem deals with a change in vision. While many people think of vision problems only in terms of either nearsightedness (*myopia*) or farsightedness (*hyperopia*), vision problems can also be much more specific in nature. For example, a patient could have blindness in half of her field of vision (*hemianopsia*).

Complaints relating to the tear glands are very common as well. Excessive tearing (*dacryorrhea*) or excessive dryness (*xerophthalmia*) can both cause a patient discomfort.

Patients may also experience problems with their eyelids. An eyelid twitch (*blepharospasm*) is not serious, but it can be very uncomfortable and distracting.

As with any part of the body, patients can experience pain in their eyes. The pain may be generalized (*ophthmalgia*) or specific to a part of the eye (*iridalgia* or *keratalgia*). Finally, patients may notice that their pupils are either large (*mydriasis*) or small (*miosis*).

The Ear

A change in hearing is a common ear complaint. A patient may complain of decreased (*hypoacusis*) or increased (*hyperacusis*) sensitivity to sound. Patients might also complain of ringing in the ears (*tinnitus*). Ear pain (*otalgia/ otodynia*) and discharge (*otorrhea*) are especially common in children with ear infections. Pain in the mastoid (*mastoidalgia*) may indicate a dangerous spread of the ear infection into the mastoid bone. *Vertigo* is a severe form of dizziness that often indicates problems with the patient's inner ear.

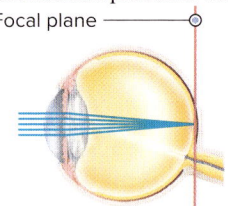

Focal plane

Emmetropia (normal)

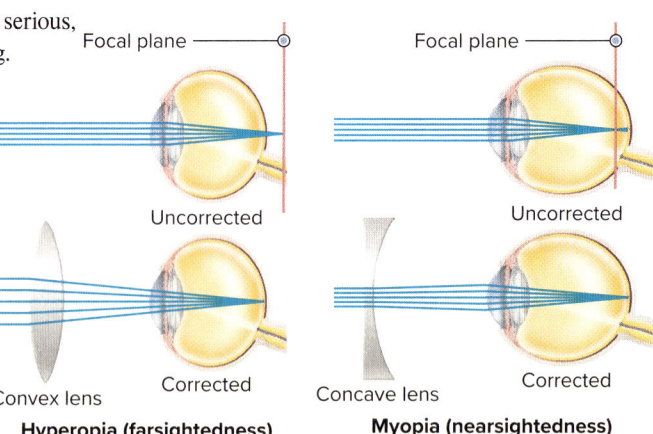

Focal plane

Uncorrected

Convex lens Corrected

Hyperopia (farsightedness)

Focal plane

Uncorrected

Concave lens Corrected

Myopia (nearsightedness)

McGraw-Hill Global Education Holdings, LLC

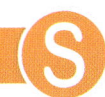

eye

TERM	WORD ANALYSIS
amblyopia AM-blih-OH-pee-ah	ambly / opia dull / vision condition

DEFINITION decreased vision; when it occurs in one eye, it is referred to as *lazy eye*

McGraw-Hill Global Education Holdings, LLC

astigmatism ah-STIG-mah-TIZ-um	a / stigmat / ism no / point / condition

DEFINITION vision problem caused by the fact that light rays entering the eye aren't focused on a single point in the back of the eye

blepharoplegia BLEF-ah-roh-PLEE-jah	blepharo / plegia eyelid / paralysis

DEFINITION paralysis of the eyelid

P. Marazzi/Science Source

blepharospasm BLEF-ah-roh-SPAZ-um	blepharo / spasm eyelid / involuntary contraction

DEFINITION involuntary contraction of an eyelid

hyperopia HAI-per-OH-pee-ah	hyper / opia over / vision condition

DEFINITION farsightedness

keratalgia KEH-rah-TAL-jah	kerat / algia cornea / pain

DEFINITION pain in the cornea

miosis mai-OH-sis	from Greek, for *to lessen*

DEFINITION abnormal contraction of the pupil

McGraw-Hill Global Education Holdings, LLC

eye *continued*

TERM	WORD ANALYSIS
mydriasis mi-DRAI-ah-sis	from Greek, for *red-hot metal*

DEFINITION abnormal dilation of pupil
NOTE: We don't really see the connection—do you?

McGraw-Hill Global Education Holdings, LLC

myopia mai-OH-pee-ah	my / opia shut / vision condition

DEFINITION nearsightedness
NOTE: The *my* root in this word is not from *myo* (muscle); instead, it's from another word that means *to shut* that is related to the word at the root of *mystery*—from something that is hidden from view until it is revealed.

ophthalmalgia awf-thal-MAL-jah	ophthalm / algia eye / pain

DEFINITION eye pain

ophthalmoplegia awf-THAL-moh-PLEE-jah	ophthalmo / plegia eye / paralysis

DEFINITION eye paralysis

McGraw-Hill Global Education Holdings, LLC

presbyopia PREZ-bee-OH-pee-ah	presby / opia old age / vision condition

DEFINITION decreased vision caused by old age

xerophthalmia ZER-awf-THAL-mee-ah	xer / ophthalm / ia dry / eye / condition

DEFINITION dry eyes

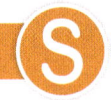

6.2 Patient History, Problems, Complaints

ear	
TERM	**WORD ANALYSIS**
otalgia oh-TAL-jah	ot / algia ear / pain
DEFINITION ear pain	
presbycusis PREZ-bih-KOO-sis	presby / cusis old age / hearing condition
DEFINITION loss of hearing in old age NOTE: The *a* in *acusis* was swallowed up by the *y* at the end of *presby*. The word is sometimes written as *presbyacusis*, but that's a lot harder to pronounce.	

ear *continued*	
TERM	**WORD ANALYSIS**
tinnitus tih-NAI-tis	from Latin, for *to ring or jingle* 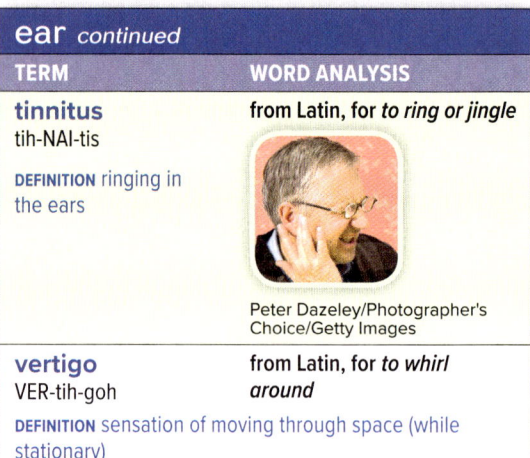 Peter Dazeley/Photographer's Choice/Getty Images
DEFINITION ringing in the ears	
vertigo VER-tih-goh	from Latin, for *to whirl around*
DEFINITION sensation of moving through space (while stationary)	

 Learning Outcome 6.2 Exercises

TRANSLATION

EXERCISE 1 Break down the following words into their component parts.

> EXAMPLE: **nasopharyngoscope**
> *naso | pharyngo | scope*

1. otalgia _____
2. hyperopia _____
3. blepharospasm _____
4. ophthalmoplegia _____
5. xerophthalmia _____

EXERCISE 2 Underline and define the word parts from this chapter in the following terms.

1. keratalgia _____
2. ophthalmalgia _____
3. myopia _____
4. presbycusis _____
5. blepharoplegia _____

EXERCISE 3 Match the term on the left with its definition on the right.

_____	1. vertigo	a. vision problem caused by the fact that light rays entering the eye aren't focused on a single point in the back of the eye
_____	2. astigmatism	b. abnormal contraction of the pupil
_____	3. amblyopia	c. abnormal dilation of the pupil
_____	4. presbyopia	d. decreased vision (when it occurs in one eye, it is referred to as *lazy eye*)
_____	5. presbycusis	e. decreased vision caused by old age
_____	6. tinnitus	f. loss of hearing in old age
_____	7. mydriasis	g. ringing in the ears
_____	8. miosis	h. the sensation of moving through space (while stationary)

EXERCISE 4 Translate the following terms as literally as possible.

> **EXAMPLE:** nasopharyngoscope *an instrument for looking at the nose and throat*

1. otalgia _____

2. ophthalmalgia _____

3. presbycusis _____

4. akinetopsia _____

5. xerophthalmia _____

6. astigmatism _____

GENERATION

EXERCISE 5 Build a medical term from the information provided.

> **EXAMPLE:** inflammation of the sinuses
> *sinusitis*

1. eye paralysis (use *ophthalm/o*) _____

2. paralysis of the eyelid _____

3. involuntary contraction of an eyelid _____

4. pain in the cornea (use *kerat/o*) _____

5. over vision condition (farsightedness) _____

6. decreased vision caused by old age _____

EXERCISE 6 Multiple-choice questions. Select the correct answer.

1. The medical term for nearsightedness is
   a. amblyopia   c. myopia
   b. tinnitus   d. vertigo

2. When this condition occurs in one eye, it is known as *lazy eye*.
   a. amblyopia   c. tinnitus
   b. myopia   d. vertigo

3. The medical term used to describe *ringing in the ears* is
   a. amblyopia   c. myopia
   b. tinnitus   d. vertigo

4. *Vertigo* is a condition of the
   a. inner ear   c. inner eye
   b. outer/middle ear   d. outer eye

EXERCISE 7 Briefly describe the difference between each pair of terms.

1. myopia, hyperopia _____

2. miosis, mydriasis _____

OBJECTIVE

6.3 Observation and Discovery

The Eye

As you might imagine, the physical exam of the eye is mainly limited to visual inspection. Often an eye exam begins with looking at the parts that surround it. An examiner might observe swelling (*blepharedema*) or drooping (*blepharoptosis*) around the eyelids. If pus is draining from the eyelids (*blepharopyorrhea*), that's a strong sign of infection.

After checking the eyelids, a health care professional might examine the position of the eye. An eye

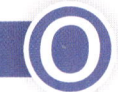
bulging from the orbit is known as *exophthalmos,* a condition commonly seen in hyperthyroidism.

The main areas of emphasis when inspecting the eye during a routine exam are the color of the sclera, the size of the pupils, and the movement of the eyes. The sclera of the eye is normally white. The blood vessels of the conjunctiva are normally so small that they are invisible. If the conjunctiva becomes inflamed, the vessels increase in size and the sclera may appear red. If one of the vessels in the conjunctiva ruptures, a small collection of blood may remain. Using a penlight or specialized light for examining eyes (*ophthalmoscope*), an examiner can check the size of a patient's pupils and determine how they react to light. They should constrict when exposed to light (*miosis*) and dilate when the light is dimmed.

Both eyes should work together. Shining a light in one eye should cause both pupils to constrict. The pupils should appear symmetric when looking straight ahead. One eye angled inward (*esotropia*) or outward (*exotropia*) is known as *strabismus.* A jittery, abnormal movement of the eye is called *nystagmus.* This may be a sign of an eye problem or a problem with the nervous system.

Further inspection of the eye may require specialized tools. An ophthalmoscope may be used to examine the back of a patient's eyes. It may show swelling of the optic nerve (*papilledema*). Other tools look at specific parts of the eye (*retinoscope, phacoscope*) or check for the pressure inside the eye (*tonometer*).

The Ear

When a patient presents with an ear problem, a health care professional is likely to first examine the outer part of the ear, including its size (*macrotia/ microtia*) and signs of inflammation, such as redness and swelling. To inspect the ear canal and eardrum, a special light known as an *otoscope* is needed.

One common finding is an excessive amount of ear wax in the ear (*ceruminosis/cerminoma*) that makes it difficult to see the eardrum. Upon visualizing the eardrum, the examiner looks for signs of fluid behind the ear. If the eardrum is red or bulging outward, an ear infection may be present. If the

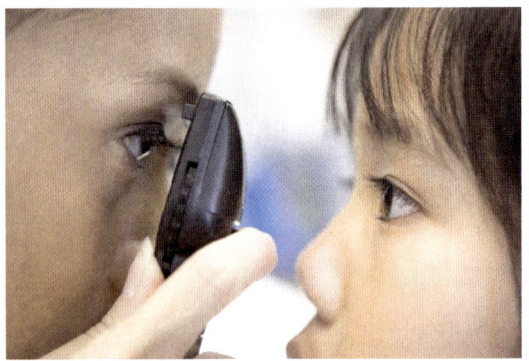

The doctor's primary instruments for observation of the eye and ear are the ophthalmoscope and the otoscope.

Fuse/Getty Images

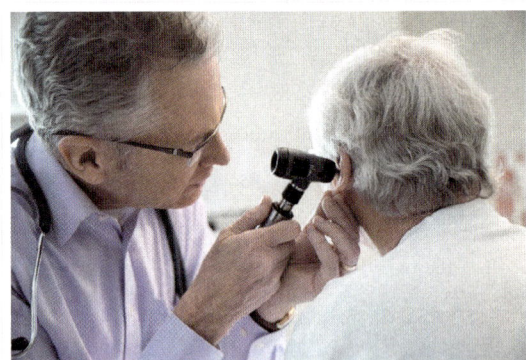

Hero Images Inc./Alamy Stock Photo

ear infection is bad enough, the eardrum may burst (*tympanic perforation*). Once the burst eardrum heals, the perforation may leave small, visible scars (*tympanosclerosis*).

The visualization of the ear canal and eardrum with an otoscope is called *otoscopy.* While very important, it can be difficult to determine the presence of an ear infection just by looking. If otoscopy alone does not reveal the presence of an ear infection, forcing air into the ear canal to see if it moves the eardrum (*pneumatic otoscopy*) may work.

Other tools to evaluate the ear include the *audiometer,* an instrument commonly used to check a patient's hearing, and the *salpingoscope,* a specialized instrument for examining the tubes that connect the middle ear to the nose and throat.

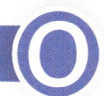

eye

TERM	WORD ANALYSIS
blepharoptosis BLEF-ar-awp-TOH-sis	blepharo / ptosis eyelid / drooping
DEFINITION drooping eyelid	

McGraw-Hill Global Education Holdings, LLC

TERM	WORD ANALYSIS
esotropia AY-soh-TROH-pee-ah	eso / trop / ia inward / turn / condition
DEFINITION inward turning of the eye, toward the nose	

McGraw-Hill Global Education Holdings, LLC

exotropia EKS-oh-TROH-pee-ah	exo / trop / ia outward / turn / condition
DEFINITION outward turning of the eye, away from the nose	

McGraw-Hill Global Education Holdings, LLC

nasolacrimal NAY-zoh-LAH-krih-mal	naso / lacrim / al nose / tear / pertaining to
DEFINITION pertaining to the nose and tear system	

nystagmus nih-STAG-mus	from Greek, for *to nod*
DEFINITION involuntary back-and-forth movement of the eyes	

ophthalmologist AWF-thal-MAW-loh-jist	ophthalmo / logist eye / specialist
DEFINITION eye specialist	

Fuse/Getty Images

eye *continued*

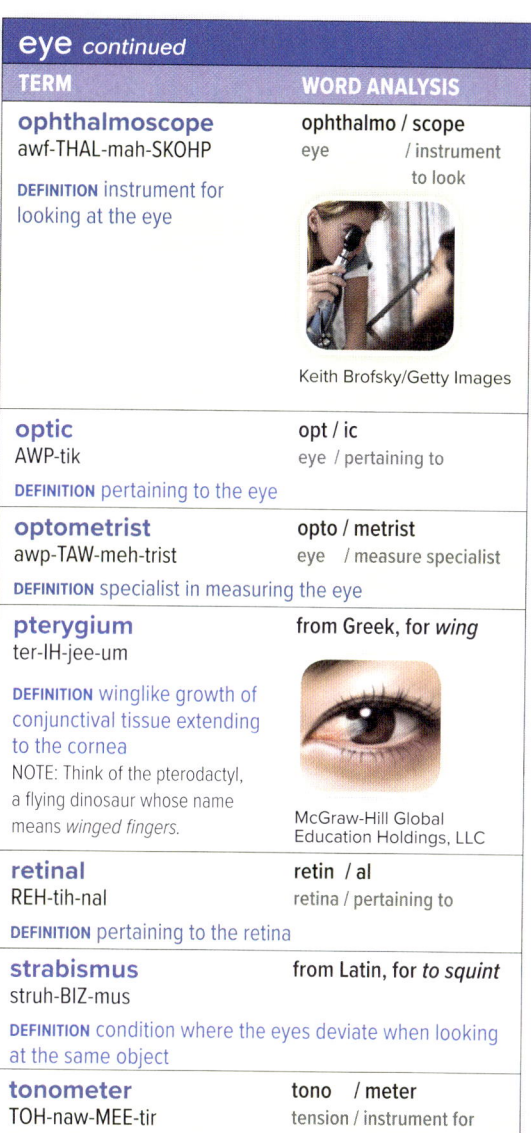

TERM	WORD ANALYSIS
ophthalmoscope awf-THAL-mah-SKOHP	ophthalmo / scope eye / instrument to look
DEFINITION instrument for looking at the eye	

Keith Brofsky/Getty Images

optic AWP-tik	opt / ic eye / pertaining to
DEFINITION pertaining to the eye	

optometrist awp-TAW-meh-trist	opto / metrist eye / measure specialist
DEFINITION specialist in measuring the eye	

pterygium ter-IH-jee-um	from Greek, for *wing*
DEFINITION winglike growth of conjunctival tissue extending to the cornea NOTE: Think of the pterodactyl, a flying dinosaur whose name means *winged fingers*.	

McGraw-Hill Global Education Holdings, LLC

retinal REH-tih-nal	retin / al retina / pertaining to
DEFINITION pertaining to the retina	

strabismus struh-BIZ-mus	from Latin, for *to squint*
DEFINITION condition where the eyes deviate when looking at the same object	

tonometer TOH-naw-MEE-tir	tono / meter tension / instrument for measuring
DEFINITION instrument for measuring tension or pressure in the eye (intraocular pressure)	

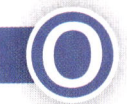
ear	
TERM	**WORD ANALYSIS**
audiogram AW-dee-oh-GRAM	audio / gram hearing / record
DEFINITION record produced by an audiometer	
audiologist aw-dee-AW-loh-jist	audio / logist hearing / specialist
DEFINITION hearing specialist	
audiometer aw-dee-AW-meh-ter	audio / meter hearing / instrument for measuring
DEFINITION instrument for measuring hearing	
McGraw-Hill Global Education Holdings, LLC	
audiometry aw-dee-AW-meh-tree	audio / metry hearing / measuring procedure
DEFINITION procedure for measuring hearing	
aural AW-ral	aur / al ear / pertaining to
DEFINITION pertaining to the ear NOTE: This word is easily confused with *oral*.	

ear *continued*	
TERM	**WORD ANALYSIS**
ceruminosis seh-ROO-min-OH-sis	cerumin / osis ear wax / condition
DEFINITION excessive formation of ear wax	
McGraw-Hill Global Education Holdings, LLC	
otolaryngologist OH-toh-LAH-rin-GAW-loh-jist	oto / laryngo / logist ear / throat / specialist
DEFINITION specialist in the ear and throat	
otorhinolaryngologist OH-toh-RAI-noh-LAH-rin-GAW-loh-jist	oto / rhino / laryngo / ear / nose / throat / logist specialist
DEFINITION specialist in the ear, nose, and throat	
otosclerosis OH-toh-skleh-ROH-sis	oto / scler / osis ear / hardening / condition
DEFINITION hearing loss caused by the hardening of the bones of the middle ear	
otoscope OH-toh-SKOHP	oto / scope ear / instrument to look
DEFINITION instrument for looking in the ear	
otoscopy oh-TAW-skoh-pee	oto / scopy ear / looking procedure
DEFINITION procedure for examining the ear	
Arthur Tilley/Getty Images	

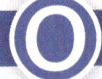

Learning Outcome 6.3 Exercises

PRONUNCIATION

EXERCISE 1   Indicate which syllable(s) is emphasized when pronounced.

EXAMPLE: bronchitis bron<u>chi</u>tis

1. retinal _____

2. otoscopy _____

3. audiometer _____

4. audiologist _____

5. strabismus _____

6. nystagmus _____

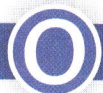

TRANSLATION

EXERCISE 2   Break down the following words into their component parts.

> EXAMPLE: nasopharyngoscope
> *naso | pharyngo | scope*

1. audiogram _____
2. audiometer _____
3. aural _____
4. optometrist _____
5. otosclerosis _____
6. ceruminosis _____
7. nasolacrimal _____
8. blepharoptosis _____
9. otolaryngologist _____
10. otorhinolaryngologist _____

EXERCISE 3   Underline and define the word parts from this chapter in the following terms.

1. optic _____
2. retinal _____
3. otoscopy _____
4. audiometry _____
5. audiologist _____
6. ophthalmologist _____
7. tonometer _____
8. ceruminoma _____
9. macrotia _____

EXERCISE 4   Match the term on the left with its definition on the right.

_____ 1. pterygium
_____ 2. exotropia
_____ 3. esotropia
_____ 4. nystagmus
_____ 5. strabismus

a. condition where the eyes deviate when looking at the same object
b. winglike growth of conjunctival tissue extending to the cornea
c. involuntary back-and-forth movement of the eyes
d. inward turning of the eye, toward the nose
e. outward turning of the eye, away from the nose

EXERCISE 5   Match the term on the left with its definition on the right.

_____ 1. otoscope
_____ 2. ophthalmoscope

a. instrument for looking at the eye
b. instrument for looking in the ear

EXERCISE 6   Translate the following terms as literally as possible.

> EXAMPLE: nasopharyngoscope   *an instrument for looking at the nose and throat*

1. tonometer _____
2. nasolacrimal _____
3. retinal _____
4. audiometer _____
5. audiometry _____
6. aural _____
7. otolaryngologist _____
8. otorhinolaryngologist _____
9. ceruminosis _____

GENERATION

EXERCISE 7 Build a medical term from the information provided.

> EXAMPLE: inflammation of the sinuses *sinusitis*

1. instrument for looking at the eye (use *ophthalm/o*) _____

2. instrument for looking in the ear (use *ot/o*) _____

_____

3. abnormal softening of the cornea (use *kerat/o*) _____

_____

4. procedure for looking in the ear (use *ot/o*) _____

_____

5. hearing record (use *audi/o*) _____

6. hearing specialist (use *audi/o*) _____

7. pertaining to the eye (use *opt/o*) _____

EXERCISE 8 Multiple-choice questions. Select the correct answer.

1. This term comes from Greek, for *wing,* and describes a winglike growth of conjunctival tissue extending to the cornea.
   a. lacrimation
   b. papilledema
   c. pterygium
   d. strabismus

2. The medical term for tear formation, or *crying,* is
   a. lacrimation
   b. nystagmus
   c. pterygium
   d. strabismus

3. A condition where the eyes deviate when looking at the same object is
   a. lacrimation
   b. nystagmus
   c. papilledema
   d. strabismus

4. Involuntary back-and-forth movement of the eyes is called
   a. lacrimation
   b. nystagmus
   c. papilledema
   d. pterygium

EXERCISE 9 Briefly describe the difference between each pair of terms.

1. optometrist, ophthalmologist _____

2. esotropia, exotropia _____

ASSESSMENT

6.4 Diagnosis and Pathology

The Eye

OUTER STRUCTURES

Structures around the eye often get inflamed. *Blepharitis* is usually caused by a mild bacterial skin infection. *Dacryoadenitis* is inflammation of the tear gland. The cause is not well understood, but it's thought to be an extension of inflammation of the conjunctiva.

More common is inflammation of the tear duct that drains the eye. In infants, this drainage system can be blocked (*dacryostenosis*) and can lead to a mild infection (*dacryocystitis*). Probably the most common eye complaint seen in most doctors' offices is inflammation of the conjunctiva (*conjunctivitis*). This can result from allergies, irritants in the eye, or infection. Infections of the conjunctiva (commonly known as *pink eye*) are usually caused by a virus or bacteria.

OUTER LAYER

The sclera has few general problems—the main one being *scleritis.* This painful, chronic illness is often

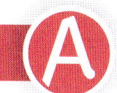

due to general inflammatory disorders such as *rheumatoid arthritis*. Problems with the cornea (*keratopathy*) include scratching from a foreign object (*corneal abrasion*) and inflammation (*keratitis*). Often caused by infection, keratitis is generally a very serious condition.

MIDDLE LAYER

The most common concern of the lens is clouding (*cataract*). The lens may also be undeveloped or absent (*aphakia*). Often aphakia is a result of surgical removal. Iridopathies, or disorders of the iris, include bleeding (*iridemia*). Inflammation of the iris (*iritis*) and iris with extension to the ciliary muscle (*iridocyclitis*) are unusual and painful.

INNER LAYER

The optic nerve is vulnerable to pressure from inside the eye (*glaucoma*) or from the brain; pressure from the brain can lead to swelling of the optic disc (*papilledema*). Like the other parts of the eye, the optic nerve can become inflamed (*optic neuritis*).

The retina can become detached from the blood supply. This emergency situation requires immediate reattachment, or blindness will occur. General retinal damage (*retinopathy*) can result from diabetes or blood disorders. Premature infants sometimes develop retinopathy after receiving oxygen as treatment for a lung disease.

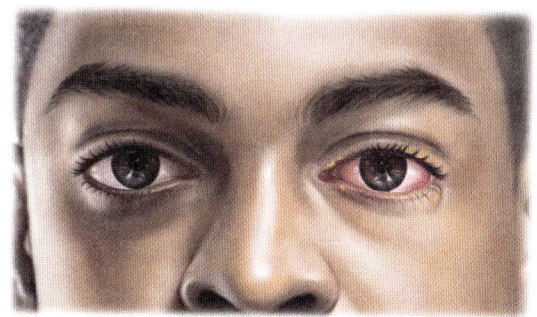

Infections of the conjunctiva are commonly known as pink eye.
McGraw-Hill Global Education Holdings, LLC

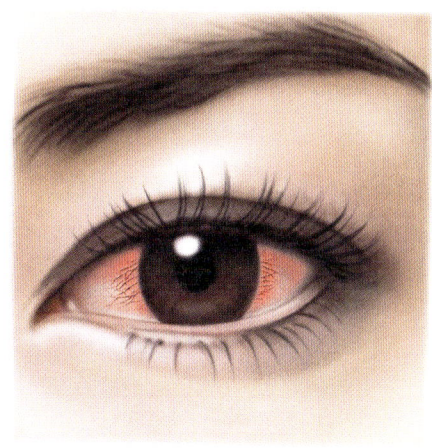

Inflamed blood vessels in the sclera
McGraw-Hill Global Education Holdings, LLC

The Ear

Many problems of the outer and middle ear involve infection. Infection of the outer ear (*otitis externa*) is a very common problem in summer, as swimmers often get water trapped in the ear canal. The common term for this illness is *swimmer's ear*. Otitis externa can also result from using a cotton swab to clean out the ears, which can push ear wax down into the ear until it forms a hard mass known as *cerumen impaction*.

Infection of the middle ear (*otitis media*) is one of the most common complaints seen in pediatric offices. Occasionally, the eardrum can be so inflamed that it blisters (*bullous myrigitis*). Less commonly, an ear infection can lead to a serious infection of the nearby skull bone (*mastoiditis*).

Inner ear problems manifest as either a loss of hearing (*sensorineural hearing loss*) or *vertigo*. Vertigo arises from inflammation of the inner ear structures (*labyrinthitis*) or the nerve that connects it to the brain (*vestibular neuritis*).

eye

TERM	WORD ANALYSIS
aphakia ah-FAY-kee-ia	a / phak / ia no / lens / condition

DEFINITION absence of a lens

NOTE: *Phak* is written with a *k* instead of a *c*. Although both are acceptable spellings, some people use a *k* to make sure the word is pronounced ah-FAY-kee-ia instead of ah-FAY-see-ia, which could be confused with other terms.

McGraw-Hill Global Education Holdings, LLC

blepharitis BLEF-ah-RAI-tis	blephar / itis eyelid / inflammation

DEFINITION eyelid inflammation

McGraw-Hill Global Education Holdings, LLC

cataract KAT-ah-RAKT	from Latin, for *waterfall*

DEFINITION opacity (cloudiness) of the lens of the eye

Photolibrary/Getty Images Plus

conjunctivitis con-JUNK-tih-VAI-tis	conjunctiv / itis conjunctiva / inflammation

DEFINITION inflammation of the conjunctiva (also known as *pink eye*)

Centers for Disease Control and Prevention

corneal abrasion KOR-nee-al a-BRAY-zhun	corne / al cornea / pertaining to
	ab / rasion away / rubbing

DEFINITION scratch on the cornea

Mediscan/Alamy Stock Photo

eye *continued*

TERM	WORD ANALYSIS
iridopathy EAR-ih-DOP-ah-thee	irido / pathy iris / disease

DEFINITION disease of the iris

iritis ai-RAI-tis	ir / itis iris / inflammation

DEFINITION inflammation of the iris

keratopathy KEH-rah-TOP-ah-thee	kerato / pathy cornea / disease

DEFINITION disease of the cornea

oculopathy AW-kyoo-LAW-pah-thee	oculo / pathy eye / disease

DEFINITION eye disease

ophthalmitis AWF-thal-MAI-tis	ophthalm / itis eye / inflammation

DEFINITION inflammation of the eye

ophthalmopathy AWF-thal-MOH-pah-thee	ophthalmo / pathy eye / disease

DEFINITION eye disease

retinopathy REH-tih-NOP-ah-thee	retino / pathy retina / disease

DEFINITION disease of the retina

ear

TERM	WORD ANALYSIS
acoustic neuroma ah-KOO-stik nir-OH-mah	acous / tic hearing / pertaining to
	neur / oma nerve / tumor

DEFINITION tumor on the acoustic nerve

McGraw-Hill Global Education Holdings, LLC

aerotitis AIR-oh-TAI-tis	aer / ot / itis air / ear / inflammation

DEFINITION inflammation of the ear caused by air

NOTE: This one is tricky because, unless you are careful, you will be tempted to miss the *ot* root in the middle. Most people want to divide the word *aero* + *itis*. The problem is the *t* in the middle. That is your clue that a root is hiding in the middle.

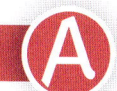

ear *continued*	
TERM	**WORD ANALYSIS**
cerumen impaction SEH-roo-men im-PAK-shun	**cerumen** ear wax
	im / pac / tion in / drive / condition
DEFINITION buildup of ear wax blocking ear canal	
conductive hearing loss con-DUK-tiv	**con / duct / ive** together / lead / pertaining to
DEFINITION hearing loss caused by sound not getting to the middle/inner ear (due to blockages)	
myringitis MIR-in-JAI-tis	**myring / itis** eardrum / inflammation
DEFINITION inflammation of the eardrum	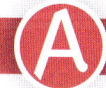 BSIP /Science Source
otitis externa oh-TAI-tis eks-TERN-nah	**ot / itis externa** ear / inflammation outside
DEFINITION inflammation of the outer ear	
otitis media oh-TAI-tis MEH-dee-ah	**ot / itis media** ear / inflammation middle
DEFINITION inflammation of the middle ear	

ear *continued*	
TERM	**WORD ANALYSIS**
otomycosis oh-toh-mai-KOH-sis	**oto / myc / osis** ear / fungus / condition
DEFINITION fungal ear condition	
otosclerosis oh-toh-skleh-ROH-sis	**oto / scler / osis** ear / hardening / condition
DEFINITION hearing loss caused by the hardening of the bones of the middle ear	
sensorineural hearing loss SEN-sor-ee-NIR-al	**sensori / neur / al** sense / nerve / pertaining to
DEFINITION hearing loss caused by sound not being transmitted from the inner ear to the brain (due to problems with the sensory organs or nerves)	

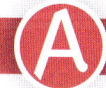 **Learning Outcome 6.4 Exercises**

PRONUNCIATION

EXERCISE 1   Indicate which syllable(s) is emphasized when pronounced.

EXAMPLE: bronchitis bron**chi**tis

1. acoustic _____

2. neuroma _____

3. iritis _____

4. aphakia _____

5. otomycosis _____

TRANSLATION

EXERCISE 2 Break down the following words into their component parts.

> EXAMPLE: nasopharyngoscope
> *naso | pharyngo | scope*

1. retinopathy _____

2. ophthalmopathy _____

3. otomycosis _____

EXERCISE 3 Underline and define the word parts from this chapter in the following terms.

1. corneal abrasion _____

2. conjunctivitis _____

3. vestibulitis _____

4. myringitis _____

5. blepharitis _____

4. otosclerosis _____

5. oculopathy _____

6. keratopathy _____

7. iridopathy _____

8. cerumen impaction _____

9. aphakia _____

EXERCISE 4 Match the term on the left with its definition on the right.

_____ 1. cataract   a. opacity (cloudiness) of the lens of the eye

_____ 2. iritis   b. inflammation of the eye

_____ 3. ophthalmitis   c. inflammation of the iris

EXERCISE 5 Match the term on the left with its definition on the right.

_____ 1. otitis media   a. inflammation of the outer ear

_____ 2. otitis externa   b. inflammation of the ear caused by air

_____ 3. aerotitis   c. hearing loss caused by sound not getting to the middle/inner ear (due to blockages)

_____ 4. conductive hearing loss   d. inflammation of the middle ear

_____ 5. sensorineural hearing loss   e. inflammation of the nose and eustachian tubes

_____ 6. acoustic neuroma   f. tumor on the acoustic nerve

_____ 7. rhinosalpingitis   g. hearing loss caused by sound not being transmitted from the inner ear to the brain (due to problems with the sense organs or nerves)

EXERCISE 6 Translate the following terms as literally as possible.

> EXAMPLE: nasopharyngoscope *an instrument for looking at the nose and throat*

1. oculopathy _____

2. ophthalmopathy _____

3. sclerokeratoiritis _____

4. acoustic neuroma _____

GENERATION

EXERCISE 7 Build a medical term from the information provided.

> EXAMPLE: inflammation of the sinuses   *sinusitis*

1. inflammation of the iris _____

2. inflammation of the eardrum (use *myring/o*)

   _____

3. inflammation of the eye (use *ophthalm/o*)

   _____

4. inflammation of the eyelid _____

EXERCISE 8 Multiple-choice questions. Select the correct answer(s).

1. Select the terms that pertain to the eye.
   a. aerotitis
   b. aphakia
   c. cataract
   d. cerumen impaction
   e. corneal abrasion
   f. otitis media

2. Select the terms that pertain to the ear.
   a. aerotitis
   b. aphakia
   c. cataract
   d. cerumen impaction
   e. corneal abrasion
   f. otitis media

3. A cataract affects what part of the eye?
   a. cornea
   b. lens
   c. optic nerve
   d. retina

4. A scratch on the cornea is called a(n)
   a. aphakia
   b. cataract
   c. corneal abrasion
   d. oculitis externa

5. Cerumen impaction is a
   a. buildup of ear wax blocking the ear canal
   b. buildup of ear wax hindering the function of the eardrum
   c. buildup of fluid causing pain in the ear canal
   d. buildup of fluid causing pain in the eardrum

6. Inflammation of the ear caused by air is
   a. aerotitis
   b. otitis externa
   c. otitis media
   d. pneumatic acoustitis

EXERCISE 9 Briefly describe the difference between each pair of terms.

1. iridopathy, keratopathy _____

2. otitis externa, otitis media _____

3. otosclerosis, otomycosis _____

   _____

4. conductive hearing loss, sensorineural hearing loss _____

P LAN

6.5 Treatments and Therapies

The Eye

Many advances have been made in eye surgery in recent years. A skilled surgeon can treat many disorders that could lead to blindness. In the outer layer, the sclera is a common site for making a cut (*sclerotomy*) in order to perform surgery in other parts of the eye.

The cornea is another common site for eye surgery. In a *corneal transplant,* a diseased cornea is removed and replaced with a donor cornea. Another type of corneal surgery, which involves making cuts in the cornea like spokes in a wheel (*radial keratotomy*), corrects myopia, hyperopia, and astigmatism.

6.5 Treatments and Therapies

Many surgeries involve the next layer of the eye. The most common eye surgery is *cataract extraction.* The modern approach involves breaking the original lens up into small pieces, aspirating the pieces out of the eye through a needle (*phacoemulsification*), and then installing a new lens (*intraocular lens implantation*). *Iridotomy* and *iridectomy* are procedures used to treat glaucoma. Retinal detachment requires immediate reattachment (*retinopexy*) in order to prevent blindness.

In the most dire situations, such as aggressive cancer, an eye may need complete removal (*enucleation*). Cosmetic surgeries of the eye usually involve the eyelid (*blepharoplasty*) to remove wrinkles.

There are limited medicines specific to ophthalmology. *Cycloplegics* are used prior to surgery to temporarily paralyze the pupil. *Mydriatics* are used prior to a thorough eye exam to dilate the eyes. *Miotics* were commonly used to treat glaucoma before more effective treatments were discovered.

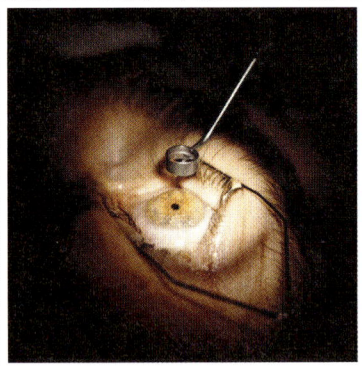

Surgery may be performed to treat a variety of eye disorders.

Penny Tweedie/The Image Bank/Getty Images

The Ear

Many treatments of the outer ear first involve a thorough cleaning of the ear canal. This can be done with washing (*ear lavage*) or inserting medicine to clear out the wax (*ceruminolytic*). One outer ear surgery (*otoplasty*) can make a deformed ear appear more normal. Another outer ear intervention is putting in a hearing aid (*auditory prosthesis*). This very common device is used to help people with hearing loss.

Middle ear procedures usually involve just the eardrum. Perhaps the most common surgery children undergo involves making a cut in the eardrum (*myringotomy*) and putting in a *tympanostomy* tube to drain fluid from the ear. Occasionally, when the tube falls out over time, it may leave a hole. In that case,

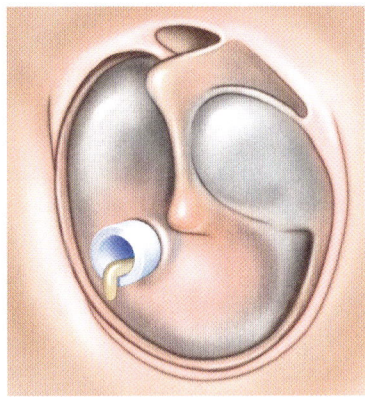

Tubes may be surgically installed in the eardrum to drain fluid from the ear.

McGraw-Hill Global Education Holdings, LLC

the eardrum will need patching (*tympanoplasty*). In the inner ear, a more advanced electronic device can be placed in the cochlea (*cochlear implant*). Another inner ear surgery, *labryinthectomy,* can be used to treat severe vertigo.

6.5 Treatments and Therapies

eye

TERM	WORD ANALYSIS
blepharoplasty BLEF-ah-roh-PLAS-tee	**blepharo / plasty** eyelid / reconstruction
DEFINITION surgical reconstruction of the eyelid	

McGraw-Hill Global Education Holdings, LLC

TERM	WORD ANALYSIS
blepharotomy BLEF-ah-RAW-toh-mee	**blepharo / tomy** eyelid / incision
DEFINITION incision into the eyelid	
corneal transplant KOR-nee-al TRANZ-plant	**corne / al** cornea / pertaining to **trans / plant** across / place
DEFINITION replacement of damaged cornea with donated tissue	
intraocular lens implant IN-trah-AW-kyoo-lar lenz IM-plant	**intra / ocul / ar** inside / eye / pertaining to **lens im / plant** lens in / place
DEFINITION insertion of a new lens inside the eye	

McGraw-Hill Global Education Holdings, LLC

TERM	WORD ANALYSIS
iridectomy EAR-id-EK-toh-mee	**irid / ectomy** iris / removal
DEFINITION removal of the iris	
iridotomy EAR-id-AW-toh-mee	**irido / tomy** iris / incision
DEFINITION incision into the iris	
keratoplasty ker-A-toh-PLAS-tee	**kerato / plasty** cornea / reconstruction
DEFINITION surgical reconstruction of the cornea	

McGraw-Hill Global Education Holdings, LLC

eye *continued*

TERM	WORD ANALYSIS
keratotomy KER-ah-TAW-toh-mee	**kerato / tomy** cornea / incision
DEFINITION incision into the cornea	
phacoemulsification FAY-koh-ee-MUL-sih-fih-KAY-shun	**phaco / emulsific / ation** lens / mix up / condition
DEFINITION fragmentation of an existing lens in order to remove and replace it	
retinopexy reh-TIH-noh-PEK-see	**retino / pexy** retina / surgical fixation
DEFINITION surgical fixation (reattachment) of a retina	

McGraw-Hill Global Education Holdings, LLC

pharmacology

TERM	WORD ANALYSIS
Eye	
miotic mai-AW-tik	**miot / ic** constriction / pertaining to
DEFINITION drug that causes the abnormal contraction of the pupil	
mydriatic MID-ree-AT-ik	**mydriat / ic** dilation / pertaining to
DEFINITION drug that causes the abnormal dilation of the pupil	
Ear	
ceruminolytic seh-ROO-min-oh-LIH-tik	**cerumino / lyt / ic** ear wax / loose / pertaining to
DEFINITION drug that aids in the breakdown of ear wax	
ototoxic OH-toh-TOK-sik	**oto / tox / ic** ear / poison / pertaining to
DEFINITION drug that is damaging to the ear/hearing	

ear	
TERM	**WORD ANALYSIS**
cochlear implant KOH-klee-ar IM-plant	cochle / ar cochlea / pertaining to
	im / plant in / place
DEFINITION electronic device that stimulates the cochlea; it can give a sense of sound to those who are profoundly deaf	 McGraw-Hill Global Education Holdings, LLC
ear lavage ee-ir lah-VAJ	from Latin, for *to wash, bathe*
DEFINITION rinsing/washing the external ear canal (usually to remove ear wax) NOTE: It's the origin of the English word *lavatory*.	
myringoplasty mir-IN-goh-PLAS-tee	myringo / plasty eardrum / reconstruction
DEFINITION surgical reconstruction of the eardrum	
myringotomy mir-in-GAW-toh-mee	myringo / tomy eardrum / incision
DEFINITION incision into the eardrum	

ear *continued*	
TERM	**WORD ANALYSIS**
otoplasty OH-toh-PLAS-tee	oto / plasty ear / reconstruction
DEFINITION surgical reconstruction of the ear	
tympanocentesis tim-PAN-oh-sin-TEE-sis	tympano / centesis eardrum / puncture
DEFINITION puncture of the eardrum	
tympanoplasty tim-PAN-oh-PLAS-tee	tympano / plasty eardrum / reconstruction
DEFINITION surgical reconstruction of the eardrum	
tympanostomy TIM-pan-AW-stoh-mee	tympano / stomy eardrum / opening procedure
DEFINITION creation of an opening in the eardrum	 McGraw-Hill Global Education Holdings, LLC

Learning Outcome 6.5 Exercises

TRANSLATION

EXERCISE 1 Break down the following words into their component parts.

> EXAMPLE: nasopharyngoscope
> *naso | pharyngo | scope*

1. keratotomy _____
2. myringotomy _____
3. blepharotomy _____
4. tympanostomy _____

EXERCISE 2 Underline and define the word parts from this chapter in the following terms.

1. iridectomy _____
2. iridotomy _____
3. blepharoplasty _____
4. otoplasty _____
5. keratoplasty _____
6. tympanoplasty _____
7. myringoplasty _____
8. tympanocentesis _____
9. intraocular lens implant _____

EXERCISE 3   Match the term on the left with its definition on the right.

_____ 1. corneal transplant

_____ 2. cochlear implant

_____ 3. ototoxic

_____ 4. ear lavage

_____ 5. ceruminolytic

_____ 6. retinopexy

_____ 7. mydriatic

_____ 8. miotic

_____ 9. phacoemulsification

a. drug that is damaging to the ear/hearing

b. electronic device that stimulates the cochlea

c. drug that causes the abnormal contraction of the pupil

d. drug that causes the abnormal dilation of the pupil

e. fragmentation of an existing lens in order to remove and replace it

f. replacement of damaged cornea with donated tissue

g. rinsing/washing the external ear canal (usually to remove ear wax)

h. surgical fixation (reattachment) of a retina

i. breakdown of ear wax

EXERCISE 4   Translate the following terms as literally as possible.

EXAMPLE: **nasopharyngoscope**   *an instrument for looking at the nose and throat*

1. ototoxic _____

2. tympanostomy _____

3. iridectomy _____

4. keratoplasty _____

5. phacoemulsification _____

GENERATION

EXERCISE 5   Build a medical term from the information provided.

EXAMPLE: **inflammation of the sinuses**   *sinusitis*

1. incision into the eardrum (use *myringo*) _____

2. incision into the cornea _____

3. incision into the iris _____

4. incision into the eyelid _____

EXERCISE 6   Multiple-choice questions. Select the correct answer(s).

1. Select the terms that pertain to the ear.
   a. blepharoplasty   d. otoplasty
   b. keratoplasty   e. tympanoplasty
   c. myringoplasty

2. Select the terms that pertain to the eye.
   a. blepharoplasty   d. otoplasty
   b. keratoplasty   e. tympanoplasty
   c. myringoplasty

EXERCISE 7   Briefly describe the difference between the pair of terms.

1. mydriatic, miotic _____

6.6 Electronic Health Records

Discharge Summary

Patient Name: Ms. Susan Cloud
Date of Admission: 6/23/15
Date of Discharge: 6/28/15

Admission Diagnosis
1. **Cataract** extraction

Discharge Diagnosis
1. Post cataract extraction
2. **Endophthalmitis**

Discharge Condition
Stable

Consultations
Infectious disease

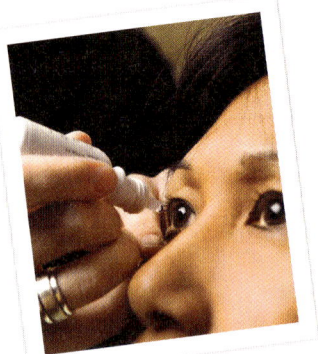

Jupiterimages/Getty Images

Procedures
1. **Extracapsular cataract** extraction with **phacoemulsification** and implantation of a posterior chamber **intraocular lens,** right eye.
2. **Vitrectomy.**

Labs
CBC: WBC 22.4 on 6/24; 18.5 on 6/25; 15.1 on 6/27; BCx. negative; **vitreous** culture: *Staphylococcus epidermidis*

Imaging
Ocular u/s: **vitreous** inflammation. No **retinal** detachment.

HPI
Ms. Cloud is a 58-year-old woman who first presented to her **ophthalmologist** with c/o **leukocoria.** She was also noted to have **nystagmus** and **strabismus.** She was diagnosed with a **cataract.** She was treated surgically with **cataract** extraction and **lens** implantation. She was admitted to the hospital on 6/23/2015 for postoperative observation.

Hospital Course
On postop day 2, Ms. Cloud began complaining of increasing right **ophthalmalgia.** She was noted to be febrile to 102.2. Exam revealed **conjunctival** infection and edema. She was presumed to have postoperative endophthalmitis. **Vitrectomy** was performed under sterile conditions, and samples were sent to lab for culture. She was given **intravitreal** antibiotics. Over the next couple of days, her fever curve trended down and her WBC count improved. Cultures came back positive for *S. epidermidis*. Infectious disease was consulted; they recommended two weeks of IV therapy. A PICC line was placed and she was discharged with care instructions.

Activity
Eye rest

Diet
No restrictions

Meds
IV vancomycin via PICC

Follow-Up Appointments
Ophthalmology outpatient clinic in 2 days
Infectious disease clinic in 1 week

—Lynn Holmes, MD

EXERCISE 1   Match the term on the left with its definition on the right.

_____ 1. conjunctival   a. condition where the eyes deviate when looking at the same object

_____ 2. retinal   b. eye specialist

_____ 3. ocular   c. fragmentation of an existing lens in order to remove and replace it

_____ 4. ophthalmologist   d. inflammation of the eye

_____ 5. ophthalmitis   e. involuntary back-and-forth movement of the eyes

_____ 6. ophthalmalgia   f. opacity (cloudiness) of the lens of the eye

_____ 7. cataract   g. pain in the eye

_____ 8. nystagmus   h. pertaining to the conjunctiva

_____ 9. strabismus   i. pertaining to the eye

_____ 10. phacoemulsification   j. pertaining to the retina

EXERCISE 2   Fill in the blanks.

1. According to the admission diagnosis, Ms. Cloud was admitted for a(n) _____.

2. The images performed on Ms. Cloud revealed that she had no *retinal detachment,* or that her _____ was still properly attached.

3. Ms. Cloud first presented to her _____ (eye specialist) with c/o leukocoria and was noted to have *nystagmus* (give definition: _____) and *strabismus* (give definition: _____).

4. During her surgery, her _____ was removed and a(n) _____ was implanted.

5. On *postop* (give definition: _____) day 2, Ms. Cloud began complaining of increasing right eye pain, or _____.

EXERCISE 3   True or false questions. Indicate true answers with a T and false answers with an F.

1. This health record was created at an ophthalmology clinic. _____

2. Ms. Cloud began complaining that her eye felt inflamed the second day after her operation. _____

3. During her second postop day, Ms. Cloud was noted to have a fever. _____

4. The cultures came back negative for an infection. _____

5. Ms. Cloud will need to follow up with an optometrist in 2 days. _____

EXERCISE 4   Multiple-choice questions. Select the correct answer(s).

1. The patient was admitted to the hospital for
   a. a cataract extraction
   b. a lens implantation
   c. ophthalmalgia and a fever
   d. postoperative observation

2. The health record indicates that the patient "was presumed to have postoperative endophthalmitis." The term *endophthalmitis* is created by combining the prefix *endo-* with the term *ophthalmitis,* which means
   a. discharge from the cornea
   b. discharge from the eye
   c. inflammation in the cornea
   d. inflammation in the eye

Quick Reference

glossary of roots

ROOT	DEFINITION	ROOT	DEFINITION
acous/o	sound	myring/o	eardrum
-acusis	hearing condition	ocul/o	eye
audi/o	sound	ophthalm/o	eye
aur/o	ear	-opia	vision condition
blephar/o	eyelid	-opsia	vision condition
cerumin/o	ear wax	opt/o	eye
conjunctiv/o	conjunctiva	ot/o	ear
corne/o	cornea	phac/o	lens
dacry/o	tear	phak/o	lens
ir/o	iris	retin/o	retina
irid/o	iris	salping/o	eustachian tube
kerat/o	cornea	scler/o	sclera (the white of the eye)
lacrim/o	tear	tympan/o	eardrum

eye abbreviations

ABBREVIATION	DEFINITION
ARMD	age-related macular degeneration
HEENT	head, eyes, ears, nose, and throat
IOL	intraocular lens
IOP	intraocular pressure
LASIK	laser-assisted in situ keratomileusis
OD	right eye (from Latin—*oculus dexter*)
OS	left eye (from Latin—*oculus sinister*)
OU	both eyes (from Latin—*oculus uterque*)
PERRLA	pupils are equal, round, and reactive to light and accommodation
VA	visual acuity
VF	visual field

ear abbreviations

ABBREVIATION	DEFINITION
AD	right ear (from Latin—*auris dextra*)
AS	left ear (from Latin—*auris sinistra*)
AOM	acute otitis media
AU	both ears (from Latin—*auris utraque*)
EENT	eye, ear, nose, and throat
ENT	ear, nose, and throat
OM	otitis media
TM	tympanic membrane

The Endocrine System—Endocrinology

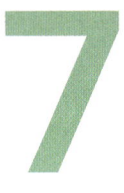

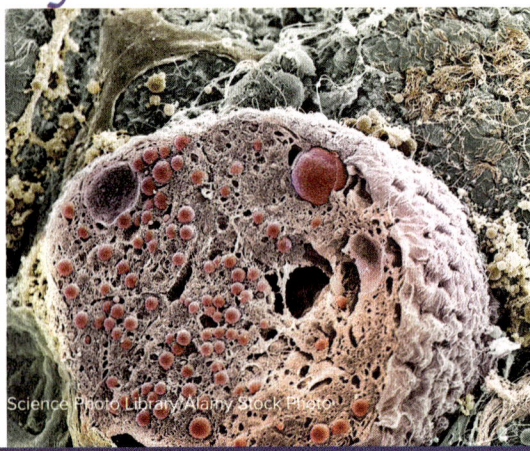

Science Photo Library/Alamy Stock Photo

Learning Outcomes

Upon completion of this chapter,
you will be able to:

7.1 Identify the **roots/word parts** associated with the **endocrine system.**

(S) **7.2** Translate the **Subjective** terms associated with the **endocrine system.**

(O) **7.3** Translate the **Objective** terms associated with the **endocrine system.**

(A) **7.4** Translate the **Assessment** terms associated with the **endocrine system.**

(P) **7.5** Translate the **Plan** terms associated with the **endocrine system.**

7.6 Distinguish terms associated with the **endocrine system** in the context of **electronic health records.**

Introduction and Overview of the Endocrine System

Any building with heating or air conditioning also has a thermostat. A thermostat watches for changes in the temperature of a space and then responds to keep it in a desired range. When the building is too warm or too cold, the thermostat sends a signal to the heater or air conditioner to turn on or off. For the human body, the endocrine system serves this function of sending signals to keep all the body's many functions in balance.

The endocrine system can be broken down into signal senders, the signals they send, and the signals' outcomes. The main signal senders are the endocrine glands, which include the hypothalamus, pituitary, thyroid, parathyroid, adrenal, pancreas, and gonads (ovaries and testicles). Endocrine glands specifically send chemical signals to different parts of the body. These chemical signals, which are hormones, generally cause slower, subtler changes than the nervous system, which uses electric signals.

The signals travel through the rest of the body via the bloodstream, but only the intended cells in the body respond to these hormonal signals. These cells are keyed with receptors that fit with the hormone—just like two matching puzzle pieces. The hormone then signals the cell to perform a desired job, such as releasing another hormone, releasing or taking in nutrients, or changing the speed at which the body makes certain proteins.

The end result is that the endocrine system can adjust the levels of nutrients in the blood, excrete excess nutrients, help the body respond to its environment, and direct growth and development. For example, the pancreas secretes hormones that help the body control the level of sugar in the blood. The adrenal glands, thyroid gland, and parathyroid glands keep critical minerals such as calcium and sodium in balance. The adrenal glands also make hormones for the fight-or-flight response to danger. Growth hormone helps the body grow to adult height and affects metabolism. The gonads make hormones that help drive sexual development. The endocrine system even stimulates milk production in new mothers.

7.1 Word Parts of the Endocrine System

Word Roots for Endocrine Glands

As you recall, the signal makers and senders of the endocrine system are called *glands.* They are located throughout your body, including in your brain, in the area above your kidneys, in your genitals, and in the front part of your neck.

The main gland that affects most of the other glands in your body is named the *hypothalamus,* because it sits just under a part of your brain known as the *thalamus.* The main role of the hypothalamus is to direct the activity of the *pituitary gland.* It can cause the pituitary to make and release its chemical signals via chemicals called *releasing hormones* (example: *gonadotropin-releasing hormone*).

The pituitary gland is made of two parts: the *anterior* (front) and *posterior* (back) pituitary. The anterior pituitary gland is the origin for many very important hormones. These hormones travel by blood and stimulate many other endocrine glands, including your *thyroid* gland, *adrenal* glands, and *gonads.*

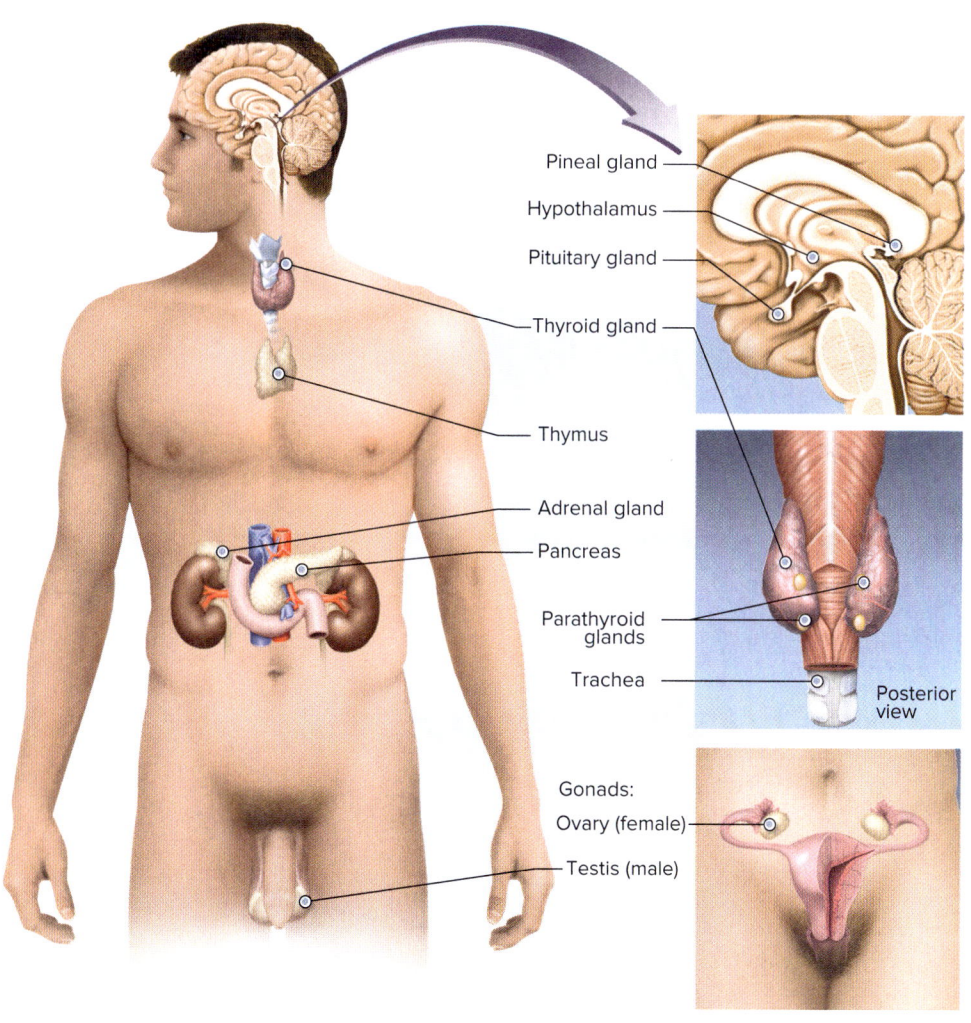

Pineal gland

Hypothalamus

Pituitary gland

Thyroid gland

Thymus

Adrenal gland

Pancreas

Parathyroid glands

Trachea

Posterior view

Gonads:

Ovary (female)

Testis (male)

Located in the front part of your neck resting just below the Adam's apple is your thyroid gland and just behind it, the *parathyroid* glands. The thyroid gland makes hormones that affect the body's metabolism, as well as a hormone that helps control the level of calcium in the blood. The parathyroid glands also make a hormone that works along with the thyroid hormone to control the blood's calcium level.

The *pancreas,* an interesting gland that sits just under your stomach, is both an endocrine gland and a gastrointestinal organ. As an endocrine gland, it sends hormones directly into the bloodstream that help keep blood sugar level in balance. As a gastrointestinal organ, it secretes enzymes by ducts (*exocrine*) directly into your intestines to help with digestion.

The adrenal gland gets its name from its location in your body, as it lies on top of your kidneys. The adrenal gland has an inner layer that makes the fight-or-flight hormone, commonly known as *adrenaline.* Its outer layer, or cortex, makes two general types of hormones. One type keeps mineral levels in balance and maintains the proper volume of water and salt in the blood. The other helps keep blood sugar levels in balance and affects your body's response to inflammation.

The gonads help with reproduction and with expression of male and female characteristics. The male gonads are the *testes.* They produce the male hormone *testosterone. Ovaries,* the female gonads, secrete *estrogens,* which help the body develop female attributes and prepare the body for pregnancy.

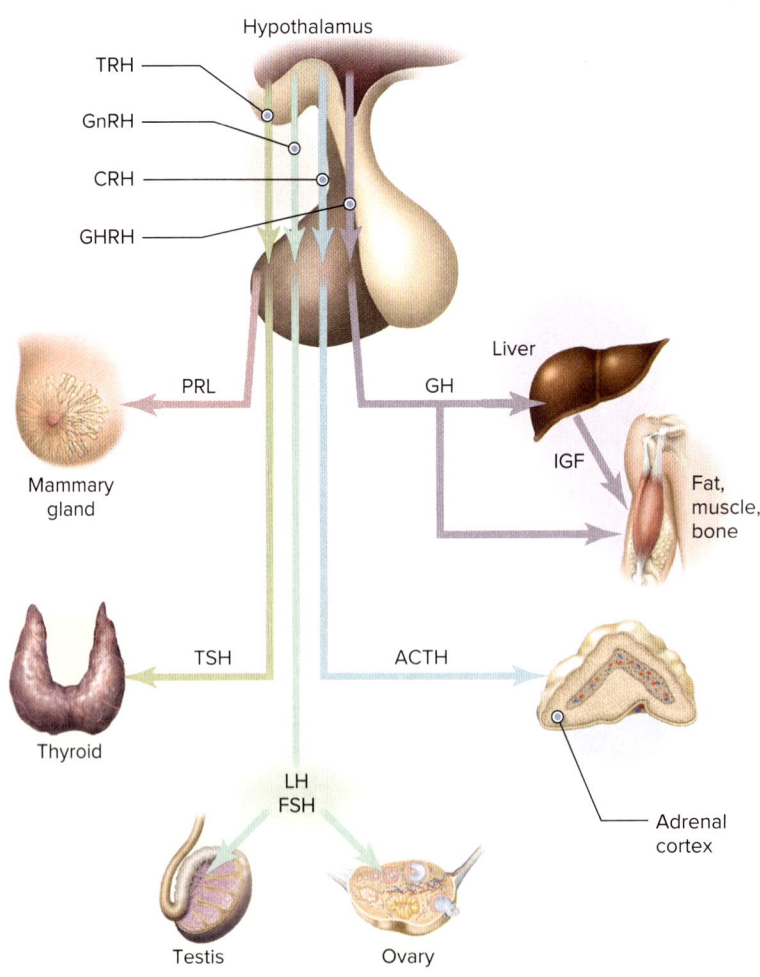

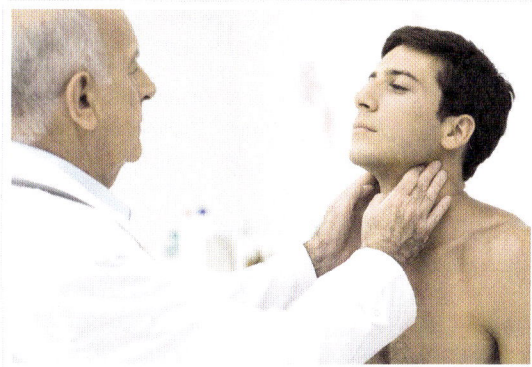

One indicator doctors use in determining health is whether or not the patient has swollen glands.

PhotoAlto sas/Alamy Stock Photo

gland

ROOT: **aden/o**

EXAMPLES: adenoma, adenopathy

NOTES: This root refers to any gland. Since the endocrine system has a lot of glands, the term comes up often.

adrenal gland

ROOTS: **adren/o, adrenal/o**

EXAMPLES: adrenarche, adrenalitis

NOTES: The name *adrenal* describes where this gland is located in the body. It literally means *on the kidney—ad* (to, on) + *renal* (kidney).

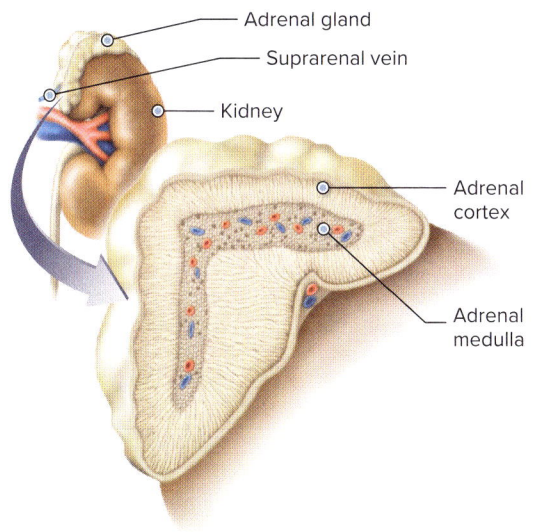

pancreas

ROOT: **pancreat/o**

EXAMPLES: pancreatitis, pancreatolith

NOTES: The term *pancreas* comes from two Greek words: *pan* (all) and *kreas* (flesh). The reasoning for this has long been debated; some people think the name stuck because of the organ's fleshy consistency.

If you ever find yourself tempted by the word *sweetbreads* on a menu, think carefully before ordering. That's the term used by chefs to mean *cooked pancreas.*

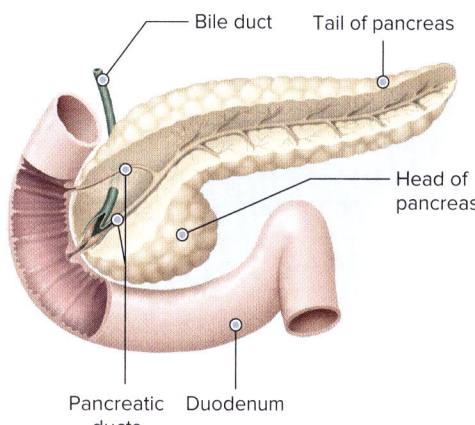

pituitary gland

ROOTS: **pituitar/o, hypophys/o**

EXAMPLES: hyperpituitarism, hypophysitis

NOTES: The word *pituitary* comes from a Latin word meaning *mucus* because the Romans believed that the pituitary gland channeled mucus from the brain to the nose.

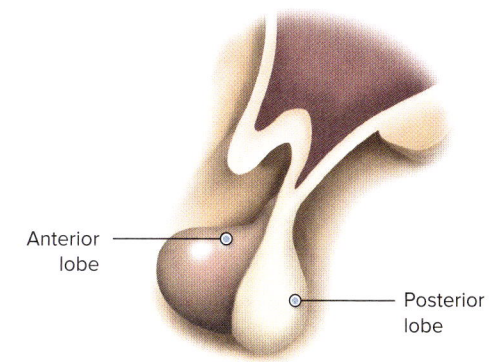

The other root, *hypophyso,* comes from the Greek words *hypo* (under) + *physis* (growth) and refers to the appearance and location of the pituitary gland, a pea-sized gland located under the brain right behind the eyes. It looks a little like an abnormal growth underneath the brain—but it is a critical part of the endocrine system.

thymus

ROOT: **thym/o**

EXAMPLES: *thymoma, thymectomy*

NOTES: The *thymus* is an organ found in the upper chest, under the sternum and in front of the heart. Its name is derived from the name of the herb *thyme.* To those who first discovered it, the organ looked like a bunch of thyme.

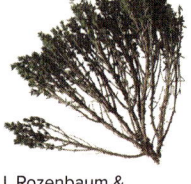

I. Rozenbaum & F. Cirou/PhotoAlto

thyroid

ROOTS: **thyr/o, thyroid/o**

EXAMPLES: thyrotoxin, thyroidectomy

NOTES: The word *thyroid* comes from the Greek word *thyros,* meaning *shield.*

Thyro (shield) + *oid* (resembling) = the gland resembling a shield. It really does look like a shield spread out over the throat, doesn't it?

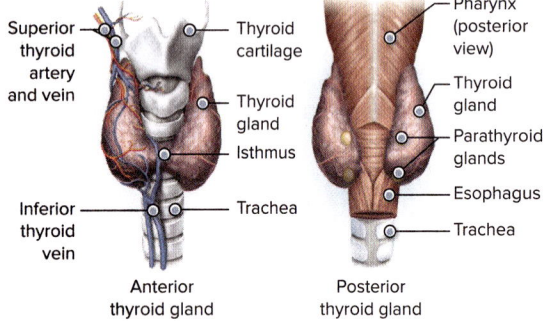

Superior thyroid artery and vein — Thyroid cartilage
Thyroid gland
Isthmus
Inferior thyroid vein — Trachea

Anterior thyroid gland

Pharynx (posterior view)
Thyroid gland
Parathyroid glands
Esophagus
Trachea

Posterior thyroid gland

Word Roots for Secretions, Chemicals, and Blood Work

Once the signals (*hormones*) are made in the endocrine organs, they wait to be secreted (*crino*) to their target body part. Endocrine signals travel via the bloodstream. The *pituitary* gland makes many hormones that encourage other endocrine glands in the body to work. *Adrenocorticotropic hormone (ACTH)* stimulates the outer part of the adrenal gland. *Thyroid-stimulating hormone (TSH)* stimulates the thyroid gland. *Luteinizing hormone (LH)* and *follicle-stimulating hormone (FSH)* stimulate the gonads. The pituitary gland also makes growth hormone and prolactin.

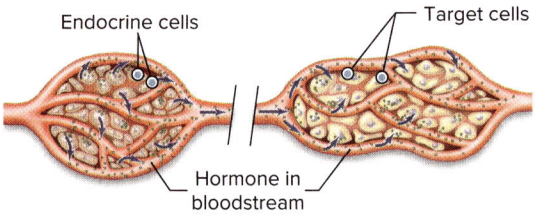

Endocrine cells
Target cells
Hormone in bloodstream

The thyroid makes three very important hormones: *T4, T3,* and *calcitonin.* T4 and T3 affect the body's metabolism. An overactive thyroid (*hyperthyroidism*) leads to a higher than normal metabolism—everything speeds up. As a result, a person suffering from hyperthyroidism experiences weight loss, increased hunger, diarrhea, and nervousness. On the opposite end, for people with *hypothyroidism,* everything slows down. They typically experience weight gain, decreased energy and appetite, and constipation.

Calcitonin is a hormone that encourages the uptake of calcium in the blood into bone. This keeps the level of calcium in the blood from getting too high.

The parathyroid glands make *parathyroid hormone.* This hormone has the opposite effect of calcitonin. It helps keep the level of calcium in the blood from getting too low by releasing calcium from bones into the blood.

As you recall, the pancreas is both a digestive organ and an endocrine organ. The endocrine part of the pancreas makes two hormones that work together to keep the level of sugar in the blood in balance. *Insulin* decreases the level of sugar in the blood. It encourages cells to open up to the blood sugar (*glucose*) and take it in. *Glucagon* works against insulin. It tells the liver to release stored sugar and thus increases the level of sugar in the blood.

The adrenal gland creates hormones in two parts—the inner part or the outer part. The inner part of the adrenal gland makes *epinephrine,* also known as adrenaline. Many people know adrenaline as the chemical that surges in danger and helps mothers lift cars off their babies. While it doesn't truly gift people with super powers, it does play an important role in the fight-or-flight response by increasing your heart rate and opening your airways to get more oxygen. Norepinephrine, also made in the adrenal gland, causes very similar changes.

The outer part of the adrenal gland (*cortex*) also makes very important hormones. ACTH stimulates the cortex to release *corticosteroids,* which are steroid hormones made in the cortex. The three types of corticosteroids are hormones dealing with mineral balance (*mineralcorticoids*), hormones dealing with sugar balance (*glucocorticoids*), and the steroid sex hormones (testosterone and estrogen). The main source of these hormones, however, is the gonads.

The gonads of men and women make different hormones. In men, the testes make testosterone. The testes trigger the production of sperm and the development of masculine body characteristics, such as increased muscle and facial hair. Ovaries, the female gonads, secrete estrogens, which cause the development and release of eggs as well as the development of feminine attributes, such as breasts and wide hips.

Measuring the level of certain hormones and how they affect the patient's blood is one way of checking the function of the endocrine system. The most common example is checking the glucose level in the blood (*glycemia*). These levels may be high (*hyperglycemia*), low (*hypoglycemia*), or normal (*euglycemia*).

Another body fluid that is often measured is a patient's *urine.* Substances such as sugar (*glucosuria*) or ketones (*ketonuria*) may be found in the urine.

sugar

ROOTS: ***gluc/o, glucos/o, glyc/o***

EXAMPLES: glucocorticoid, glucosuria, hypoglycemia

NOTES: Three common types of sugar are sucrose, glucose, and fructose. *Sucrose* is a complex molecule made up of glucose and fructose. *Glucose* and *fructose* have the same chemical composition but different molecular structures. Glucose (which requires insulin to break it down) is the universal fuel of all living things and is also used in brain functions. Neurologists often use glucose consumption as an indicator of brain activity. When the brain lacks glucose, certain mental functions, such as self-control and decision making, become more difficult.

Glucose

Fructose

Sucrose

to secrete

ROOT: *crin/o*

EXAMPLES: endocrine, exocrine

NOTES: *Endocrine* means *to secrete internally;* it refers to chemicals secreted into the bloodstream. The opposite of this is *exocrine,* which means *to secrete externally* and refers to chemicals secreted through ducts to the surface of an organ. Examples of this include sweat glands and salivary glands. Next time you find yourself sweating through a workout or drooling over some food, you can say that you're having an excessive exocrine response.

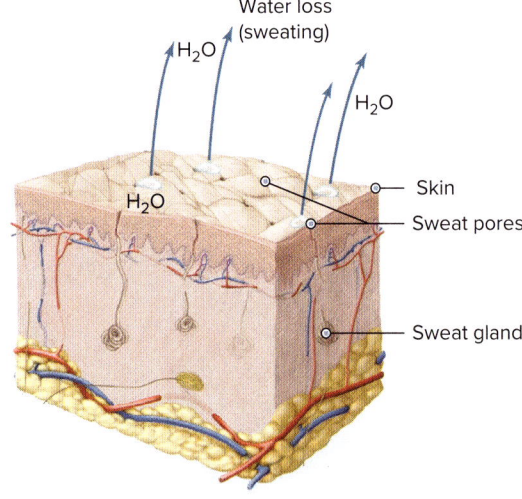

Water loss (sweating)

H_2O

H_2O

H_2O

Skin

Sweat pores

Sweat gland

Suffixes for Secretions, Chemicals, and Blood Work

stimulating hormone

SUFFIX: *-tropin*

EXAMPLES: thyrotropin, gonadotropin

NOTES: If a term has the suffix *-tropin,* it refers to a hormone that has a stimulating effect on a target organ. The suffix comes from a Greek word meaning *to turn*—perhaps because it turns the target organ on and tells it to start working.

-Tropin has the same root as the word *trophy.* In ancient Greece, a *trophy* was a monument built on a battlefield to mark the spot where the battle *turned* in the victor's favor.

blood condition

SUFFIX: *-emia*

EXAMPLES: glycemia, calcemia

NOTES: Because the endocrine system deals with internal secretions, blood analysis (which is, of course, analysis of a secretion of the body) is usually the best way to detect problems.

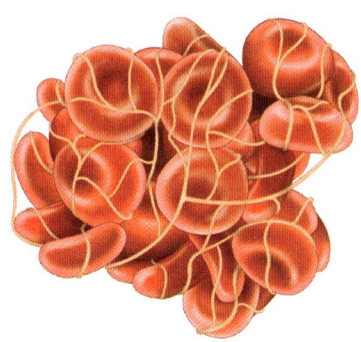

urine condition

SUFFIX: **-uria**

EXAMPLE: polyuria

NOTES: Substances in the urine can be useful clues in diagnosing endocrine problems.

For example, in 1889, Oscar Minkowski and Joseph von Mering removed the pancreas of a healthy dog. Several days after the dog's pancreas was removed, the researchers noticed that flies were feeding on the dog's urine—something that was not the case prior to the removal of the pancreas. Analysis of the dog's urine revealed the presence of sugar—a discovery that helped establish the relationship between the pancreas and diabetes.

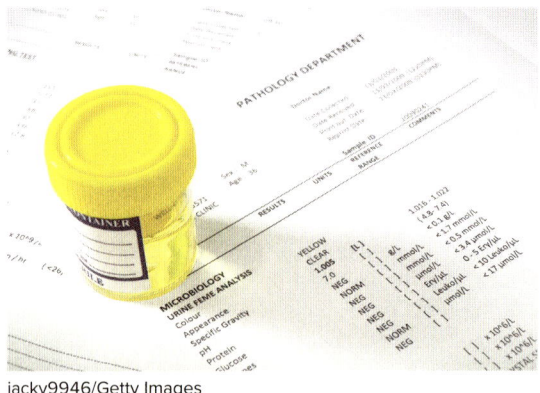

jacky9946/Getty Images

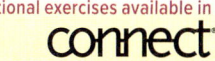
TRANSLATION

EXERCISE 1 Match the root on the left with its definition on the right.

_____ 1. pancreat/o   a. adrenal gland

_____ 2. pituitar/o   b. gland

_____ 3. adren/o   c. pancreas

_____ 4. thym/o   d. pituitary gland

_____ 5. thyr/o   e. thymus

_____ 6. aden/o   f. thyroid

EXERCISE 2 Translate the following roots.

1. adrenal/o _____

2. pancreat/o _____

3. thyroid/o _____

4. thym/o _____

5. aden/o _____

6. hypophys/o _____

EXERCISE 3 Break down the following words into their component parts and translate.

> EXAMPLE: **sinusitis**   *sinus | itis*
> *inflammation of the sinuses*

1. thyroidectomy _____

2. thymectomy _____

3. adrenalectomy _____

4. pancreatectomy _____

5. hypophysectomy _____

6. hypopituitarism _____

7. adenopathy _____

EXERCISE 4 Match the word part on the left with its definition on the right. Some definitions will be used more than once.

_____ 1. glyc/o   a. blood condition

_____ 2. gluc/o   b. stimulating hormone

_____ 3. -emia   c. sugar

_____ 4. -uria   d. to secrete

_____ 5. -tropin   e. urine condition

_____ 6. crin/o

EXERCISE 5 Translate the following word parts.

1. glucos/o _____

2. crin/o _____

3. glyc/o _____

4. -uria _____

5. -emia _____

6. -tropin _____

EXERCISE 6 Break down the following words into their component parts and translate.

> EXAMPLE: **sinusitis**   *sinus | itis*
> *inflammation of the sinuses*

1. hyperglycemia _____

2. euglycemia _____

3. glucosuria _____

4. endocrine _____

GENERATION

EXERCISE 7   Identify the word parts from this chapter for the following terms.

1. adrenomegaly _____
2. pancreatalgia _____
3. hypophysitis _____
4. thymoma _____
5. polyadenopathy _____
6. panhypopituitarism _____
7. thyrotoxicosis _____
8. hypothyroidism _____

EXERCISE 8   Build a medical term from the information provided.

1. inflammation of the pancreas _____
2. inflammation of the thyroid _____
3. inflammation of a gland _____
4. good thyroid _____

EXERCISE 9   Identify the word parts from this chapter for the following terms.

1. polyuria _____
2. exocrine _____
3. glucogenesis _____
4. endocrinologist _____
5. hyperphosphatemia _____
6. euglycemia (2 parts) _____

EXERCISE 10   Build a medical term from the information provided.

1. sugar urine condition (use *glucoso*) _____

_____

2. low blood sugar condition (use *glyco*) _____

_____

3. thyroid-stimulating hormone (use *thyro*) _____

_____

(S)UBJECTIVE

7.2 Patient History, Problems, Complaints

The symptoms a patient experiences from an endocrine problem all depend on which organ is affected. Patients with pituitary problems may present to a health care provider with growth disturbances. This can be on either extreme, from the abnormally large (*pituitary gigantism*) to the small (*pituitary dwarfism*). If the extra growth is disproportionate in the face and long bones of the body, it is known as *acromegaly.*

Patients with an overactive thyroid (*hyperthyroidism*) have higher-than-normal metabolism—everything speeds up. As a result, a person suffering from hyperthyroidism experiences weight loss, increased hunger, diarrhea, and nervousness. Some also have bulging eyes (*exophthalmos*).

On the opposite end, for someone with *hypothyroidism,* everything slows down. Patients with this disease typically experience weight gain, decreased energy, hair loss, decreased appetite, and constipation. They may also experience swelling and puffiness in the hands and face. This grouping of symptoms is called *myxedema.* Both hyperthyroidism and hypothyroidism can present with an enlarged thyroid (*goiter*).

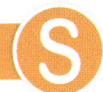
Decreased pancreatic endocrine activity leads to diabetes. Patients with diabetes may complain of excessive thirst (*polydipsia*), excessive urination (*polyuria*), and constant hunger (*polyphagia*), with an unexpected weight loss.

Premature sexual traits may represent a problem with the adrenal gland or the gonads. Males may experience premature puberty from an overactive adrenal gland (*adrenal virilism*). Females with the same problem may report facial hair (*hirsutism*). When a female has a hyperactive gonad (*hypergonadism*), she may present with periods (*menarche*) or breast development (*thelarche*) at a premature age. Females with underfunctioning gonads may complain of lack of menstruation (*amenorrhea*). Males may experience breast development (*gynecomastia*). This is very common in puberty.

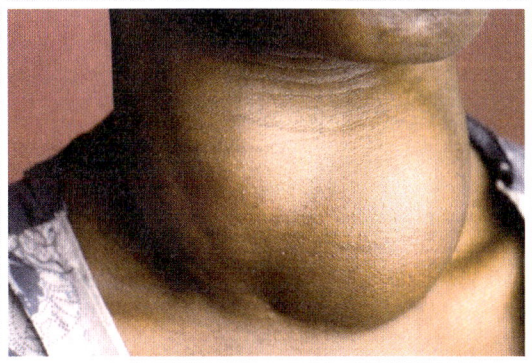

Goiter, or swollen thyroid gland, is most commonly caused by iodine deficiency. The easy solution to this, and to other health problems caused by low iodine, is to add iodine to salt. Check the container of table salt in your home. Chances are good that it's iodized salt.

Medicimage/Shutterstock

glands

TERM	WORD ANALYSIS	
acromegaly AK-roh-MEH-gah-lee	acro	/ megaly
	extremities /	abnormal enlargement
DEFINITION abnormal enlargement of the extremities NOTE: The term *acro* can mean *top* or *high,* as in *acrophobia,* the fear of heights, or it can mean *the end* or *extremity,* as it does here.		
adrenal virilism a-DREE-nal VIR-il-izm	adrenal viril	/ ism
	adrenal man /	condition
DEFINITION development of male secondary sexual characteristics caused by excessive secretion of the adrenal gland		
exophthalmos EKS-of-THAL-mohs	ex / ophthalmos	
	out / eye	
DEFINITION protrusion of the eyes out of the eye socket		

glands *continued*

TERM	WORD ANALYSIS		
goiter GOY-ter	from Latin, for *gutter (meaning throat)*		
DEFINITION swollen thyroid gland NOTE: The most common cause of goiter is iodine deficiency. The easy solution to this, and to other health problems caused by low iodine, is to add iodine to salt.			
hypoglycemic HAI-poh-glai-SEE-mik	hypo / glyc	/ em	/ ic
	under / sugar	/ blood /	pertaining to
DEFINITION pertaining to low blood sugar			
myxedema MIX-eh-DEE-mah	myx	/ edema	
	mucus /	swelling	
DEFINITION swelling of the skin caused by deposits under the skin NOTE: Though the deposits under the skin aren't mucus, they appear to have the consistency of mucus, so that's the root that was used to describe it.			

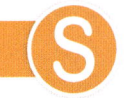

glands *continued*	
TERM	**WORD ANALYSIS**
pituitary dwarfism pih-TOO-ih-TER-ee DWAR-fizm	pituitary dwarfism
DEFINITION abnormally short height caused by undersecretion of growth hormone from the pituitary gland	
pituitary gigantism pih-TOO-ih-TER-ee jai-GAN-tizm	pituitary gigantism
DEFINITION abnormally tall height caused by oversecretion of growth hormone from the pituitary gland	

glands *continued*	
TERM	**WORD ANALYSIS**
polydipsia PAW-lee-DIP-see-ah	poly / dips / ia excessive / thirst / condition
DEFINITION excessive thirst NOTE: You might expect *hyperdipsia,* but the term uses *poly* instead. The reason is because this word is not first a medical word but the ancient Greek term for *excessively thirsty.* In Greek, *poly* can mean *excessive* as well as *many.*	
polyuria PAW-lee-YOO-ree-ah	poly / uria excessive / urine condition
DEFINITION excessive urination	

Learning Outcome 7.2 Exercises

PRONUNCIATION

EXERCISE 1 Indicate which syllable(s) is emphasized when pronounced.

> EXAMPLE: bronchitis bron<u>chi</u>tis

1. hypoglycemic _____
2. myxedema _____
3. polydipsia _____

TRANSLATION

EXERCISE 2 Underline and define the word parts from this chapter in the following terms.

1. polyuria _____
2. adrenal virilism _____
3. pituitary dwarfism _____
4. pituitary gigantism _____
5. exophthalmos _____

EXERCISE 3 Match the term on the left with its definition on the right.

_____	1. polyuria	a. abnormal enlargement of the extremities
_____	2. polydipsia	b. excessive thirst
_____	3. goiter	c. excessive urination
_____	4. acromegaly	d. swelling of the skin caused by deposits under the skin
_____	5. myxedema	e. swollen thyroid gland

EXERCISE 4 Translate the following terms as literally as possible.

> EXAMPLE: **nasopharyngoscope** *an instrument for looking at the nose and throat*

1. polyuria _____

2. exophthalmos _____

GENERATION

EXERCISE 5 Build a medical term from the information provided.

> EXAMPLE: **inflammation of the sinuses** *sinusitis*

1. excessive urination _____

2. pertaining to low blood sugar _____

EXERCISE 6 Multiple-choice questions. Select the correct answer.

1. In the condition known as *adrenal virilism,* the adrenal gland secretes excess hormones causing the development of
   a. a swollen thyroid gland
   b. abnormal enlargement of the extremities
   c. breast tissue in males
   d. male secondary sexual characteristics
   e. all of these

2. A term that describes the swelling of the skin caused by deposits under the skin is called
   a. goiter
   b. exophthalmos
   c. myxedema
   d. polydipsia
   e. none of these

EXERCISE 7 Briefly describe the difference between the pair of terms.

1. polydipsia, polyuria _____

O BJECTIVE

7.3 Observation and Discovery

When a patient is examined for endocrine problems, many of the findings are the same things that the patient noticed and reported. The examiner may notice that the patient is much taller or shorter than average, or that he or she is overweight or underweight. Patients may have incorrect sexual traits, such as a male with breast development. Patients may have swelling or fat that is more pronounced in certain parts of their bodies.

Much of what is left for data collection relates to laboratory testing. There are numerous tests in endocrinology. The tests check either the level of hormones in the blood or their effect. Many of the hormones take on similar names to the gland that made them. For example, one of the hormones that the parathyroid gland makes is parathyroid hormone. Adrenal glands make adrenaline (also known as *epinephrine*). They may take on the name from the part of the gland in which they are made. Cortisol is made in the cortex of the adrenal gland. Other hormones are named for the organ they "turn on." These types of hormones are known as *-tropins*. For example, adrenocorticotropic hormone stimulates the cortex of the adrenal gland. Other -tropins include gonadotropins (*LH* and *FSH*) and thyrotopin (*TSH*).

There are two general fluids that can be checked to see the results of hormones: blood and urine. Any lab level that represents a substance in the blood ends in *-emia*. For instance, magnesemia is the level of magnesium in the blood. If the level is higher than normal, it has the prefix *hyper-*, and if it is lower than normal, it has the prefix *hypo-*. For example, if a patient has a lower than expected level of magnesium in his or her blood, the patient has hypomagnesemia. Any lab level for a substance in

the urine ends with *-uria*. If a patient has calcium in his or her urine, the patient has calciuria. One specific nutrient the endocrine system manages is the sugar level in the blood. It controls how fast sugar is being made (*gluconeogenesis*) and how fast it is broken down (*glycolysis*). If someone has low blood sugar (*hypoglycemia*), then the body releases a hormone to increase the production of sugar and slow the breakdown of sugar. Ketones are a by-product of this.

conditions	
TERM	**WORD ANALYSIS**
euglycemia YOO-glai-SEE-mee-ah	eu / glyc / emia good / sugar / blood condition
DEFINITION good blood sugar	
glucosuria GLOO-koh-SOO-ree-ah	glucos / uria sugar / urine condition
DEFINITION sugar in the urine	
hyperglycemia HAI-per-glai-SEE-mee-ah	hyper / glyc / emia excessive / sugar / blood condition
DEFINITION high blood sugar	
hypoglycemia HAI-poh-glai-SEE-mee-ah	hypo / glyc / emia under / sugar / blood condition
DEFINITION low blood sugar	

Testing blood is central to gathering data on the endocrine system. A finger prick is the easiest and least invasive path when only a little blood is needed.

Purestock/SuperStock

conditions continued

TERM	WORD ANALYSIS
polyuria PAW-lee-YOO-ree-ah	poly / uria excessive / urine condition
DEFINITION excessive urination	
uremia yoo-REE-mee-ah	ur / emia urine / blood condition
DEFINITION presence of urinary waste in the blood	

hormones

TERM	WORD ANALYSIS
adrenaline a-DREN-ah-lin	adrenal / ine adrenal / chemical
DEFINITION hormone secreted by the adrenal gland	
corticotropin KOR-tih-koh-TROH-pin	cortico / tropin cortex / stimulating
DEFINITION shorter name for adrenocorticotropic hormone	
epinephrine EH-pee-NEF-rin	epi / nephr / ine upon / kidney / chemical
DEFINITION hormone secreted by the adrenal gland NOTE: Both *adrenaline* and *epinephrine* mean the same thing and can be used interchangeably. *Adrenaline* comes from Latin and *epinephrine* from Greek. In America, health care professionals prefer *epinephrine*.	
gonadotropin goh-NAD-oh-TROH-pin	gonado / tropin gonad / stimulating
DEFINITION hormone that stimulates the gonads	

hormones continued

TERM	WORD ANALYSIS
insulin IN-suh-lin	insul / in island / chemical
DEFINITION hormone secreted by the pancreas that controls the metabolism and uptake of sugar and fats NOTE: The root used to name this hormone comes from the fact that insulin is secreted by a cluster or *island* of cells in the pancreas called the *islet of Langerhans*.	
thyrotropin THAI-roh-TROH-pin	thyro / tropin thyroid / stimulating
DEFINITION hormone that stimulates the thyroid	

professional terms

TERM	WORD ANALYSIS
endocrine EN-doh-krin	endo / crine inside / secretion
DEFINITION to secrete internally (i.e., into the bloodstream)	
endocrinologist EN-doh-krih-NAW-loh-jist	endo / crino / logist inside / secretion / specialist
DEFINITION specialist in internal secretions	
euthyroid YOO-thai-royd	eu / thyroid good / thyroid
DEFINITION normal functioning thyroid	

Learning Outcome 7.3 Exercises

PRONUNCIATION

EXERCISE 1 Indicate which syllable(s) is emphasized when pronounced.

EXAMPLE: bronchitis bron<u>chi</u>tis

1. uremia _____

2. insulin _____

3. adrenaline _____

4. endocrine _____

5. euthyroid _____

TRANSLATION

EXERCISE 2 Break down the following words into their component parts.

EXAMPLE: synesthesia *syn | es | the | sia*

1. euthyroid _____

2. endocrinologist _____

3. adrenocorticotropic hormone _____

EXERCISE 3 Underline and define the word parts from this chapter in the following terms.

1. glucosuria _____

2. endocrine _____

3. adrenaline _____

4. gonadotropin _____

5. corticotropin _____

6. thyrotropin _____

EXERCISE 4 Match the term on the left with its definition on the right.

_____ 1. hypoglycemia a. excessive urination

_____ 2. polyuria b. good blood sugar

_____ 3. euglycemia c. low blood sugar

_____ 4. uremia d. presence of urinary waste in the blood

_____ 5. glucosuria e. sugar in the urine

EXERCISE 5 Fill in the blank.

1. hyperglycemia = excessive _____ in the blood

EXERCISE 6 Translate the following terms as literally as possible.

EXAMPLE: nasopharyngoscope *an instrument for looking at the nose and throat*

1. euthyroid _____

2. endocrinologist _____

GENERATION

EXERCISE 7 Build a medical term from the information provided.

EXAMPLE: inflammation of the sinuses *sinusitis*

1. sugar in the urine (use *glucos/o*) _____

2. high blood sugar _____

3. low blood sugar _____

4. good blood sugar _____

5. presence of urinary waste in the blood _____

_____

6. a hormone that stimulates the gonads _____

_____

7. a hormone that stimulates the thyroid _____

_____

EXERCISE 8 Multiple-choice questions. Select the correct answer(s).

1. Select all of the terms below that pertain to blood conditions.
   a. chloremia   e. hyperphosphatemia
   b. glucosuria   f. polyuria
   c. hypomagnesemia g. uremia
   d. hypernatremia

2. Select all of the terms below that pertain to urine conditions.
   a. chloremia   e. hyperphosphatemia
   b. glucosuria   f. polyuria
   c. hypomagnesemia g. uremia
   d. hypernatremia

7.4 Diagnosis and Pathology

The main types of disorders of the endocrine system result from an organ either making too much of a hormone or not enough of it. When a gland is producing too much hormone, it is labeled with the prefix *hyper-*. An overactive thyroid gland, for example, causes *hyperthyroidism.* A gland that doesn't make enough hormone is labeled with the prefix *hypo-*. When a patient's thyroid gland does not make enough thyroid hormone, the patient develops *hypothyroidism.*

Another way of saying a gland doesn't make enough hormone is to call it *insufficient.* When the cortex of the adrenal gland doesn't make enough cortisol, the condition is called *adrenocortical insufficiency.*

The pancreas is a bit different from many of the other glands in this regard. It produces competing hormones that work against each other: *glucagon* and *insulin.* While problems can occur with either hormone, underproduction of insulin is the most common disorder. This condition leads to *diabetes.*

Many times, overproduction of a hormone is caused by a tumor in the gland that causes it to secrete too much hormone. When a tumor on a gland is benign, it is called an *adenoma;* when a tumor is malignant, it is called an *adenocarcinoma.*

Another cause for the change in the function of a gland is *inflammation.* A patient with *thyroiditis* may initially have high levels of thyroid hormone in his or her blood, followed by hypothyroidism. This initial thyroid hormone is not from overproduction, however. Instead, it originates from the release of already-made hormones. This condition is called *thyrotoxicosis.*

Bleeding into a gland, which causes cells in the gland to die, can also lead to common gland problems. This happens in the case of *pituitary infarctions.* Bleeding into the pituitary decreases the number of gland cells available to make the hormones, thus causing it to function abnormally.

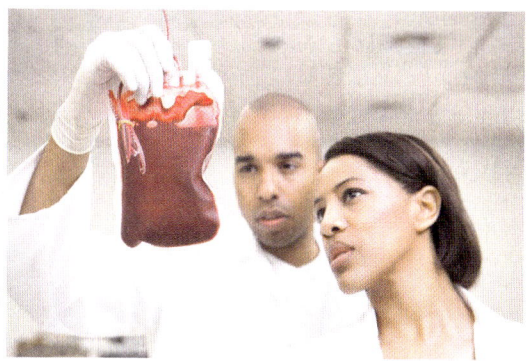

Analyzing blood and urine provides key information about the functioning of the endocrine system.
ERproductions Ltd/Blend Images LLC

general terms

TERM	WORD ANALYSIS
adenitis	aden / itis
AD-en-AI-tis	gland / inflammation
DEFINITION inflammation of a gland	

oncology

TERM	WORD ANALYSIS
adenoma	aden / oma
AD-eh-NOH-mah	gland / tumor
DEFINITION glandular tumor	
insulinoma	insulin / oma
IN-suh-lin-OH-mah	insulin / tumor
DEFINITION tumor that secretes insulin (found in the insulin-producing cells in the pancreas)	

glands

TERM	WORD ANALYSIS
adrenalitis a-DREE-nah-LAI-tis	adrenal / itis adrenal / inflammation
DEFINITION inflammation of the adrenal gland	
diabetes mellitus DAI-ah-BEE-teez MEH-lih-tis	diabetes mellitus pass through honey
DEFINITION metabolic disease characterized by excessive urination and hyperglycemia NOTE: *Diabetes* is an ancient Greek word that refers to any condition that causes excessive urination. *Mellitus* (which means *honey*) was added to describe a specific kind of diabetes characterized by excessive sugar in the urine.	
hyperparathyroidism HAI-per-PAR-ah-THAI-roid-IZM	hyper / para / thyroid over / beside / thyroid / ism / condition
DEFINITION overproduction by the parathyroid glands	
hyperpituitarism HAI-per-pih-TOO-ih-tar-IZM	hyper / pituitar / ism over / pituitary / condition
DEFINITION overfunctioning of the pituitary gland	
hyperthyroidism HAI-per-THAI-roid-IZM	hyper / thyroid / ism over / thyroid / condition
DEFINITION overproduction by the thyroid	
hypoparathyroidism HAI-poh-PAR-ah-THAI-roid-IZM	hypo / para / thyroid under / beside / thyroid / ism / condition
DEFINITION underproduction by the parathyroid	
hypopituitarism HAI-poh-pih-TOO-ih-tar-IZM	hypo / pituitar / ism under / pituitary / condition
DEFINITION condition caused by the undersecretion of the pituitary gland	

glands *continued*

TERM	WORD ANALYSIS
hypothyroidism HAI-poh-THAI-roid-IZM	hypo / thyroid / ism under / thyroid / condition
DEFINITION underproduction by the thyroid	
pancreatitis PAN-kree-ah-TAI-tis	pancreat / itis pancreas / inflammation
DEFINITION inflammation of the pancreas	
panhypopituitarism PAN-HAI-poh-pih-TOO-ih-tar-IZM	pan / hypo / pituitar / ism all / under / pituitary / condition
DEFINITION defective or absent function of the entire pituitary gland	
thyroiditis THAI-roid-AI-tis	thyroid / itis thyroid / inflammation
DEFINITION inflammation of the thyroid	
thyrotoxicosis THAI-roh-TOKS-ih-KOH-sis	thyro / toxic / osis thyroid / poison / condition
DEFINITION condition caused by the exposure of body tissue to excessive levels of thyroid hormone (an extreme version of this is known as "thyroid storm")	

TRANSLATION

EXERCISE 1   Break down the following words into their component parts.

EXAMPLE:	nasopharyngoscope
	*naso	pharyngo	scope*

1. adrenalitis _____
2. thyroiditis _____
3. pancreatitis _____
4. adenoma _____
5. insulinoma _____
6. hypopituitarism _____
7. panhypopituitarism _____
8. hyperparathyroidism _____
9. hypoparathyroidism _____

EXERCISE 2   Underline and define the word parts from this chapter in the following terms.

1. adenitis _____
2. hyperpituitarism _____
3. hyperthyroidism _____
4. hypothyroidism _____
5. thyrotoxicosis _____

EXERCISE 3   Multiple-choice question. Select the correct answer.

1. *Diabetes mellitus* is a metabolic disease characterized by
   a. excessive urination
   b. hyperglycemia
   c. high blood sugar
   d. polyuria
   e. all of these

EXERCISE 4   Translate the following terms as literally as possible.

EXAMPLE:	nasopharyngoscope *an instrument for looking at the nose and throat*

1. hyperthyroidism _____
2. hypothyroidism _____
3. hyperpituitarism _____
4. hypopituitarism _____
5. panhypopituitarism _____
6. hyperparathyroidism _____
7. hypoparathyroidism _____
8. thyrotoxicosis _____

GENERATION

EXERCISE 5   Build a medical term from the information provided.

EXAMPLE:	inflammation of the sinuses *sinusitis*

1. inflammation of the thyroid _____
2. inflammation of the pancreas _____
3. inflammation of the adrenal gland _____
4. inflammation of a gland _____
5. a glandular tumor _____
6. a tumor that secretes insulin _____

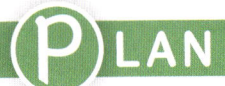

7.5 Treatments and Therapies

Most treatments of endocrine problems involve correcting abnormal hormone levels. If the level of a particular hormone, such as insulin, is too low, the proper treatment involves giving the patient supplemental hormones to bring the levels to normal (*hormone replacement therapy*). There are many routes for delivering the supplemental hormones, including injection, oral, and topical. An even more advanced method is continuous subcutaneous insulin infusion, which is an insulin pump that injects insulin under the skin as needed.

When the hormone level disorder is caused by a tumor or an overactive organ, more aggressive measures may be needed. This can involve taking a medicine that destroys all or part of the problematic gland or undergoing surgery to partially or completely remove the gland (i.e., *adenectomy*).

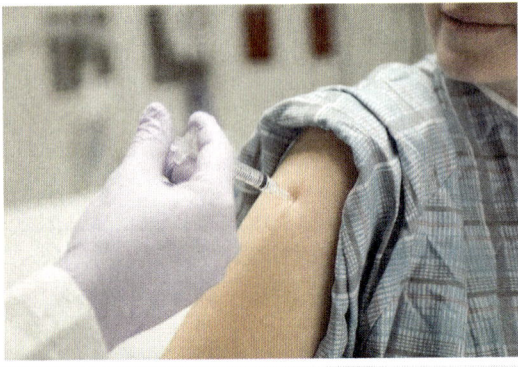

Once an endocrine imbalance has been diagnosed, sometimes the treatment is as easy as supplying the needed hormone.

M. Constantini /PhotoAlto

glands

TERM	WORD ANALYSIS
adenectomy AD-en-EK-toh-mee	aden / ectomy gland / removal
DEFINITION removal of a gland	
adrenalectomy a-DREE-nal-EK-toh-mee	adrenal / ectomy adrenal / removal
DEFINITION removal of the adrenal gland	
hypophysectomy hai-POF-is-EK-toh-mee	hypophys / ectomy pituitary / removal
DEFINITION removal of the pituitary gland	
pancreatectomy PAN-kree-ah-TEK-toh-mee	pancreat / ectomy pancreas / removal
DEFINITION removal of the pancreas	
parathyroidectomy PAR-ah-THAI-roid-EK-toh-mee	para / thyroid / ectomy beside / thyroid / removal
DEFINITION removal of the parathyroid	
thymectomy thai-MEK-toh-mee	thym / ectomy thymus / removal
DEFINITION removal of the thymus	
thyroid function tests THAI-roid FUNK-shun TESTS	thyroid function tests
DEFINITION tests performed to evaluate the function of the thyroid	
thyroidectomy THAI-roid-EK-toh-mee	thyroid / ectomy thyroid / removal
DEFINITION removal of the thyroid	
thyroidotomy THAI-roid-AW-toh-mee	thyroido / tomy thyroid / incision
DEFINITION incision into the thyroid	

pharmacology

TERM	WORD ANALYSIS
thyroidotoxin thai-ROI-doh-TOK-sin	thyroido / toxin thyroid / poison
DEFINITION substance poisonous to the thyroid gland	

TRANSLATION

EXERCISE 1   Break down the following words into their component parts.

> EXAMPLE: nasopharyngoscope
> *naso | pharyngo | scope*

1. thymectomy _____

2. adenectomy _____

3. adrenalectomy _____

4. thyroidectomy _____

5. parathyroidectomy _____

EXERCISE 2   Underline and define the word parts from this chapter in the following terms.

1. thyroid function tests _____

2. thyroidotomy _____

3. thyroidotoxin _____

4. pancreatectomy _____

5. hypophysectomy _____

EXERCISE 3   Translate the following terms as literally as possible.

> EXAMPLE: nasopharyngoscope   *an instrument for looking at the nose and throat*

1. thyroidotomy _____

2. thyroidotoxin _____

3. adrenalectomy _____

4. pancreatectomy _____

GENERATION

EXERCISE 4   Build a medical term from the information provided.

> EXAMPLE: inflammation of the sinuses   *sinusitis*

1. removal of the pituitary gland (use *hypophys/o*) _____

2. removal of the pancreas _____

3. removal of the thymus _____

4. removal of the adrenal gland _____

5. removal of a gland _____

6. removal of the thyroid _____

7. removal of the parathyroid _____

7.6 Electronic Health Records

Surgery Follow-Up Note

Subjective

Mr. Shield presented to our office today for follow-up from his **thyroidectomy**. He initially presented to his primary care physician with concerns over a **goiter**. His PCP noticed mild **exophthalmos** and an enlarged thyroid with palpable nodules. He had thyroid **scintigraphy** and **TFTs** that both revealed active nodules. After discussion with Dr. Sharp during a consultation, Mr. Shield elected for surgical correction. Dr. Sharp performed a thyroidectomy 2 weeks ago. Mr. Shield had postoperative **hypocalcemia** but otherwise had an unremarkable hospital stay. Since discharge, Mr. Shield has done very well.

Objective

Temp: 98.6; HR 60; RR: 16; BP 102/62; Wt: 176.

General: No acute distress. Alert and oriented.

HEENT: PERRLA. No conjunctival injection. Mucous membranes moist and pink. TMs normal.

Neck: Postop incision site is clean, dry and intact. No erythema induration or discharge. No goiter.

Resp: CTA. w/o wheezes, rales, or rhonchi.

CV: RRR without murmur.

Gen: Soft, nontender, nondistended.

Ext: No c/c/e. Labs: Mildly elevated **TSH** and low T4. Calcium—normal.

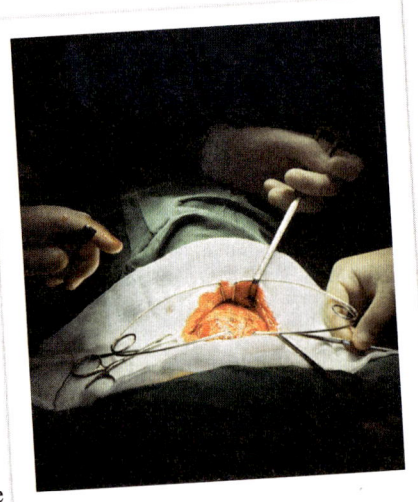

Image Source/Getty Images

Impression/Plan

Mr. Shield's thyroid labs are still not where I want them to be. We will increase his medicine to help get him **euthyroid**.

No lasting **hypoparathyroidism** from the surgery.

Return for follow-up visit including labs in 1 month.

—Sue Stenson, NP

EXERCISE 1   Match the term on the left with its definition on the right.

_____ 1. hypocalcemia   a. "good thyroid"

_____ 2. thyroidectomy   b. swollen thyroid gland

_____ 3. euthyroid   c. low calcium levels in the blood

_____ 4. exophthalmos   d. removal of the thyroid

_____ 5. hypoparathyroidism   e. protrusion of the eyes out of the eye socket

_____ 6. goiter   f. underproduction by the parathyroid

EXERCISE 2   Fill in the blanks.

1. Mr. Shield is at the office today to follow up from his *thyroidectomy* (give definition: _____
   _____).

2. Using the data recorded at the patient's discharge physical examination, fill in the following blanks.
   a. The patient's temperature: _____
   b. The patient's heart rate: _____
   c. The patient's respiratory rate: _____
   d. The patient's blood pressure: _____
   e. HEENT (_____):
   _____ (pupils equal, round, and reactive to light and accommodation).
   f. Resp: CTA (_____ to _____).
   g. CV: _____ (regular rate and rhythm).

EXERCISE 3   True or false questions. Indicate true answers with a T and false answers with an F.

1. The patient recently had his thyroid removed. _____

2. He initially presented to his PCP with concerns over a swollen thyroid gland. _____

3. His thyroid function tests revealed active nodules. _____

4. After Mr. Shield's operation, he had normal blood sugar. _____

5. According to the patient's labs, he has low thyroxin levels. _____

EXERCISE 4   Multiple-choice questions. Select the correct answer.

1. The patient suffered from postoperative *hypocalcemia*. Which of the following is a correct breakdown of the term?
   a. *hypo* (over) + *calc* (calcium) + *-emia* (blood condition)
   b. *hypo* (over) + *calc* (calcium) + *-emia* (urine condition)
   c. *hypo* (under) + *calc* (calcium) + *-emia* (blood condition)
   d. *hypo* (under) + *calc* (calcium) + *-emia* (urine condition)

2. The patient has no lasting *hypoparathyroidism*. Which of the following is a correct breakdown of the term?
   a. *hypo* (over) + *para* (beside) + *thyroid* (the thyroid gland) + *-ism* (condition)
   b. *hypo* (over) + *parathyroid* (the parathyroid gland) + *-ism* (condition)
   c. *hypo* (under) + *parathyroid* (the parathyroid gland) + *-ism* (condition)
   d. *hypo* (under) + *para* (beside) + *thyroid* (the thyroid gland) + *-ism* (condition)

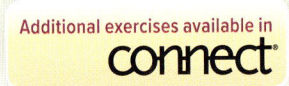

Chapter Review exercises, along with additional practice items, are available in Connect!

Quick Reference

glossary of roots

ROOT	DEFINITION	ROOT	DEFINITION
aden/o	gland	pancreat/o	pancreas
adren/o, adrenal/o	adrenal gland	pituitar/o	pituitary gland
crin/o	secrete	thym/o	thymus
-emia	blood condition	thyr/o, thyroid/o	thyroid
gluc/o, glucos/o, glyc/o	sugar	-tropin	stimulating hormone
hypophys/o	pituitary gland	-uria	urine condition

endocrine system abbreviations

ABBREVIATION	WORD ANALYSIS
ACTH	adrenocorticotropic hormone
BS	blood sugar
CGM	continuous glucose monitor
CSII	continuous subcutaneous insulin infusion
DI	diabetes insipidus
DM	diabetes mellitus
FBS	fasting blood sugar
GDM	gestational diabetes mellitus
GH	growth hormone
GTT	glucose tolerance test
IDDM	insulin-dependent diabetes mellitus (type 1)
NIDDM	noninsulin-dependent diabetes mellitus (type 2)
TFT	thyroid function test
TSH	thyroid-stimulating hormone (also known as thyrotropin)
T3	triiodothyronine (one of two primary hormones produced by the thyroid)
T4	thyroxine (one of two primary hormones produced by the thyroid)

The Blood and Lymphatic Systems–Hematology and Immunology

8

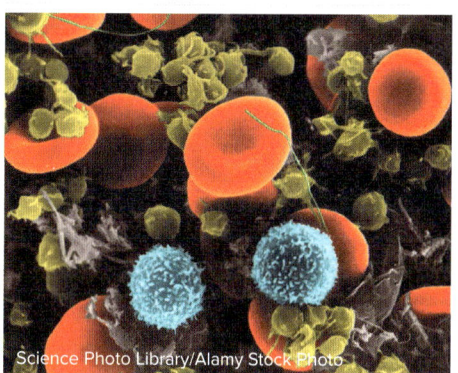
Science Photo Library/Alamy Stock Photo

Learning Outcomes

Upon completion of this chapter, you will be able to:

8.1 Identify the **roots/word parts** associated with the **hematological/ immunological systems.**

(S) 8.2 Translate the **Subjective** terms associated with the **hematological/ immunological systems.**

(O) 8.3 Translate the **Objective** terms associated with the **hematological/ immunological systems.**

(A) 8.4 Translate the **Assessment** terms associated with the **hematological/ immunological systems.**

(P) 8.5 Translate the **Plan** terms associated with the **hematological/ immunological systems.**

8.6 Distinguish terms associated with the **hematological/immunological systems** in the context of **electronic health records.**

Introduction and Overview of Hematology and Immunology

People who live together in a community, such as an apartment complex or neighborhood, all need certain services. A community needs energy, such as electricity, to provide power for all its lights and appliances. A community needs ways to communicate, such as phones or mail service. A community needs recycling and garbage removal systems. Finally, a community needs protection, such as the services rendered by police officers and firefighters.

In many ways, the body is a collection of many communities. The blood and lymphatic systems provide many of these valuable services and resources to the body's communities. These services are absolutely critical to life. If blood flow stops even for a few minutes, hazardous waste will accumulate, and cells will starve. For example, the blood provides energy by delivering sugar and oxygen. The blood carries signals from other parts of the body, allowing for communication. The blood also takes away the waste made by the body's cells.

The lymphatic system provides constant protection by repairing injuries and fighting infections.

8.1 Word Parts Associated with the Hematological/Immunological Systems

Word Roots of the Hematological System

Blood has three main types of cells (*cytes*). Red blood cells (*erythrocytes*) are the transport trucks that bring oxygen to all the cells of the body and take away the waste. White blood cells (*leukocytes*) fight infection. Platelets (*thrombocytes*) are the small scab-makers of the body. They patch things up.

Red blood cells are the most common cells in the blood (*hemo/hemato*). They contain a substance called *hemoglobin.* Hemoglobin grabs on to oxygen when the surrounding oxygen levels are high and releases it when the ambient oxygen levels are low. In this way, it helps carry fresh oxygen from the lungs to all the parts of the body that need it.

White blood cells protect the body from invasion. The blood contains different types of white blood cells that fight different types of infections (*neutrophils, lymphocytes, basophils,* and *eosinophils*). Each carries out a different job.

These white blood cells aren't the body's only defense, though. The body also makes special protective proteins as well. These proteins are called *immunoglobulins.* Just like the white blood cells, different types of immunoglobulins are designed for specific tasks. In fact, immunizations are means of forcing the body to make immunoglobulins against dangerous illnesses.

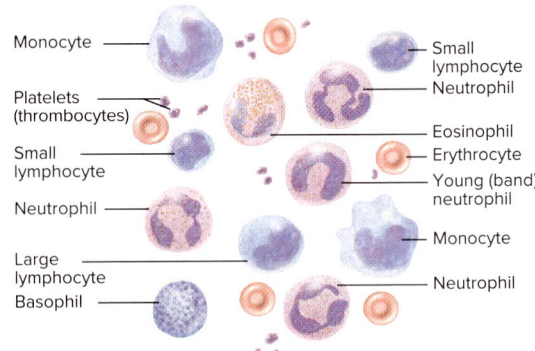

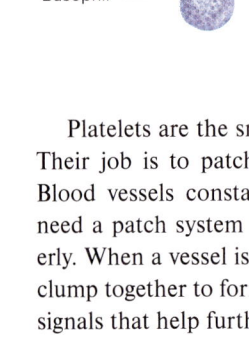

Platelets are the smallest of the cells in the blood. Their job is to patch up any broken blood vessels. Blood vessels constantly develop small leaks. They need a patch system to keep them functioning properly. When a vessel is injured, it attracts platelets that clump together to form a sticky patch. They also send signals that help further form a permanent clot.

BLOOD

clot

ROOT:	*thromb/o*
EXAMPLES:	thrombocyte, thrombosis
NOTES:	The blood's ability to clot can be both life saving and life threatening. When the body is wounded, clotting enables the body to stop the bleeding and begin the healing process. *Hemophilia* is a disease in which the blood doesn't clot well, potentially causing minor cuts to become life-threatening injuries. Clots become life threatening when they form in the bloodstream in places where they aren't needed, which could block blood flow to vital organs.

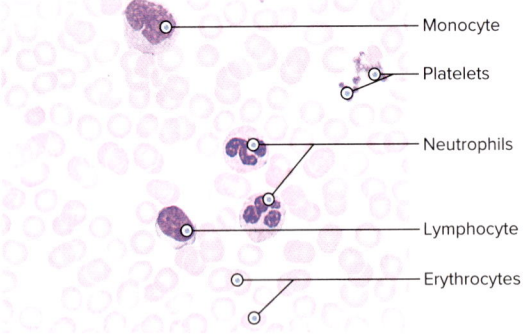

Ed Reschke

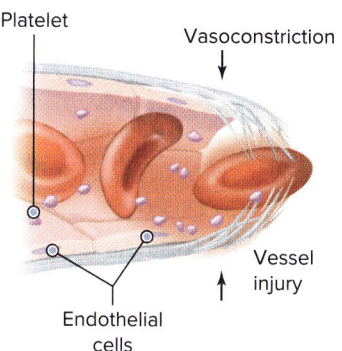
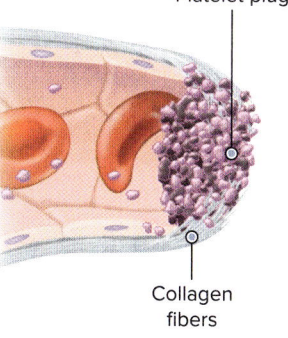
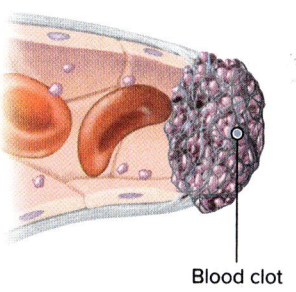

Platelet

Vasoconstriction

Vessel injury

Endothelial cells

Platelet plug

Collagen fibers

Blood clot

(a) Vascular spasm **(b) Platelet plug formation** **(c) Coagulation**

This shows the process of coagulation and the formation of a clot.

blood

ROOTS: *hem/o, hemat/o*

EXAMPLES: hemolysis, hematology

NOTES: The average-sized man has almost 6 quarts of blood in his body. The average-sized woman has almost 4 quarts.

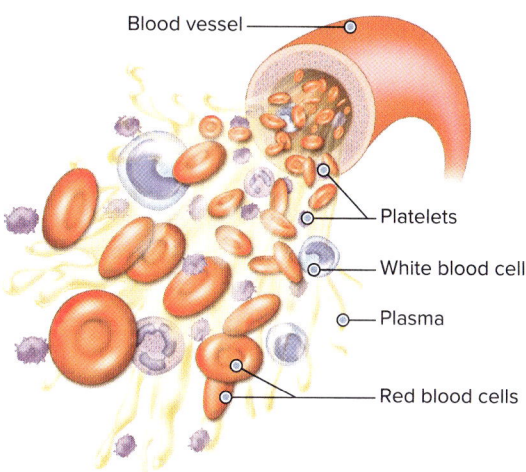

Blood vessel

Platelets

White blood cell

Plasma

Red blood cells

white

ROOT: *leuk/o*

EXAMPLES: leukocytes, leukemia

NOTES: Leukocytes, which are white blood cells, act as the bloodstream's police force and garbage collectors. They are the primary responders to infection and tissue damage. They also remove debris from the bloodstream through a process called *phagocytosis* (remember: *phago* means *to eat*) and begin the process of cell repair.

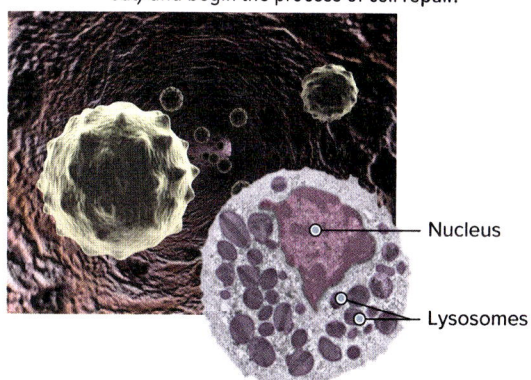

Nucleus

Lysosomes

Purestock/SuperStock

cell

ROOT: *cyt/o*

EXAMPLES: erythrocyte, thrombocytosis

NOTES: *Cyto* comes from a Greek word meaning *jar* or *basket*. The word in Greek can also refer to the individual units of a beehive, which is probably where the connection with human cells comes from.

SCIEPRO/Getty Images

vein

ROOTS: *phleb/o, ven/o*

EXAMPLES: phlebotomy, venospasm

NOTES: The term *phlebotomy* comes from *phlebo* (vein) and *tomy* (incision). It is the term used for drawing blood. But make sure you pronounce the word carefully: You don't want to get some blood drawn (*phlebotomy*) and end up having a portion of your brain removed (*lobotomy*).

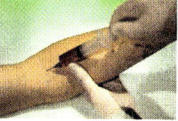

Stockbyte/Getty Images

Word Roots of the Immunological System

LYMPHATIC SYSTEM

Runoff water from mountains collects into small tributaries that collect into larger streams, then into rivers, and eventually into the ocean.

The lymphatic system works in a similar way. Excess fluid from body tissues collects into lymph vessels that pour into larger vessels. This fluid then eventually pours back into the "ocean" of the body's blood supply. Along with lymphatic vessels, the lymph system includes lymph nodes, tonsils, a spleen, and a thymus.

Together, the lymphatic system plays a large role in the body's immune system. Lymph vessels carry immune proteins to all parts of the body. Lymph nodes and the spleen act as filters in the body, filtering out dangerous things such as infectious agents and cancerous cells.

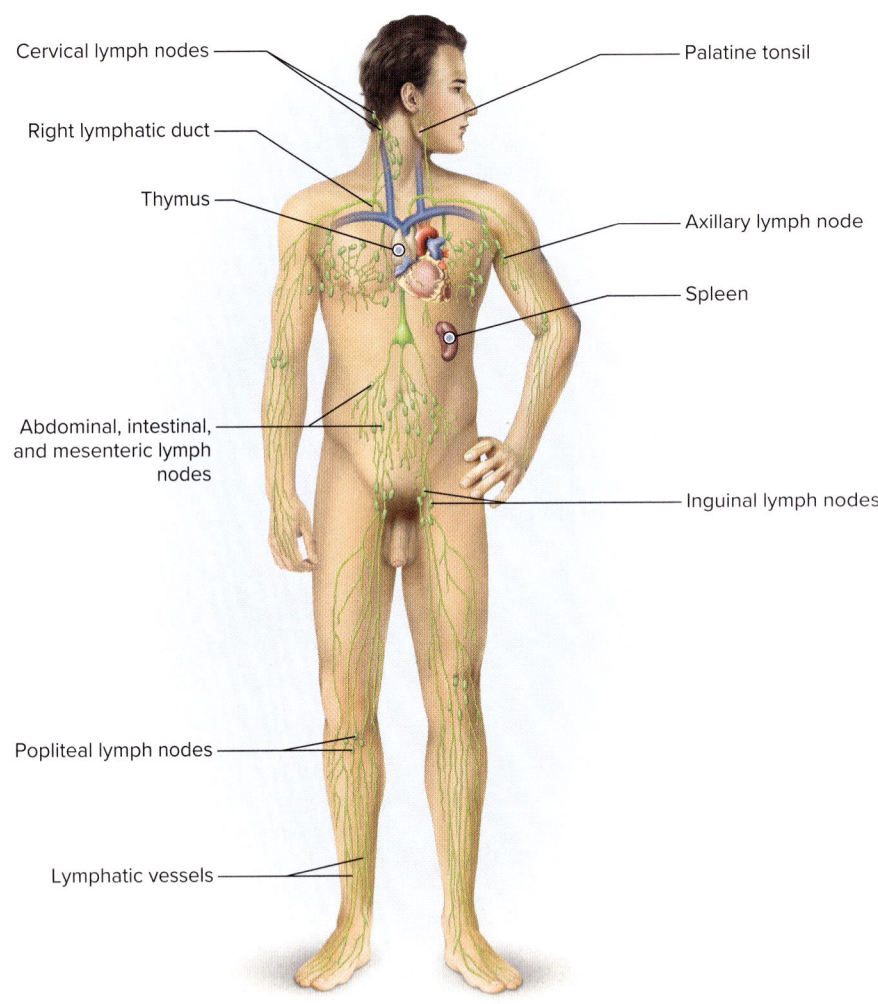

Cervical lymph nodes

Right lymphatic duct

Thymus

Abdominal, intestinal, and mesenteric lymph nodes

Popliteal lymph nodes

Lymphatic vessels

Palatine tonsil

Axillary lymph node

Spleen

Inguinal lymph nodes

lymph

ROOT: *lymph/o*

EXAMPLES: lymphadenitis, lymphoma

NOTES: *Lymph* comes from a Latin word meaning *water* or *spring* and refers to a clear liquid that circulates in the body, providing nutrients to cells and removing waste from them.

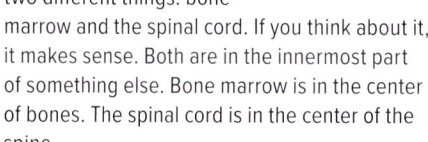

bone marrow, spine

ROOT: *myel/o*

EXAMPLES: myelitis, myelodysplasia

NOTES: This root comes from a Greek word meaning *the innermost part* and is used in medicine to refer to two different things: bone marrow and the spinal cord. If you think about it, it makes sense. Both are in the innermost part of something else. Bone marrow is in the center of bones. The spinal cord is in the center of the spine.

blood condition

SUFFIX: *-emia*

EXAMPLES: anemia, leukemia

NOTES: *-Emia* comes from a combination of *hemo,* meaning *blood,* and *-ia,* meaning *condition.* The *h* at the beginning of *hemo* got dropped because it is hard to pronounce when added to the end of a word. Think about it. Which is easier to say: *anemia* or *anhemia?*

On occasion, the *h* makes a comeback, in words such as *polycythemia.* So watch out.

tonsils

ROOT: *tonsill/o*

EXAMPLES: tonsillitis, tonsillectomy

NOTES: The *tonsils* are masses of lymphoid tissue located in the back of the mouth at the top of the throat. The word *tonsil* comes from the Latin word meaning *almond,* no doubt because of its appearance. The fact that the root has two letter *l*s, not just one, is not a spelling mistake. The English word *tonsil* has one *l*, but its root form has two. That's why the words *tonsillitis* and *tonsillectomy* have two.

lynx/iconotec.com/ Glow Images

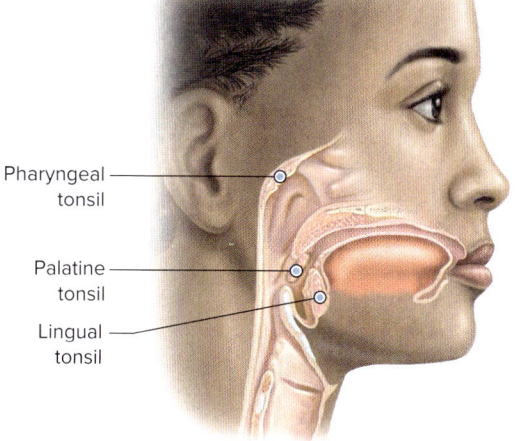

Pharyngeal tonsil

Palatine tonsil

Lingual tonsil

spleen

ROOT: *splen/o*

EXAMPLES: splenomegaly, splenectomy

NOTES: The spleen is an organ in the upper left portion of your abdomen. One of its jobs is to filter old red blood cells out of your blood. A human can live without a spleen with no adverse effects, which is good news for motocross and BMX bikers, who have a high rate of spleen injury and removal. Why? Because when they have accidents, their abdomens often crash into the handlebars of their bikes.

thymus

ROOT: *thym/o*

EXAMPLES: thymoma, thymectomy

NOTES: The *thymus* is an organ found at the base of the neck. Its name is derived from the herb *thyme.* Evidently, the organ looked like a bunch of thyme to the folks who first discovered it.

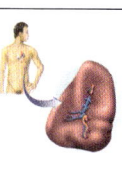

deficiency

SUFFIX: *-penia*

EXAMPLE: cytopenia

NOTES: *-Penia* comes from a Greek word meaning *poverty* or *famine.* It is related to the English word *penury,* which means *poverty.* But that's a word that doesn't get used much these days.

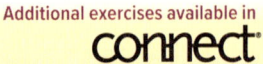
TRANSLATION

EXERCISE 1 Match the root on the left with its definition on the right. Some definitions will be used more than once.

_____ 1. leuk/o   a. blood

_____ 2. cyt/o   b. cell

_____ 3. ven/o   c. clot

_____ 4. hem/o   d. vein

_____ 5. hemat/o   e. white

_____ 6. thromb/o

_____ 7. phleb/o

EXERCISE 2 Translate the following roots.

1. leuk/o _____

2. cyt/o _____

3. ven/o _____

4. hem/o _____

5. hemat/o _____

6. thromb/o _____

7. phleb/o _____

EXERCISE 3 Underline and define the word parts from this chapter for the following terms.

1. leukemia _____

2. hematopoiesis _____

3. hemoglobinopathy _____

4. thromboembolism _____

5. phlebarteriectasia _____

6. phagocytosis _____

7. thrombophlebitis (2 parts) _____

EXERCISE 4 Break down the following words into their component parts and translate.

> EXAMPLE: **sinusitis**   *sinus | itis*
>   *inflammation of the sinuses*

1. leukocyte _____

2. thrombocyte _____

3. phlebotomy _____

4. hematoma _____

5. hemolysis _____

EXERCISE 5 Match the word part on the left with its definition on the right.

_____ 1. tonsill/o   a. blood condition

_____ 2. lymph/o   b. bone marrow

_____ 3. splen/o   c. deficiency

_____ 4. thym/o   d. lymph

_____ 5. -emia   e. spleen

_____ 6. myel/o   f. thymus

_____ 7. -penia   g. tonsil

EXERCISE 6 Translate the following word parts.

1. tonsill/o _____

2. lymph/o _____

3. splen/o _____

4. thym/o _____

5. myel/o _____

6. -emia _____

7. -penia _____

EXERCISE 7 Underline and define the word parts from this chapter for the following terms.

1. tonsillectomy _____

2. thymic hyperplasia _____

3. hypervolemia _____

4. myelodysplasia _____

5. lymphangiectasia _____

6. laparosplenectomy _____

7. pancytopenia (2 roots) _____

EXERCISE 8   Break down the following words into their component parts and translate.

> EXAMPLE: **sinusitis**   *sinus | itis*
> *inflammation of the sinuses*

1. tonsillectomy _____

2. thymectomy _____

3. lymphedema _____

4. splenalgia _____

5. myeloma _____

6. lymphocyte _____

7. leukopenia _____

8. hypercholesterolemia _____

GENERATION

EXERCISE 9   Identify the word parts for the following terms.

1. white _____

2. cell _____

3. clot _____

4. blood (2 roots) _____

5. vein (2 roots) _____

EXERCISE 10   Build a medical term from the information provided.

1. normal-sized cell (use the prefix *normo-*)

   _____

2. the study of the blood _____

3. the study of veins _____

4. white cell _____

5. clot cell _____

EXERCISE 11   Multiple-choice questions. Select the correct answer.

1. What are the names of the body's three different types of blood cells?
   a. leukocytes, red blood cells, white blood cells
   b. leukocytes, thrombocytes, white blood cells
   c. leukocytes, platelets, thrombocytes
   d. platelets, red blood cells, white blood cells
   e. platelets, red blood cells, thrombocytes

2. The function of a red blood cell is to
   a. bring oxygen to cells and remove waste
   b. fight infection
   c. patch up broken blood vessels
   d. all of these
   e. none of these

3. The function of a white blood cell is to
   a. bring oxygen to cells and remove waste
   b. fight infection
   c. patch up broken blood vessels
   d. all of these
   e. none of these

4. The function of a platelet is to
   a. bring oxygen to cells and remove waste
   b. fight infection
   c. patch up broken blood vessels
   d. all of these
   e. none of these

5. A scab is formed by which type of blood cell?
   a. erythrocyte   d. red blood cell
   b. leukocyte   e. white blood cell
   c. platelet

6. Neutrophils, lymphocytes, basophils, and eosinophils are all types of
   a. erythrocytes   d. thrombocytes
   b. platelets   e. white blood cells
   c. red blood cells

7. The type of blood cell that contains *hemoglobin* is a
   a. leukocyte   d. thrombocyte
   b. platelet   e. white blood cell
   c. red blood cell

8. Another name for *red blood cell* is
   a. erythrocyte   d. thrombocyte
   b. leukocyte   e. white blood cell
   c. platelet

9. Another name for *white blood cell* is
   a. erythrocyte
   b. leukocyte
   c. platelet
   d. red blood cell
   e. thrombocyte

10. Another name for *platelet* is
    a. erythrocyte
    b. leukocyte
    c. red blood cell
    d. thrombocyte
    e. white blood cell

11. Which of the following substances assists a cell in grabbing oxygen where levels are low and then releasing them when the levels are high?
    a. hemoglobin
    b. immunoglobulin
    c. leukocyte
    d. thrombocyte
    e. none of these

12. Which of the following substances is a protein that assists white blood cells in fighting infection?
    a. hemoglobin
    b. immunoglobulin
    c. leukocyte
    d. thrombocyte
    e. none of these

EXERCISE 12   Identify the word parts for the following terms.

1. tonsil _____

2. lymph _____

3. thymus _____

4. spleen _____

5. bone marrow _____

6. blood condition _____

7. deficiency _____

EXERCISE 13   Build a medical term from the information provided.

1. inflammation of the tonsil _____

2. inflammation of the spleen _____

3. disease of the thymus _____

4. bone marrow tumor _____

5. lymph cell _____

6. lymph tumor _____

7. white blood condition _____

(S)UBJECTIVE

8.2 Patient History, Problems, Complaints

Patients with blood disorders normally present with the same general symptoms. They usually seek medical care because they suffer from secondary effects of having a low amount of a specific blood cell type.

A patient with anemia may feel weak and run down, and may look paler than normal. If patients' *platelet* levels are too low, they may notice that they bruise easily (*ecchymosis*) or that they develop small, flat, red spots on their body (*petechiae*). They may also complain that they tend to bleed (*hemorrhage*) more easily than most people. This can also result from *hemophilia*.

A patient who has a low white blood cell count is more vulnerable to infection; thus, he or she will suffer from more infections than normal. A patient may even present with the chief concern of possible immune deficiency.

Disorders of the lymphatic system also have few symptoms. Most commonly, a patient will present with swollen lymph nodes (*lymphadenopathy*). This can be a sign of many different types of illnesses, which range from mild to serious. Another concern may be swelling in their extremities (*lymphedema*), which can also have serious or harmless causes.

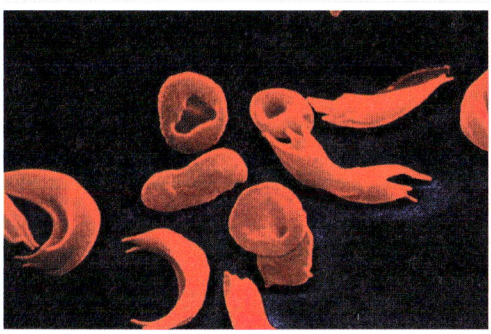

A common type of anemia is sickle-cell anemia, called that because affected red blood cells develop a hard, rigid "sickle" shape that can cause frequent clots in the sufferer.

Science History Images/Alamy Stock Photo

blood *continued*

TERM	WORD ANALYSIS
hemophilia HEE-moh-FEE-lee-ah	hemo / phil / ia blood / love / condition
DEFINITION condition in which the blood doesn't clot, thus causing excessive bleeding	
hemorrhage HIM-or-rij	hemo / rrhage blood / burst forth
DEFINITION excessive blood loss	
petechia puh-TEE-kee-yah **DEFINITION** small bruise	from Latin, for *freckle* or *spot*

DaVIDa S/Shutterstock

blood

TERM	WORD ANALYSIS
anemia ah-NEE-mee-ah	an / emia no / blood condition
DEFINITION reduction of red blood cells noticed by the patient as weakness and fatigue.	
ecchymosis eh-kih-MOH-sis	from Greek, for *to pour out*
DEFINITION large bruise	
hematoma HEE-mah-TOH-mah	hemat / oma blood / tumor
DEFINITION mass of blood within an organ, cavity, or tissue	

lymph

TERM	WORD ANALYSIS
lymphadenopathy lim-FAD-eh-NAW-pah-thee	lymph / adeno / pathy lymph / gland / disease
DEFINITION any disease of a lymph gland (node); used to refer to noticeably swollen lymph nodes, especially in the neck	
lymphedema LIMF-ah-DEE-mah	lymph / edema lymph / swelling
DEFINITION swelling caused by abnormal accumulation of lymph, usually in the extremities	
splenalgia splee-NAL-jah	splen / algia spleen / pain
DEFINITION pain in the spleen	
splenodynia SPLEE-noh-DAI-nee-ah	spleno / dynia spleen / pain
DEFINITION pain in the spleen	

TRANSLATION

EXERCISE 1   Break down the following words into their component parts.

> EXAMPLE: nasopharyngoscope
> *naso | pharyngo | scope*

1. hematoma _____

2. hemorrhage _____

3. splenodynia _____

4. splenalgia _____

5. lymphedema _____

6. hemophilia _____

7. anemia _____

8. lymphadenopathy _____

EXERCISE 2   Underline and define the word parts from this chapter in the following terms.

1. hemophilia _____

2. hemorrhage _____

3. hematoma _____

4. splenodynia _____

5. splenalgia _____

6. lymphedema _____

7. anemia _____

EXERCISE 3   Match the term on the left with its definition on the right. Some definitions may be used more than once.

_____ 1. anemia

_____ 2. hemophilia

_____ 3. hemorrhage

_____ 4. hematoma

_____ 5. splenalgia

_____ 6. splenodynia

_____ 7. lymphedema

_____ 8. ecchymosis

a. a condition in which the blood doesn't clot, thus causing excessive bleeding

b. a mass of blood within an organ, cavity, or tissue

c. excessive blood loss

d. large bruise

e. pain in the spleen

f. reduction of red blood cells noticed by the patient as weakness and fatigue

g. swelling caused by abnormal accumulation of lymph

EXERCISE 4   Translate the following terms as literally as possible.

> EXAMPLE: nasopharyngoscope   *an instrument for looking at the nose and throat*

1. splenodynia _____

2. splenalgia _____

3. hematoma _____

4. hemorrhage _____

5. anemia _____

6. lymphedema _____

GENERATION

EXERCISE 5 Build a medical term from the information provided.

EXAMPLE: inflammation of the sinuses *sinusitis*

1. spleen pain (use *-dynia*) _____

2. spleen pain (use *-algia*) _____

3. blood tumor _____

4. lymph swelling _____

5. no blood condition _____

6. any disease of a lymph gland (node) _____

OBJECTIVE

8.3 Observation and Discovery

There are two ways of looking at blood cells. The first is to count them. A *complete blood count (CBC)* is one of the most common tests in medicine. A machine counts the number of each type of cells in the blood.

A lower-than-normal number of red blood cells is known as *anemia.* It is the most common blood problem and has a variety of causes. A higher-than-normal number of red blood cells (*erythrocytosis* or *polycythemia*) is much less common. When it is severe, it can be dangerous because the blood becomes too thick to flow well.

A low number of white blood cells (*leukopenia*) can be caused by an infection. If the number is too low, however, it may mean the patient has a weakened immune system (*immunodeficiency*). In general, people are more at risk if they are low in a specific type of white blood cell, neutrophils (*neutropenia*). Having a high number of white blood cells in the blood (*leukocytosis*) is a common marker for infection. Less commonly, it can indicate cancer.

Low platelet numbers (*thrombocytopenia*) can lead to easy bleeding and bruising. Having too many platelets in the blood (*thrombocytosis*) indicates inflammation. If platelet levels are too high, the patient runs the risk of experiencing abnormal blood clotting and forming a floating clot (*thromboembolism*).

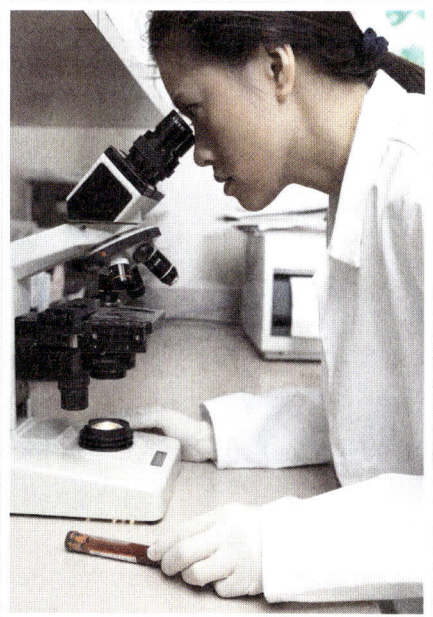

In hematology, a great deal of information is gathered through microscopic analysis of blood samples.
ERproductions Ltd/Blend Images LLC

Another way of evaluating blood cells is by looking at their size and shape. The size of red blood cells helps distinguish among different causes for anemia. In fact, it is generally the first step in diagnosing the cause.

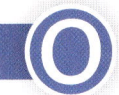

Causes for anemia with small red blood cells (*microcytosis*) include iron deficiency and lead poisoning. Anemias with enlarged blood cells (*macrocytosis*) can be a result of folate deficiency or B_{12} deficiency. Normal-sized blood cell (*normocytic*) anemias include bleeding and anemia from chronic disease. Some problems with the makeup of a red blood cell can cause it to assume abnormal shapes. *Spherocytes* and *elliptocytes* are two types of blood cells with abnormal shapes.

The physical exam of the lymphatic system focuses mainly on the few organs of the system, including the lymph nodes and the spleen. The lymph nodes may be swollen and painful (*lymphadenopathy*). The spleen may also be enlarged (*splenomegaly*). When lymph vessels become swollen, they can cause swelling in arms and legs (*lymphedema*).

There are no lab tests specific to the lymphatic system, but there is a special type of image that examines the lymph vessels (*lymphangiogram*). Most other lymphatic system issues, such as the absence of a spleen (*asplenia*), can be seen on a CT scan.

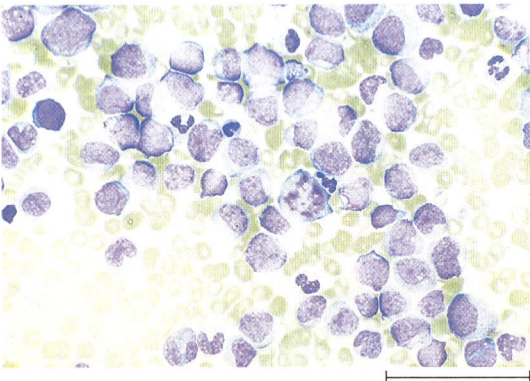

Blood from a patient with acute monocytic leukemia. Note the abnormally high number of white blood cells, especially monocytes.

Ed Reschke

blood

TERM	WORD ANALYSIS
embolism EM-boh-LIZ-um	embol / ism embolus / condition
DEFINITION blockage in a blood vessel caused by an embolus	
embolus EM-boh-lus	em / bolus in / throw
DEFINITION mass of matter present in the blood NOTE: In Greek, this word means *stopper*, as in a cap for a bottle.	
erythrocyte eh-RIH-throh-SAIT	erythro / cyte red / cell
DEFINITION red blood cell	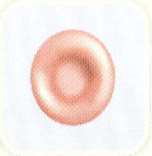
hematopoiesis heh-MAH-toh-poh-EE-sis	hemato / poiesis blood / formation
DEFINITION formation of blood cells	
hemolysis hee-MAW-lih-sis	hemo / lysis blood / breakdown
DEFINITION breakdown of blood cells	
leukocyte LOO-koh-sait	leuko / cyte white / cell
DEFINITION white blood cell	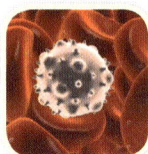 MedicalRF.com/Getty Images
leukopenia LOO-koh-PEE-nee-ah	leuko / penia white / deficiency
DEFINITION deficiency in white blood cells	
thrombocyte THROM-boh-sait	thrombo / cyte clot / cell
DEFINITION cell that helps blood clot; also known as a platelet	

75 μm

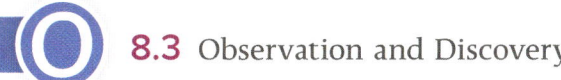

blood *continued*

TERM	WORD ANALYSIS
thromboembolism THROM-boh-EM-boh-LIZ-um	thrombo / embol / ism clot / embolus / condition

DEFINITION blockage of a vessel (embolism) caused by a clot that has broken off from where it formed

| **thrombosis**
throm-BOH-sis | thromb / osis
clot / condition |

DEFINITION the formation of a blood clot

Steve Gschmeissner/Science Photo Library RF/Getty Images

| **thrombus**
THROM-bus | from Greek, for *lump, clot,* or even *curd of milk* |

DEFINITION blood clot

NOTE: The difference between a thrombus and an embolus is twofold. A thrombus is a clot of blood and is stationary. An embolus is foreign material and is in motion. When a thrombus breaks off, it becomes a *thromboembolus.*

lymph

TERM	WORD ANALYSIS
hepatosplenomegaly heh-PAT-oh-SPLEE-noh-MEH-gah-lee	hepato / spleno / megaly liver / spleen / enlargement

DEFINITION enlargement of the liver and spleen

Dr. M.A. Ansary/Science Source

| **lymphocyte**
LIM-foh-SAIT | lympho / cyte
lymph / cell |

DEFINITION lymph cell

| **splenomegaly**
SPLEE-noh-MEH-gah-lee | spleno / megaly
spleen / enlargement |

DEFINITION enlargement of the spleen

Boilershot Photo/Science Source

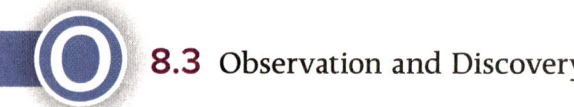
professional terms

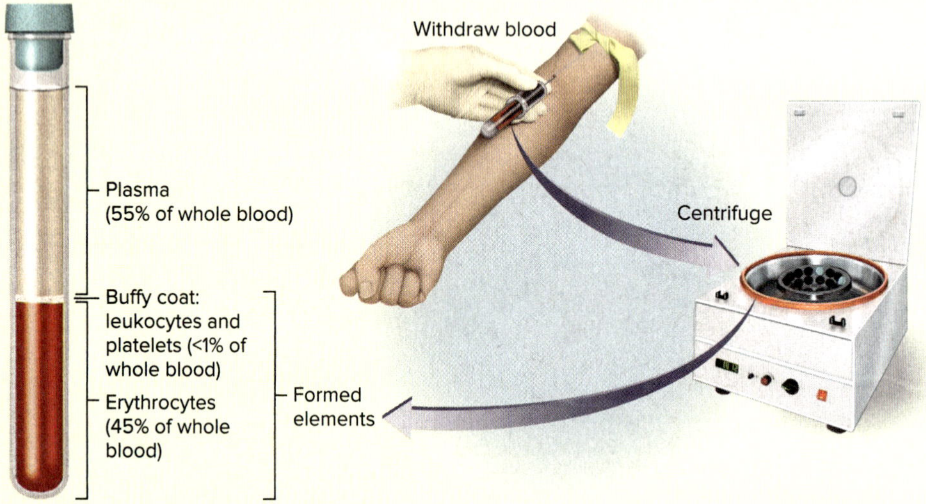

TERM	WORD ANALYSIS

hematocrit
hee-MAT-oh-krit

hemato / crit
blood   / judge (separate)

DEFINITION test to judge or separate the blood; it is used to determine the ratio of red blood cells to total blood volume
NOTE: The root *crit* comes from the Greek word that is the basis of the English word *critic*.

Withdraw blood

Plasma
(55% of whole blood)

Centrifuge

Buffy coat:
leukocytes and
platelets (<1% of
whole blood)

Erythrocytes
(45% of whole
blood)

Formed
elements

hematology
HEE-mah-TAW-loh-jee

hemato / logy
blood   / study

DEFINITION study of the blood

phlebotomist
fleh-BAW-toh-mist

phlebo / tom / ist
vein   / cut   / specialist

DEFINITION specialist in drawing blood

phlebotomy
fleh-BAW-toh-mee

phlebo / tomy
vein   / incision

DEFINITION incision into a vein; another name
for drawing blood

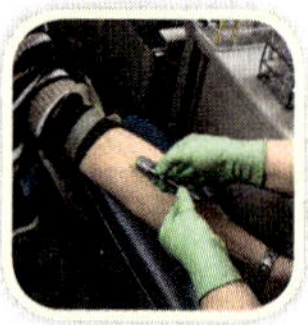

liquidlibrary/Getty Images

sphygmomanometer
SFIG-moh-mah-NAW-meh-ter

sphygmo / mano / meter
strangle   / thin   / instrument for measuring

DEFINITION fancy name for the device used to measure
blood pressure

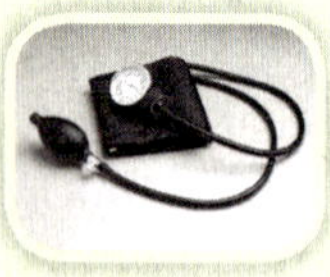

Creatas/Getty Images

radiology

TERM	WORD ANALYSIS
lymphangiography lim-FAN-jee-AW-grah-fee	lymph / angio / graphy lymph / vessel / writing procedure
DEFINITION procedure to study the lymph vessels	

Learning Outcome 8.3 Exercises

PRONUNCIATION

EXERCISE 1   Indicate which syllable(s) is emphasized when pronounced.

> EXAMPLE: bronchitis bron<u>chi</u>tis

1. embolus _____
2. thrombus _____

3. thrombosis _____
4. leukocyte _____
5. phlebotomy _____
6. hemolysis _____

TRANSLATION

EXERCISE 2   Break down the following words into their component parts.

> EXAMPLE: nasopharyngoscope
> *naso | pharyngo | scope*

1. hemolysis _____
2. hematocrit _____
3. thrombosis _____
4. hepatosplenomegaly _____
5. splenomegaly _____
6. lymphangiography _____

7. phlebotomist _____
8. sphygmomanometer _____

EXERCISE 3   Underline and define the word parts from this chapter in the following terms.

1. hematology _____
2. phlebotomy _____
3. hematopoiesis _____
4. lymphangiography _____
5. leukopenia (2 parts) _____

EXERCISE 4 Match the term on the left with its definition on the right.

_____ 1. lymphocyte   a. cell that helps blood clot (platelet)

_____ 2. leukocyte   b. lymph cell

_____ 3. thrombocyte   c. red blood cell

_____ 4. erythrocyte   d. white blood cell

EXERCISE 5 Match the term on the left with its definition on the right.

_____ 1. thrombus   a. blockage in a blood vessel caused by an embolus

_____ 2. embolism   b. blockage of a vessel (embolism) caused by a blood clot (thrombus) that has broken off from where it formed

_____ 3. embolus   c. a mass of matter present in the blood; from the Greek word for _stopper_, as in the cap on a bottle

_____ 4. thromboembolism   d. stationary blood clot

GENERATION

EXERCISE 6 Build a medical term from the information provided.

> EXAMPLE: inflammation of the sinuses   _sinusitis_

1. study of blood   _____

2. lymph cell   _____

3. white blood cell   _____

4. clot cell   _____

5. red blood cell   _____

6. enlargement of the spleen   _____

EXERCISE 7 Multiple-choice questions. Select the correct answer(s).

1. A _sphygmomanometer_ measures
   a. blood pressure   c. white blood cells
   b. red blood cells   d. none of these

2. An _embolism_ is
   a. a blockage in a blood vessel caused by a foreign material in motion
   b. a cell capable of producing a blood clot
   c. the formation of a blood clot
   d. none of these

3. A blockage of a vessel caused by a clot that has broken off from where it formed is a(n)
   a. embolism   c. thrombosis
   b. thromboembolism   d. thrombus

4. The formation of a blood clot is a(n)
   a. embolism   c. thrombosis
   b. thromboembolism   d. thrombus

EXERCISE 8 Briefly describe the difference between each pair of terms.

1. phlebotomist, phlebotomy   _____

2. hematopoiesis, hemolysis   _____

3. embolus, thrombus   _____

_____

8.4 Diagnosis and Pathology

Diseases affecting the blood often affect one specific blood cell type. The most common type of red blood cell problem is not having enough of them to do their job (*anemia*), which results from the body not being able to make enough of them. Iron is a necessary mineral for generating blood cells. As a result, a low level of iron can cause a decreased production of red blood cells *(iron deficiency anemia).* The available red blood cells may also be low because they break too easily (*hemolytic anemia*).

Even if there are enough red blood cells, there may be a problem with the blood's *hemoglobin,* the protein that actually carries oxygen. In less common situations, a patient may have too many red blood cells (*polycythemia*). This condition can make the blood thicker, making the flow of blood more difficult.

As with red blood cells, an insufficient number of white blood cells in the body can cause serious problems. A deficiency of white blood cells may cause the patient to be more vulnerable to infections (*immune deficiency*). Sometimes this can be caused by an outside force (*immunosuppression*) such as a medication or illness. When the body has a problem with making white blood cells, it may make way too many of them. This is what happens in people who have *leukemia.*

Not having enough platelets in the blood (*thrombocytopenia*) can cause problems with bleeding. It can be mild, causing bruising and bloody noses, or it can be more severe, creating risk for bleeding into major organs such as the brain.

On the other hand, if the blood has too many platelets, spontaneous clots (*thrombosis*) may occur. Problems also arise when other parts of the body's clotting team are not working well—whether the blood is not clotting enough (*coagulopathy*) or clotting too easily (*hypercoagulability*).

Finally, blood diseases can be caused by things that are carried in the blood along with blood cells.

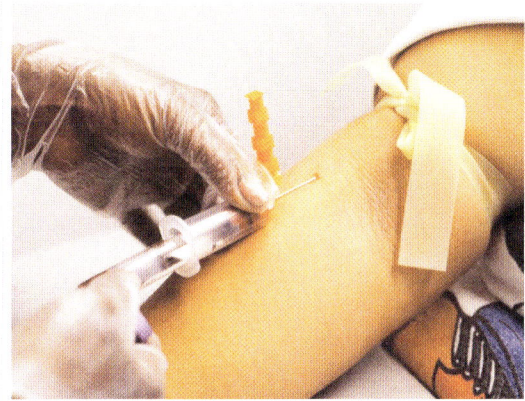

Often, a phlebotomy is the first step in diagnosing blood conditions.

Pixtal/AGE Fotostock

Infection can spread to the bloodstream (*septicemia*), which can be very dangerous. Fat floats in the blood as well. Too much fat (*hyperlipidemia*) in the blood can eventually lead to heart problems. Another thing that may be seen in the blood is the recycled blood product *bilirubin.* Too much bilirubin in the blood may cause the skin to appear yellow.

Problems in the lymphatic system are mainly seen in lymph nodes. Lymph nodes can become sore (*lymphadenopathy*) when overworked or infected (*lymphadenitis*). They are also a common site for cancer (*lymphoma*). The main spleen condition patients encounter is an enlarged spleen (*splenomegaly*), which can happen when it is overactive (*hypersplenism*) or, more commonly, as a result of an infection. The most common infection that affects the spleen is *mononucleosis.*

Bone marrow can become infected (*osteomyelitis*) from the bloodstream or from an injury to the bone. These infections are hard to treat and require a long course of antibiotics.

blood

TERM	WORD ANALYSIS
immunocompromised ih-MYOO-noh-COM-proh-MAIZD	**immuno / compromised** immune / compromised
DEFINITION having an immune system incapable of responding normally and completely to a pathogen or disease	
immunodeficiency ih-MYOO-noh-deh-FIH-shin-see	**immuno / deficiency** immune / deficiency
DEFINITION having an immune system with decreased or compromised response to disease-causing organisms	Bettman/Contributor/Getty Images
immunosuppression ih-MYOO-noh-suh-PREH-shun	**immuno / suppression** immune / suppression
DEFINITION reduction in the activity of the body's immune system	
thrombophlebitis THROM-boh-fleh-BAI-tis	**thrombo / phleb / itis** clot / vein / inflammation
DEFINITION inflammation of vein caused by a clot	

blood conditions *continued*

TERM	WORD ANALYSIS
hyperlipidemia HAI-per-LIH-pid-EE-mee-ah	**hyper / lipid / emia** over / fat / blood condition
DEFINITION excessive fat in the blood	
iron deficiency anemia AI-ern deh-FIH-shin-see ah-NEE-mee-ah	**iron deficiency** iron deficiency **an / emia** no / blood condition
DEFINITION anemia caused by inadequate iron intake	
septicemia SEP-tih-SEE-mee-ah	**septic / emia** rotting / blood condition
DEFINITION presence of disease-causing microorganisms in the blood	

blood conditions

TERM	WORD ANALYSIS
anemia ah-NEE-mee-ah	**an / emia** no / blood condition
DEFINITION reduced red blood cells	
aplastic anemia AY-plas-tik ah-NEE-mee-ah	**a / plas / tic** no / formation / pertaining to **an / emia** no / blood condition
DEFINITION anemia caused by red blood cells not being formed in sufficient quantities	
hemolytic anemia HEE-moh-LIH-tiok ah-NEE-mee-ah	**hemo / lytic** blood / breakdown **an / emia** no / blood condition
DEFINITION anemia caused by the destruction of red blood cells	

lymph

TERM	WORD ANALYSIS
lymphadenitis LIM-fad-eh-NAI-tis	**lymph / aden / itis** lymph / gland / inflammation
DEFINITION inflammation of a lymph gland (node)	
lymphangitis LIM-fan-JAI-tis	**lymph / ang / itis** lymph / vessel / inflammation
DEFINITION inflammation of lymph vessels	

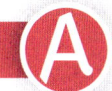
lymph *continued*

TERM	WORD ANALYSIS
mononucleosis MAW-noh-NOO-klee-OH-sis	mono / nucle / osis one / nucleus / condition
DEFINITION condition characterized by an abnormally large number of mononuclear leukocytes	
splenitis splee-NAI-tis	splen / itis spleen / inflammation
DEFINITION inflammation of the spleen	
splenorrhexis SPLEE-noh-REK-sis	spleno / rrhexis spleen / rupture
DEFINITION rupture of the spleen	
tonsillitis TON-sil-AI-tis	tonsill / itis tonsil / inflammation
DEFINITION inflammation of a tonsil	

Source: Centers for Disease Control and Prevention

oncology

TERM	WORD ANALYSIS
leukemia loo-KEE-mee-ah	leuk / emia white / blood condition
DEFINITION cancer of the blood or bone marrow characterized by the abnormal increase in white blood cells	

Ed Reschke

lymphoma lim-FOH-mah	lymph / oma lymph / tumor
DEFINITION cancerous tumor originating in lymphocytes	

Source: Robert S. Craig/CDC

myeloma MAI-eh-LOH-mah	myel / oma bone marrow / tumor
DEFINITION cancerous tumor of the bone marrow; when the tumors are present in several bones, it is called multiple myeloma	

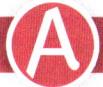

Learning Outcome 8.4 Exercises

TRANSLATION

EXERCISE 1 Break down the following words into their component parts.

> EXAMPLE: **nasopharyngoscope**
> *naso | pharyngo | scope*

1. splenitis _____
2. immunocompromised _____
3. immunosuppression _____
4. lymphangitis _____

EXERCISE 2 Underline and define the word parts from this chapter in the following terms.

1. tonsillitis _____
2. immunodeficiency _____
3. lymphoma _____
4. myeloma _____
5. lymphadenitis _____
6. anemia _____
7. splenorrhexis _____
8. leukemia (2 parts) _____
9. thrombophlebitis (2 roots) _____

EXERCISE 3   Match the term on the left with its definition on the right.

_____ 1. iron deficiency anemia
_____ 2. hemolytic anemia
_____ 3. aplastic anemia
_____ 4. hyperlipidemia
_____ 5. septicemia

a. anemia caused by inadequate iron intake
b. anemia caused by red blood cells not being formed in sufficient quantities
c. anemia caused by the destruction of red blood cells
d. excessive fat in the blood
e. the presence of disease-causing microorganisms in the blood

EXERCISE 4   Translate the following terms as literally as possible.

EXAMPLE: **nasopharyngoscope**   *an instrument for looking at the nose and throat*

1. thrombophlebitis _____

2. anemia _____

3. septicemia _____

4. lymphadenitis _____

5. lymphangitis _____

6. splenitis _____

7. splenorrhexis _____

8. tonsillitis _____

GENERATION

EXERCISE 5   Build a medical term from the information provided.

EXAMPLE: **inflammation of the sinuses**   *sinusitis*

1. lymph tumor _____

2. white blood condition _____

3. excessive fat in the blood _____

EXERCISE 6   Multiple-choice questions. Select the correct answer.

1. The root word in *immunocompromised* is
    a. *compromo*—the lymph system
    b. *compromo*—to protect
    c. *immuno*—the immune system
    d. *immuno*—the platelets and white cells of the body
    e. none of these

2. An immune system with decreased or compromised response to disease-causing organisms is called /experiencing
    a. autoimmune   d. immunosuppression
    b. immunogenic   e. none of these
    c. immunodeficiency

3. Anemia caused by inadequate iron intake is known as
    a. aplastic anemia   d. iron deficiency anemia
    b. hematopenia   e. none of these
    c. hemolytic anemia

4. A cancer of the blood or bone marrow characterized by the abnormal increase in white blood cells is known as
    a. leukemia   d. osteomyelitis
    b. myeloma   e. none of these
    c. lymphoma

EXERCISE 7   Briefly describe the difference between the pair of terms.

1. aplastic anemia, hemolytic anemia _____

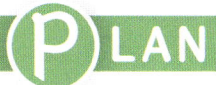

8.5 Treatments and Therapies

Treatment for blood problems generally involves both medicine and transfusions. With red blood cell problems, the treatment often involves blood transfusions (for severe problems) and then fixing the cause. Many times, iron supplements can also be helpful.

White blood cell problems—in particular, severely low white blood cell counts—can be treated with transfusions too. A patient with leukemia is treated with chemotherapy.

When the problem is significant enough, patients with very low platelet levels often are treated with transfusions as well. Other medicines that can help with platelet problems include medicines to break clots (*thrombolytics*) and those that prevent clots (*anticoagulants*).

Treating diseases of the lymphatic system generally involves surgery. Organs of the lymphatic system may be removed, such as the spleen (*splenectomy*) or the thymus (*thymectomy*). Lymph nodes may need removal (*lymphadenectomy*) as well, usually for the purpose of a biopsy.

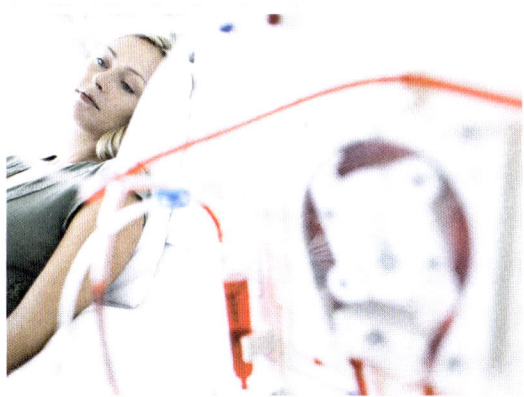

Transfusions and apheresis are important components of treating blood problems.

Science Photo Library/Getty Images

pharmacology

TERM	WORD ANALYSIS		
anticoagulant AN-tee-coh-AG-yoo-lant	anti against	/ coagul / coagulation	/ ant / agent
DEFINITION drug that prevents the coagulation of blood			
thrombolytic THROM-boh-LIH-tik	thrombo clot	/ lytic / breakdown	
DEFINITION drug that breaks down blood clots			

surgery

TERM	WORD ANALYSIS		
lymphadenectomy lim-FAD-eh-NEK-toh-mee	lymph lymph	/ aden / gland	/ ectomy / removal
DEFINITION surgical removal of a lymph gland (node)			
splenectomy spleh-NEK-toh-mee	splen spleen	/ ectomy / removal	
DEFINITION surgical removal of the spleen			
thymectomy thai-MEK-toh-mee	thym thymus	/ ectomy / removal	
DEFINITION surgical removal of the thymus			
tonsillectomy TON-sil-EK-toh-mee	tonsill tonsil	/ ectomy / removal	
DEFINITION surgical removal of a tonsil			

transfusions

TERM	WORD ANALYSIS
apheresis AH-fer-EE-sis	from Greek, for *separation* NOTE: This is the same word that was the origin of the word *heretic,* meaning one who has separated from the traditional teachings of a group.
DEFINITION general term for a process, similar to dialysis, that draws out a patient's blood, removes something from it, then returns the rest of the blood to the patient's body NOTE: *Apheresis* can also refer to the use of this process to remove unwanted or disease-causing components from the blood.	

Ismael Alonso/Contributor/ Getty Images

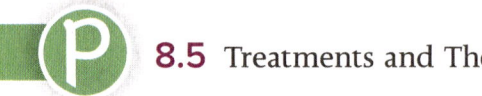
transfusions *continued*

TERM	WORD ANALYSIS
cytapheresis SAI-tah-fer-EE-sis	cyt / apheresis cell / separation
DEFINITION apheresis to remove cellular material	
plasmapheresis PLAZ-mah-fer-EE-sis	plasm / apheresis plasma / separation
DEFINITION apheresis to remove plasma	
plateletpheresis PLAYT-let-fer-EE-sis	platelet / pheresis platelet / separation
DEFINITION apheresis to remove platelets (for the purpose of donating them to patients in need of platelets)	

NOTE: Where did the *a* in *apheresis* go? Probably, this term was developed from the term *plasmapheresis.* But because the first root in that word is *plasma,* someone thought that the *a* in *apheresis* went with it, so when they made this new word, they left the *a* out. Either that, or *platelet-AH-pheresis* didn't sound as good.

transfusions *continued*

TERM	WORD ANALYSIS
transfusion tranz-FYOO-zhun	trans / fusion across / pour
DEFINITION infusion into a patient of blood from another source	

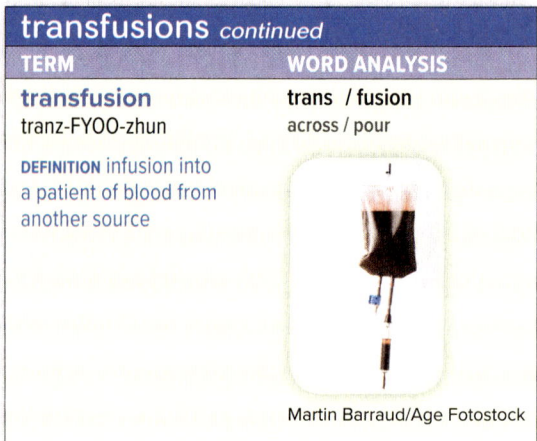

Martin Barraud/Age Fotostock

 **Learning Outcome 8.5 Exercises**

PRONUNCIATION

EXERCISE 1   Indicate which syllable(s) is emphasized when pronounced.

> EXAMPLE: bronchitis bron<u>chi</u>tis

1. transfusion _____
2. thymectomy _____
3. splenectomy _____

TRANSLATION

EXERCISE 2   Break down the following words into their component parts.

> EXAMPLE: nasopharyngoscope
> *naso | pharyngo | scope*

1. thymectomy _____
2. transfusion _____

3. plasmapheresis _____
4. plateletpheresis _____

EXERCISE 3 Underline and define the word parts from this chapter in the following terms.

1. tonsillectomy _____

2. thymectomy _____

3. splenectomy _____

4. thrombolytic _____

5. anticoagulant _____

6. cytapheresis _____

7. lymphadenectomy (2 parts) _____

EXERCISE 4 Match the term on the left with its definition on the right.

_____ 1. transfusion

_____ 2. apheresis

_____ 3. plasmapheresis

_____ 4. cytapheresis

a. apheresis to remove cellular material

b. apheresis to remove plasma

c. general term for a process, similar to dialysis, that draws blood, removes something from it, then returns the rest of the blood to the patient

d. infusion into a patient of blood from another source

EXERCISE 5 Translate the following terms as literally as possible.

> EXAMPLE: **nasopharyngoscope** *an instrument for looking at the nose and throat*

1. thrombolytic _____

2. cytapheresis _____

3. plateletpheresis _____

4. plasmapheresis _____

GENERATION

EXERCISE 6 Build a medical term from the information provided.

> EXAMPLE: **inflammation of the sinuses** *sinusitis*

1. surgical removal of the spleen _____

2. surgical removal of the thymus _____

3. surgical removal of the tonsil _____

4. a drug that prevents the coagulation of blood

_____

EXERCISE 7 Multiple-choice questions. Select the correct answer(s).

1. Select all of the statements that apply to the term *apheresis*.
   a. a process similar to dialysis
   b. can refer to the removal of unwanted or disease-causing components from the blood
   c. from the Greek word meaning *separation*
   d. requires a transfusion
   e. the blood is not returned to the patient once removed

2. After a patient has undergone *plateletpheresis,*
   a. the patient receives a transfusion to replace lost blood
   b. the plasma is cleaned and then returned to the patient
   c. the platelets are often donated to another person in need
   d. the platelets are then returned to the patient
   e. none of these

8.6 Electronic Health Records

Hospital Progress Note

Subjective

Mrs. Campos was admitted last night for fever and elevated WBC. Initial blood culture came back positive from gram-positive cocci. She has been on antibiotics for 10 hours now. Last night, the nurses noted hemorrhages. She had **hematuria, hemoptysis,** and **epistaxis.** In addition, she developed painful swelling in her right calf. She remains febrile, but the fever is improving since admission. She is still very tired. She denies vomiting.

Objective

RR: 18; HR: 70; Temp 101.2; BP: 102/74.
General: Sleeping. Tired but responsive to questions.
HEENT: NCAT, dried bloody crusts in nostrils, mucous membranes moist and pink; PERRLA, EOMI, conjunctivae clear.
Neck: Supple, no **adenopathy,** no JVD.
Resp: No increased effort, clear breath sounds.
CV: Regular, S1, S2, no murmur/rub; pedal pulses 2+ .
Abd: Soft, nontender, nondistended, normoactive bowel sounds, no **HSM.**
Lymph: No enlarged cervical, axillary, or inguinal lymph nodes.
Skin: Scattered **petechiae,** CR 2 seconds.
Ext: Right swelling with tender subcutaneous nodule.
Neuro: Alert and oriented, CN II-XII grossly intact, normal and symmetric strength in UEs and LEs, DTRs 2+ and symmetric.
Labs
Total bilirubin: 6.2
Hgb: 9.2; **WBC:** 20.2; **PLT:** 24.
PT and **PTT** both elevated.
Microangiopathic hemolysis seen on peripheral smear.

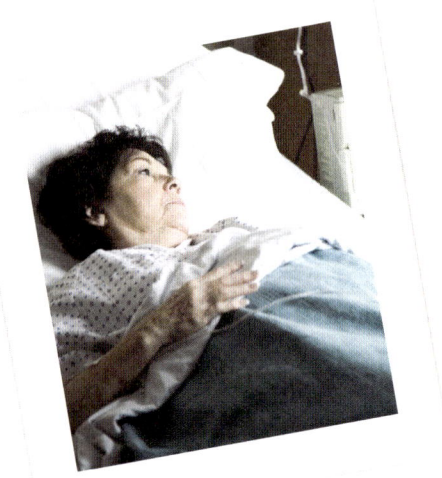

Rubberball/Nicole Hill/Getty Images

Assessment/Plan

1. **Septicemia:** Fever down slightly and WBC decreased from 25.4 to 20.2. Continue current IV antibiotics.

2. **Anemia/Coagulopathy/Thrombocytopenia:** Clinically consistent with DIC. We will transfuse a unit of platelets and follow labs in 6 hours.

3. **Calf swelling:** Suspect superficial thromboembolism. We will consult hematology/oncology in regard to their opinion on beginning anticoagulant medicine.

4. **Hyperbilirubinemia:** I suspect the etiology is liver dysfunction from DIC. Follow labs in the AM.

   —Linda Lovegood, MD

EXERCISE 1 Match the term on the left with its definition on the right.

_____ 1. anemia

_____ 2. transfusion

_____ 3. hematology

_____ 4. hemorrhage

_____ 5. hemolysis

_____ 6. anticoagulant

_____ 7. septicemia

_____ 8. hepatosplenomegaly

_____ 9. thromboembolism

a. a blockage of a vessel (embolism) caused by a clot that has broken off from where it formed

b. a drug that prevents the coagulation of blood

c. breakdown of blood cells

d. enlargement of the spleen and liver

e. excessive blood loss

f. reduction of red blood cells noticed by the patient as weakness and fatigue

g. the infusion into a patient of blood from another source

h. the presence of disease-causing microorganisms in the blood

i. the study of the blood

EXERCISE 2 Fill in the blanks.

1. Using the data recorded at the patient's physical examination, fill in the following blanks.
   a. The patient's temperature: _____
   b. The patient's heart rate: _____
   c. The patient's respiratory rate: _____
   d. The patient's blood pressure: _____
   e. Abdomen: no HSM (give definition for abbreviation: _____)

2. Using the patient's laboratory data, fill in the following blanks.
   a. Hemoglobin: _____
   b. White blood count: _____
   c. Platelet count: _____

3. According to the physician's assessment/plan,
   a. *septicemia* (give definition: _____
      _____);
      WBC (give definition for abbreviation:
      _____)
      decreased from 25.4 to 20.2.
   b. For suspected _____
      (a blockage of a vessel [embolism] caused by a clot that has broken off from where it formed), the hematology/oncology department will be consulted before beginning *anticoagulants* (give definition: _____).

EXERCISE 3 True or false questions. Indicate true answers with a T and false answers with an F.

1. The patient was admitted for an elevated red blood count. _____

2. The patient's spleen and liver are enlarged.
   _____

3. The patient will receive blood and/or blood components from another source. _____
   _____

EXERCISE 4 Multiple-choice questions. Select the correct answer.

1. The patient has *hematuria,* which is
   a. blood in the urine
   b. a condition of the liver and blood
   c. decreased blood volume
   d. none of these

2. The patient had *hemoptysis,* which comes from the root *ptysis,* which means cough, and *hemo,* which means
   a. blood
   b. bone marrow
   c. liver
   d. lymph system

3. The patient's peripheral blood smear revealed *microangiopathic hemolysis.* The term *microangiopathic* refers to a disease of the small blood vessels. The term *hemolysis* refers to
   a. breakdown of blood cells
   b. breakdown of clotting cells
   c. creation of blood cells
   d. creation of clotting cells

Quick Reference

glossary of roots

ROOT	DEFINITION	ROOT	DEFINITION
cyt/o	cell	phleb/o	vein
-emia	blood condition	splen/o	spleen
hem/o, hemat/o	blood	thromb/o	clot
leuk/o	white	thym/o	thymus
lymph/o	lymph	tonsill/o	tonsils
myel/o	bone marrow	ven/o	vein
-penia	deficiency		

blood and lymph abbreviations

ABBREVIATION	DEFINITION
AIDS	acquired immunodeficiency syndrome
BMT	bone marrow transplant
CBC	complete blood count
DIC	disseminated intravascular coagulopathy
EBV	Epstein-Barr virus
ESR	erythrocyte sedimentation rate
Hct	hematocrit
Hgb	hemoglobin
HIV	human immunodeficiency virus
HSM	hepatosplenomegaly
IV	intravenous
IVIG	intravenous immunoglobulin
LAD	lymphadenopathy
NCAT	no cervical adenopathy or tenderness
PLT	platelet count
RBC	red blood count Ingram Publishing
WBC	white blood count

The Cardiovascular System–Cardiology

9

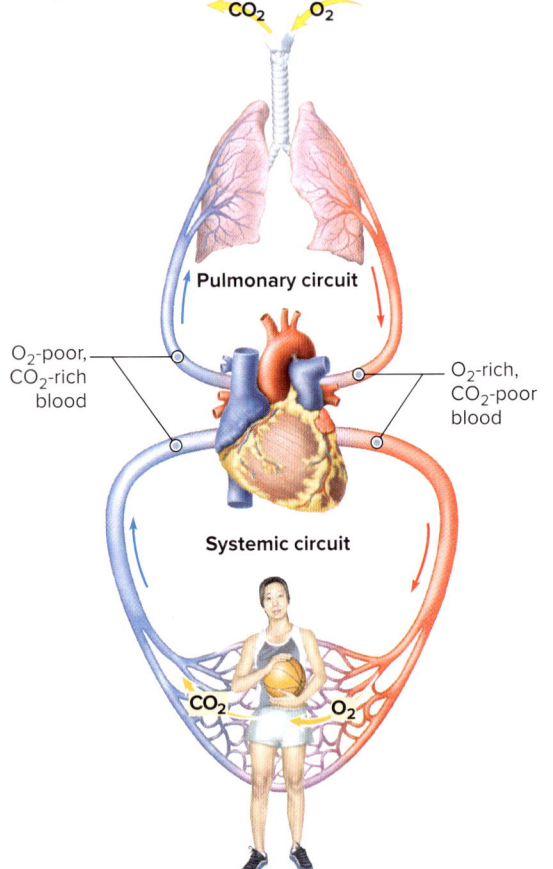

Pulmonary circuit

O_2-poor, CO_2-rich blood

O_2-rich, CO_2-poor blood

Systemic circuit

CO_2 O_2

CO_2 O_2

Introduction and Overview of the Cardiovascular System

Imagine a large city without roads or transportation of any type. There would be no way for food to get to stores, no access for emergency services to get to people in need of rescue, and no means for trash to be collected. It wouldn't take long for the city to fall into chaos.

The body is much the same. It needs a system to continually deliver fresh supplies to the cells of the body and remove waste. The body also needs a means to deliver chemical messages from one part of the body to another. The cardiovascular system is the body's transport system that provides nourishment, cleanup services, and communication.

There are two parts to the cardiovascular system: the *cardio* (heart) and the *vascular* (blood vessels). The heart is a big pump that squeezes blood out to the body, and the vessels are the tubes that carry the blood. Together, they transport all manner of essential nutrients, blood cells, and chemical signals. They also work together to help rid the body of waste.

Learning Outcomes

Upon completion of this chapter, you will be able to:

9.1 Identify the **roots/word parts** associated with the **cardiovascular system.**

(S) **9.2** Translate the **Subjective** terms associated with the **cardiovascular system.**

(O) **9.3** Translate the **Objective** terms associated with the **cardiovascular system.**

(A) **9.4** Translate the **Assessment** terms associated with the **cardiovascular system**.

(P) **9.5** Translate the **Plan** terms associated with the **cardiovascular system.**

9.6 Distinguish terms associated with the **cardiovascular system** in the context of **electronic health records**.

9.1 Word Parts of the Cardiovascular System

Heart

The heart is the workhorse of this critical transport system. It constantly pumps, getting blood moving to where it needs to go. The heart is divided into four "rooms" or chambers: the left and right receiving rooms (*atria*) and the left and right sending rooms (*ventricles*). The left side of the heart handles oxygen-rich blood, and the right side handles the oxygen-poor blood. A thick wall of muscle, the *septum,* divides the left and right sides.

Blood constantly cycles between the body and the heart, and it collects in the atria. Blood that has nourished the body and is ready to go to the lungs for more oxygen collects in the right atrium. After getting a fresh supply of oxygen, blood returns to the heart via the left atrium. From the atria, blood—on both sides—passes through the one-way doors of the valves into the ventricles.

In a normal heart, there is no blood flow between the left and right side. There are connections between the atria and ventricles, and between the ventricles and the blood vessels. The connection between each atrium and ventricle is a valve that allows blood to flow in one direction. On the left side, the *mitral valve* connects the left atrium and ventricle. Then the *aortic valve* connects the left ventricle to the outgoing blood vessel, the *aorta.*

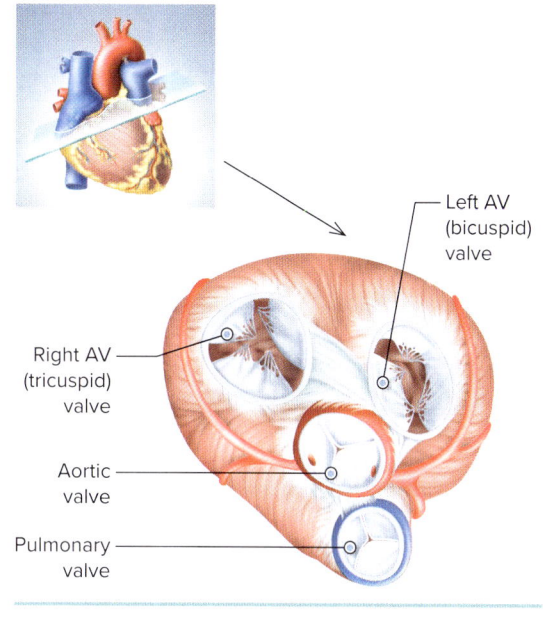

Left AV (bicuspid) valve

Right AV (tricuspid) valve

Aortic valve

Pulmonary valve

On the right side, the connector between the atrium and ventricle is the *tricuspid valve.* The *pulmonic valve* connects the right ventricle and the outgoing blood vessel, the *pulmonary artery.*

Ventricles are strong and muscular. When the heart compresses, the ventricles force the blood out into the outgoing blood vessels (*arteries*). The right ventricle sends blood to the lungs to get fresh oxygen and to discard excess carbon dioxide. The fresh blood is sent out from the heart by the left ventricle to the rest of the body to provide oxygen and collect the body's carbon dioxide waste.

---

valve

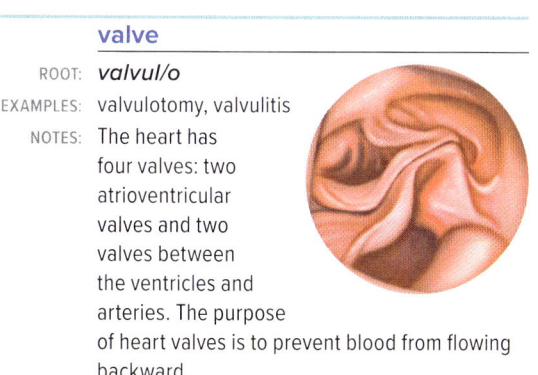

ROOT: *valvul/o*

EXAMPLES: valvulotomy, valvulitis

NOTES: The heart has four valves: two atrioventricular valves and two valves between the ventricles and arteries. The purpose of heart valves is to prevent blood from flowing backward.

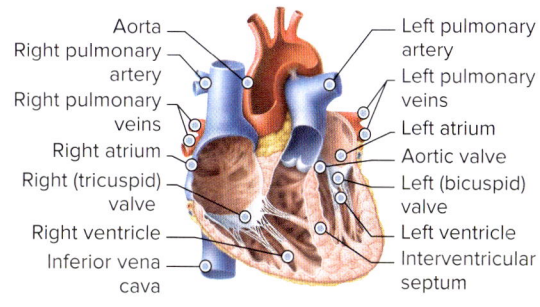

Aorta
Right pulmonary artery
Right pulmonary veins
Right atrium
Right (tricuspid) valve
Right ventricle
Inferior vena cava

Left pulmonary artery
Left pulmonary veins
Left atrium
Aortic valve
Left (bicuspid) valve
Left ventricle
Interventricular septum

atrium (upper chamber)

ROOT: *atri/o*

EXAMPLES: atrium, atrial fibrillation

NOTES: The *atrium* is the upper portion of each side of the heart. The term comes from Roman architecture, where it referred to the large open area that was characteristic of most Roman houses; typically, all the other rooms of the house would branch off from this center space. Even today, a large central area in a building is often called its *atrium*.

septum (plural: septa)

ROOT: *sept/o*

EXAMPLES: atrial septal defect, septoplasty

NOTES: *Septum* comes from a Latin word meaning *partition* or *dividing structure* and can refer to any wall dividing two cavities. There are numerous septa throughout the body, including between the two sides of the heart. The easiest to find is the nasal septum. If you place an index finger in each nostril and try to make them touch, what you are feeling is the nasal septum. If you find that your nasal septum leans to one side, you have a deviated septum.

ventricle (lower chamber)

ROOT: *ventricul/o*

EXAMPLE: ventriculotomy

NOTES: The ventricle is the lower portion of each side of the heart. The word is a combination of *venter* (stomach) plus the diminutive suffix *-icle* and means *little stomach*.

heart

ROOT: *cardi/o*

EXAMPLES: cardiology, cardiac arrest, myocarditis

NOTES: The root *cardio* can be tricky because it ends in the double vowel *io*. You expect the *o* to go away sometimes, but when a suffix beginning with an *i* is added to this root, not just the *o*, but also an *i* disappears as well. For example: *myo* (muscle) + *cardio* (heart) + *itis* (inflammation) = myocard-*i*-itis.

heart

ROOT: *coron/o*

EXAMPLES: coronary artery, coronary thrombosis

NOTES: The term *corona* literally means crown and refers to the way the blood vessels that supply the heart descend and support the heart like a crown. The term *coronary* is used in medical language to refer specifically to the heart's blood supply.

Circulation

There are miles of blood vessels in the body. From vessels the size of a garden hose down to tiny capillaries much thinner than a human hair, blood vessels make up a large transportation network that acts like a road system. This system is a closed loop.

The left ventricle forces blood into the main outgoing vessel (*aorta*). The aorta branches into smaller arteries, just as highways have exits to smaller roads. These branches break off further still. Eventually, they reach their destinations: the brain, stomach, muscles, and so on.

By this point, the blood is flowing in tiny vessels known as *capillaries*. The oxygen and other nutrients pass out into the tissues that need it, and they give back their waste.

Once the blood has made the delivery and picked up the waste, it begins its journey back to the heart through veins. Smaller veins collect into larger veins, which collect into the upper (*superior*) and lower (*inferior*) *vena cava*. These main veins return blood to the right atrium.

At the same time that the left ventricle pumps blood into the aorta, the right ventricle pumps blood into the *pulmonary artery*. The pulmonary artery carries blood to the lungs to obtain oxygen and discard carbon dioxide. Once these gases are traded, the blood returns to the heart through a system of veins that lead to the main *pulmonary vein*. The pulmonary vein dumps the oxygen-rich blood into the left atrium. When the valve opens between the left atrium and left ventricle, the blood fills the ventricle and the cycle continues.

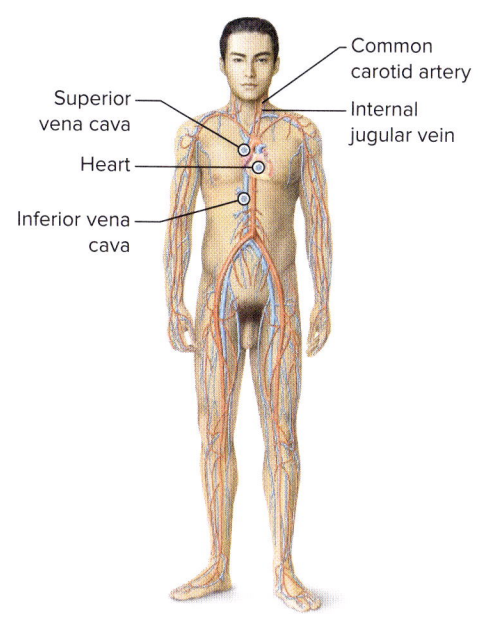

Common carotid artery

Superior vena cava

Internal jugular vein

Heart

Inferior vena cava

vessel

ROOTS: *angi/o, vas/o, vascul/o*

EXAMPLES: angioplasty, angiogram, vasodilator, vasculitis

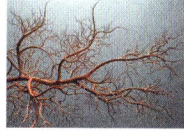
Storman/Getty Images

NOTES: All these roots come from words meaning *jar* or *pitcher. Angio* comes from Greek, and *vaso* and *vasculo* come from Latin. Although blood vessels don't look like jars, they do hold a lot of liquid—almost 6 quarts in the average man and almost 4 quarts in the average woman.

aorta

ROOT: *aort/o*

EXAMPLES: aortitis, aortolith

Aortic valve

NOTES: The *aorta* is the main artery leaving the heart and distributing oxygenated blood throughout the body. Its name means *to rise up* and refers to the fact that as the aorta leaves the heart, it rises up briefly and branches off into the arteries that supply the upper body before making what is called the *arch of the aorta* and descending into the lower body.

artery

ROOT: *arteri/o*

EXAMPLES: arteriosclerosis, endarterectomy

NOTES: Arteries are the large blood vessels that carry oxygenated blood from heart to body tissue. It's funny that the word *artery* is actually a Greek word for *trachea* or *windpipe,* a reference to the fact that some of the body's arteries are so large that early students of anatomy thought they carried air.

fatty plaque

ROOT: *ather/o*

EXAMPLE: atherosclerosis

NOTES: This root comes from Greek, for *gruel* or *porridge.* Be careful: This root is easily confused with *arterio,* especially in the words *arteriosclerosis* and *atherosclerosis.* There's another reason for the confusion: atherosclerosis is actually a form of arteriosclerosis. Arteriosclerosis means *hardening of an artery,* and atherosclerosis means *hardening of an artery due specifically to a buildup of fatty plaque.*

Complicated plaque   Artery wall

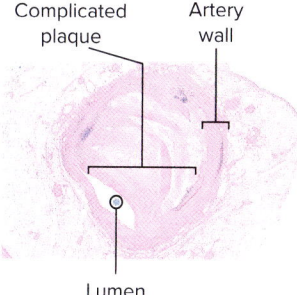

Lumen

Ed Reschke

vein

ROOTS: *phleb/o, ven/o*

EXAMPLES: phlebotomy, venospasm

NOTES: The term *phlebotomy* comes from *phlebo* (vein) and *tomy* (incision). It's the term used for drawing blood. But always make sure you pronounce the word carefully. You don't want to go to the hospital to get some blood drawn (*phlebotomy*) and end up having a portion of your brain removed (*lobotomy*).

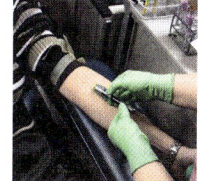
liquidlibrary/Getty Images

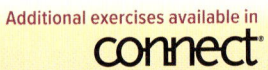
TRANSLATION

EXERCISE 1 Match the word part on the left with its definition on the right.

_____ 1. valvul/o

a. from Latin, for *partition* or *dividing structure;* can refer to any wall dividing two cavities

_____ 2. atri/o

b. literally means *crown* and refers to the way the blood vessels that supply the heart descend and support the heart like a crown; the term is used in medical language to refer specifically to the heart's blood supply

_____ 3. ventricul/o

c. lower chamber of the heart

_____ 4. sept/o

d. upper chamber of the heart

_____ 5. coron/o

e. valve

EXERCISE 2 Translate the following word parts.

1. cardi/o _____
2. atri/o _____
3. valvul/o _____
4. ventricul/o _____
5. sept/o _____
6. coron/o _____

EXERCISE 3 Underline and define the word parts from this chapter in the following terms.

1. cardiac arrest _____
2. endocarditis _____
3. valvuloplasty _____
4. coronary thrombosis _____

5. ventricular septal defect (2 roots) _____
6. atrial septal defect (2 roots) _____

EXERCISE 4 Break down the following words into their component parts and translate.

EXAMPLE: sinusitis   *sinus | itis*
inflammation of the sinuses

1. cardiology _____
2. valvulotomy _____
3. cardiomegaly _____
4. coronary circulation _____
5. atrial septal defect _____
6. ventricular septal defect _____

EXERCISE 5 Match the word part on the left with its definition on the right. Some definitions will be used more than once.

_____ 1. ven/o

a. blood vessel

_____ 2. aort/o

b. fatty plaque

_____ 3. phleb/o

c. large blood vessels that carry oxygenated blood from heart to body tissue

_____ 4. vas/o

d. main artery leaving the heart and distributing oxygenated blood throughout the body

_____ 5. vascul/o

e. vein

_____ 6. arteri/o

_____ 7. angi/o

_____ 8. ather/o

EXERCISE 6 Translate the following word parts.

1. arteri/o _____
2. aort/o _____

3. ven/o _____

4. vas/o _____

5. vascul/o _____

6. angi/o _____

7. phleb/o _____

8. ather/o _____

EXERCISE 7 Underline and define the word parts from this chapter in the following terms.

1. angiosclerosis _____

2. venosclerosis _____

3. atherosclerosis _____

4. phlebosclerosis _____

5. arteriectomy _____

6. aortolith _____

7. vasoconstrictor _____

8. vascular endoscopy _____

9. aortic stenosis _____

10. thrombophlebitis _____

11. superior vena cava _____

12. cardiovascular (2 roots) _____

13. angiocarditis (2 roots) _____

14. coronary artery bypass surgery (2 roots)
_____

EXERCISE 8 Break down the following words into their component parts and translate.

EXAMPLE: sinusitis   *sinus | itis*
inflammation of the sinuses

1. angioplasty _____

2. aortotomy _____

3. arterioplasty _____

4. atherectomy _____

5. coronary arterectomy _____

6. phlebotomy _____

7. vasculitis _____

8. vasodilator _____

9. venectomy _____

GENERATION

EXERCISE 9 Identify the roots for the following definitions.

1. septum _____

2. valve _____

3. ventricle _____

4. atrium _____

5. upper chamber of the heart _____

6. lower chamber of the heart _____

7. heart (2 roots) _____

EXERCISE 10 Build a medical term from the information provided.

1. inflammation of the heart (use *cardi/o*) _____
_____

2. inflammation of a heart valve _____

3. heart specialist (use *cardi/o*) _____

4. inflammation of the tissue around the heart (use *cardi/o*) _____

EXERCISE 11 Identify the roots for the following definitions.

1. aorta _____

2. artery _____

3. fatty plaque _____

4. vein (2 roots) _____

5. vessel (3 roots) _____

EXERCISE 12 Build a medical term from the information provided.

1. record of a vessel (use *angi/o*) _____

2. record of a vein (use *ven/o*) _____

3. record of the aorta _____

4. record of an artery _____

5. inflammation of a vein _____

6. involuntary contraction of a vessel (use *vas/o*) _____

7. the formation of a fatty plaque (use *-genesis*) _____

SUBJECTIVE

9.2 Patient History, Problems, Complaints

The most common heart problem patients report is chest pain (*pectoralgia*). The causes can range from minor issues, such as muscle soreness, to the pain associated with a heart attack (*angina pectoris*). Patients can occasionally feel pain in their blood vessels. This is most common with enlarged surface veins (*phlebalgia*).

While the heart never stops beating, we are rarely aware of its rhythm. When the heart beats out of pace, a patient might feel a jumping sensation (*palpitation*). If the heart continues to beat in an odd rhythm (*arrhythmia, dysrhythmia*), a patient may notice this as well.

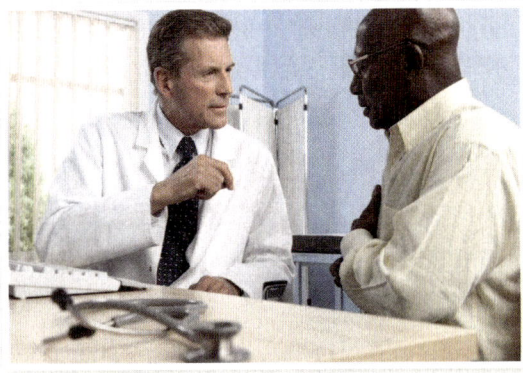

Science Photo Library/Getty Images

heart

TERM	WORD ANALYSIS
angina pectoris an-JAI-nah PEK-tor-is	angina — pectoris to choke — chest
DEFINITION oppressive pain in the chest caused by irregular blood flow to the heart	
arrhythmia ay-RITH-mee-ah	a / rrhythm / ia no / rhythm / condition
DEFINITION irregular heartbeat	
dysrhythmia dis-RITH-mee-ah	dys / rhythm / ia bad / rhythm / condition
DEFINITION irregular heartbeat (*arrhythmia* is more common)	
palpitation PAL-pih-TAY-shun	from Latin, for *to flutter*
DEFINITION rapid or irregular beating of the heart	
pectoralgia PEK-tor-AL-jah	pector / algia chest / pain
DEFINITION chest pain	

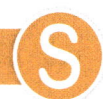

circulation

TERM	WORD ANALYSIS
aortalgia AY-or-TAL-jah	**aort / algia** aorta / pain
DEFINITION pain in the aorta	
diaphoresis DAI-ah-for-EE-sis	**dia / phoresis** through / carry
DEFINITION profuse sweating NOTE: It may seem odd to mention sweating in the heart chapter, but this is a common symptom of a heart attack.	

circulation *continued*

TERM	WORD ANALYSIS
hemorrhage HEM-oh-RIJ	**hemo / rrhage** blood / burst forth
DEFINITION loss of blood	
phlebalgia fleh-BAL-jah	**phleb / algia** vein / pain
DEFINITION pain in a vein	

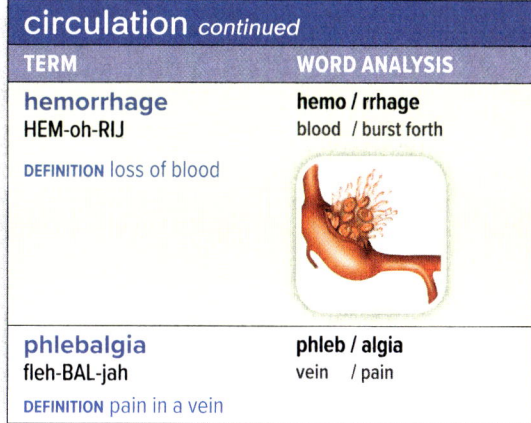

S Learning Outcome 9.2 Exercises

PRONUNCIATION

EXERCISE 1   Indicate which syllable(s) is emphasized when pronounced.

> EXAMPLE: bronchitis bron<u>chi</u>tis

1. phlebalgia _____
2. dysrhythmia _____
3. arrhythmia _____
4. angina pectoris _____

EXERCISE 2   Underline and define the word parts from this chapter in the following terms.

1. aortalgia _____
2. phlebalgia _____
3. hemorrhage _____

TRANSLATION

EXERCISE 3   Match the term on the left with its definition on the right. Some definitions may be used more than once.

_____   1. aortalgia

_____   2. phlebalgia

_____   3. pectoralgia

_____   4. arrhythmia

_____   5. dysrhythmia

_____   6. palpitation

_____   7. hemorrhage

_____   8. angina pectoris

_____   9. diaphoresis

a. oppressive pain in the chest caused by irregular blood flow to the heart

b. chest pain

c. irregular heartbeat

d. loss of blood

e. pain in a vein

f. pain in the aorta

g. profuse sweating

h. rapid or irregular beating of the heart

EXERCISE 4   Break down the following words into their component parts.

> EXAMPLE: nasopharyngoscope
> *naso | pharyngo | scope*

1. pectoralgia   _____

2. aortalgia   _____

3. phlebalgia   _____

4. arrhythmia   _____

5. dysrhythmia   _____

6. hemorrhage   _____

EXERCISE 5   Translate the following terms as literally as possible.

> EXAMPLE: nasopharyngoscope   *an instrument for looking at the nose and throat*

1. aortalgia   _____

2. phlebalgia   _____

3. pectoralgia   _____

4. arrhythmia   _____

5. dysrhythmia   _____

6. angina pectoris   _____

GENERATION

EXERCISE 6   Build a medical term from the information provided.

> EXAMPLE: inflammation of the sinuses   *sinusitis*

1. pain in a vein (use *phleb/o*)   _____

2. chest pain   _____

3. pain in the aorta   _____

4. no rhythm condition   _____

5. bad rhythm condition   _____

EXERCISE 7   Multiple-choice questions. Select the correct answer(s).

1. Select the terms that pertain to heartbeat (select all that apply).
   a. angina pectoris
   b. aortalgia
   c. arrhythmia
   d. diaphoresis
   e. hemorrhage
   f. palpitation
   g. pectoralgia
   h. phlebalgia

2. Select all the terms that pertain to pain in the heart or chest.
   a. angina pectoris
   b. aortalgia
   c. arrhythmia
   d. diaphoresis
   e. hemorrhage
   f. palpitation
   g. pectoralgia
   h. phlebalgia

3. Which of the following types of pain in the chest is caused by irregular blood flow to the heart?
   a. angina pectoris
   b. diaphoresis
   c. hemorrhage
   d. palpitation
   e. phlebalgia

4. Which of the following terms is from Latin, for *to flutter?*
   a. angina pectoris
   b. diaphoresis
   c. hemorrhage
   d. palpitation
   e. phlebalgia

5. Which of the following terms means *profuse sweating?*
   a. angina pectoris
   b. diaphoresis
   c. hemorrhage
   d. palpitation
   e. phlebalgia

6. Which of the following terms literally means *blood burst forth?*
   a. angina pectoris
   b. diaphoresis
   c. hemorrhage
   d. palpitation
   e. phlebalgia

OBJECTIVE

9.3 Observation and Discovery

During a patient consultation about a heart or circulation problem, the first thing the examiner might notice is a change in the color of the patient's skin. Patients with very poor circulation or low oxygen in their blood may appear a bit blue (*cyanosis*). Generally, cyanosis is seen in emergency situations; it signals the need for immediate action.

While skin color change may not be noted in most cardiac patients, hearts will almost always be examined by measuring patients' vital signs. The two vital signs most closely related to the heart are pulse and blood pressure. As a patient's heart squeezes, it is possible to feel throbbing when placing a finger over certain blood vessels. This is the *pulse.* A pulse is described as either strong or weak and can be a very helpful indicator in heart health. When a pulse is very weak, it may be an indication of dangerously low blood pressure (*hypotension*).

A pulse reading can also indicate how fast the patient's heart is beating (*heart rate*). If the patient's heart is beating too fast (*tachycardia*) or too slow (*bradycardia*), this may be an indication of disease. The rate at which a heart beats is controlled by electrical signals. The signals travel throughout the heart muscle fibers to get them to work together.

Have you ever noticed that in some houses the water comes out of the shower faster and harder than in others? This is due to differences in water pressure. Blood pressure works in the same way—it measures how strong the flow of blood is in the body. When a patient's heart muscle fibers are contracting and sending blood out of the ventricles, the pressure in the arteries is at its highest. This arterial pressure, the *systole,* is the first number of a blood pressure reading.

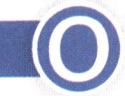

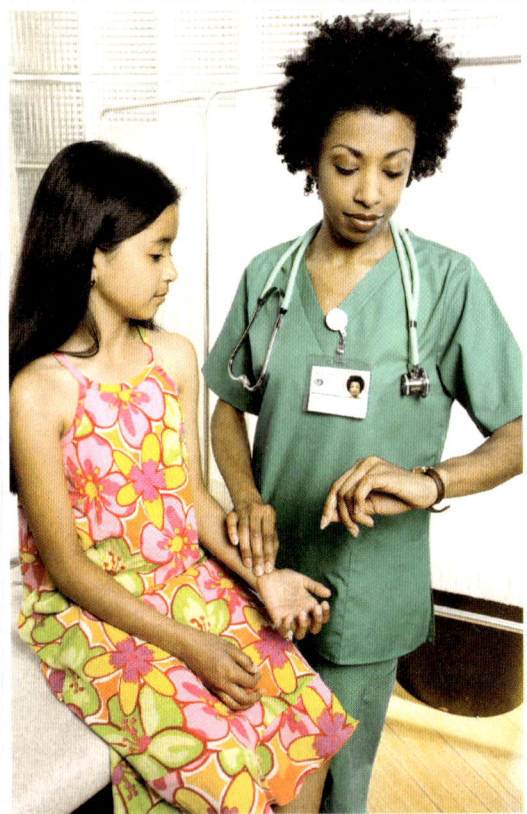

The most basic piece of observable data about the heart is the heart rate, discovered most easily through taking the patient's pulse at the wrist.

Custom Medical Stock Photo/Alamy Stock Photo

The second number of a blood pressure reading is called the *diastole*. It refers to the pressure on the vessels when the heart is relaxed and filling with blood. When a patient's blood vessels are caked with hard deposits, higher pressure is needed to force blood through them. This is the most common cause of high blood pressure *(hypertension)*. The blood pressure is another vital sign and is measured by listening to changes in the sound of blood flow through an artery as a special cuff is constricted.

Chief among the means of evaluating the heart is listening directly to the heartbeat. There are two heart sounds that are caused by the closing of valves in the heart. The first heart sound (S1) is due to the closing of the valves between the atria and ventricles. This represents the beginning of heart contraction *(systole)*. Systole ends with closing of the pulmonary and aortic valves, which creates the second heart sound (S2). When listening to the heart, the examiner listens for abnormal sounds *(murmurs)* or a disturbance in the rhythm.

Two very common tests are used to observe the heart: *electrocardiograms* and *echocardiograms.* An electrocardiogram measures the electrical signals in the heart. During the test, electrodes are placed on different parts of a patient's body and measure electrical signals from the heart. One important reason for this test is to check for signs of decreased blood flow to the heart *(ischemia)*. Sometimes a patient must exercise in order to exhibit these signs *(stress electrocardiogram)*.

An echocardiogram uses ultrahigh sound frequencies *(ultrasound)* to watch the heart as it works. With an echocardiogram, it is possible to view the layers of the heart *(pericardium, myocardium,* and *endocardium)*, the *valves,* and the wall of the heart *(septum)*. An examiner can also visualize the flow of blood through the heart. The flow through the valves may be tight *(stenosis)* or may flow back the wrong direction *(regurgitation)*.

The most common way to examine blood vessels is to inject dye into the blood and view the results using an x-ray *(angiogram)*. This type of study can show all sorts of problems, including deposits of fat *(atherosclerosis)*, a floating object that blocks blood flow *(embolus)*, a cutoff in blood flow *(occlusion)*, or the dilation of a vessel *(ectasia)*.

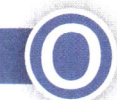
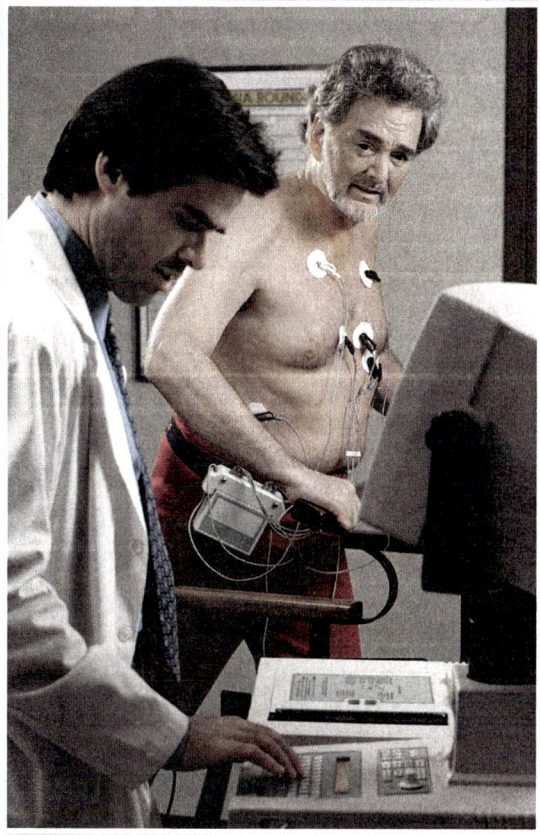

A stress electrocardiogram observes the patient's heart while the patient exercises.

Comstock/Getty Images

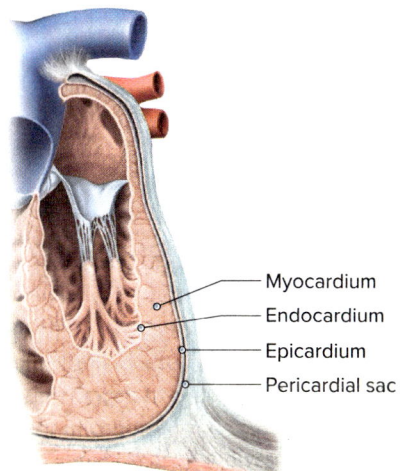

Myocardium
Endocardium
Epicardium
Pericardial sac

heart and circulation—structure

TERM	WORD ANALYSIS
endocardium EN-doh-KAR-dee-um	endo / card / ium inside / heart / tissue
DEFINITION tissue lining the inside of the heart	
epicardium EH-pee- KAR-dee-um	epi / card / ium upon / heart / tissue
DEFINITION tissue lining the outside of the heart	
myocardium MAI-oh-KAR-dee-um	myo / card / ium muscle / heart / tissue
DEFINITION heart muscle tissue	
pericardium PER-ee- KAR-dee-um	peri / card / ium around / heart / tissue
DEFINITION tissue around the heart	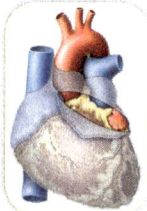
vena cava VEE-nah CAY-vah	vena cava vein hollow
DEFINITION large-diameter vein that gathers blood from the body and returns it to the heart	

heart

TERM	WORD ANALYSIS
bradycardia BRAY-dih- KAR-dee-ah	brady / card / ia slow / heart / condition
DEFINITION slow heartbeat	
cardiomegaly KAR-dee-oh-MEH-gah-lee	cardio / megaly heart / enlargement
DEFINITION enlarged heart	
murmur MIR-mir	from Latin, for *to grumble or hum*
DEFINITION abnormal heart sound	
tachycardia TAK-ih- KAR-dee-ah	tachy / card / ia fast / heart / condition
DEFINITION rapid heartbeat	

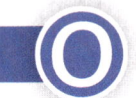

circulation

TERM	WORD ANALYSIS
aortic stenosis ay-OR-tik stih-NOH-sis	aort / ic sten / osis aorta / pertaining to narrow / condition

DEFINITION narrowing of the aorta

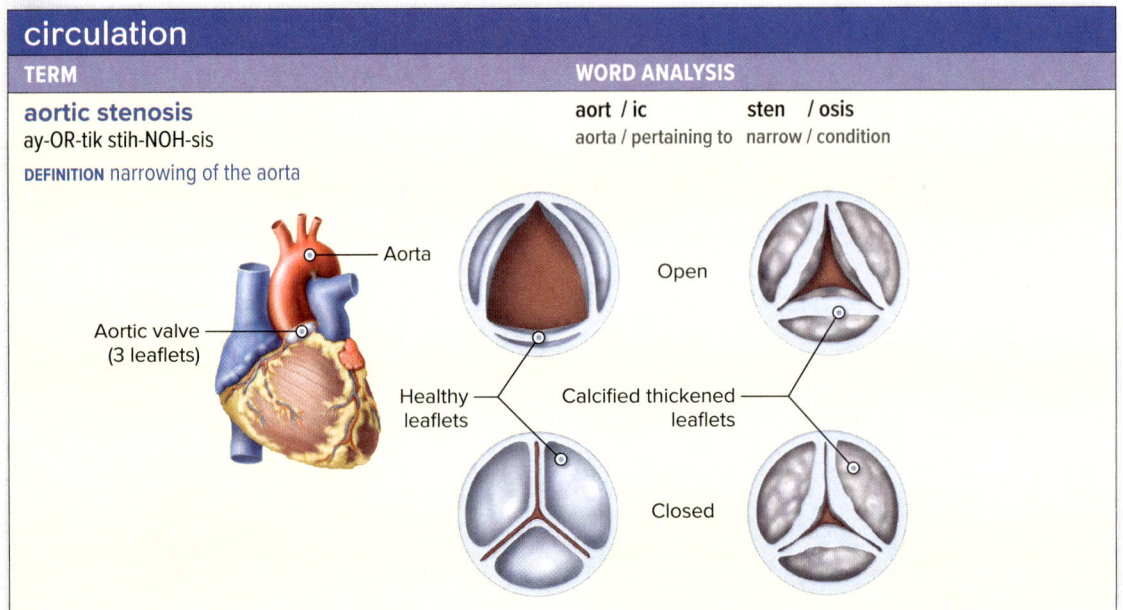

Aorta

Aortic valve
(3 leaflets)

Healthy
leaflets

Calcified thickened
leaflets

Open

Closed

---

circulation *continued*

TERM	WORD ANALYSIS
arteriorrhexis ar-TER-ee-oh-REK-sis	arterio / rrhexis artery / rupture

DEFINITION rupture of an artery

TERM	WORD ANALYSIS
arteriosclerosis ar-TER-ee-oh-skleh-ROH-sis	arterio / scler / osis artery / hard / condition

DEFINITION hardening of an artery

TERM	WORD ANALYSIS
atherosclerosis A-ther-oh-skleh-ROH-sis	athero / scler / osis fatty plaque / hard / condition

Normal   Plaque

DEFINITION hardening of an artery due to buildup of fatty plaque

---

circulation *continued*

TERM	WORD ANALYSIS
embolus EM-boh-lus	em / bolus in / throw

DEFINITION mass of matter present in the blood
NOTE: In Greek, this word was used to mean *stopper,* as in the opening of a bottle.

TERM	WORD ANALYSIS
embolism EM-boh-LIZ-um	embol / ism embolus / condition

DEFINITION blockage in a blood vessel caused by an embolus

TERM	WORD ANALYSIS
ischemia ih-SKEE-mee-ah	isch / emia hold back / blood condition

DEFINITION blockage of blood flow to an organ

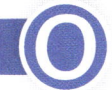

circulation *continued*

TERM	WORD ANALYSIS
occlusion oh-KLOO-zhun	from Latin, for *to close off*

DEFINITION closing or blockage of a passage

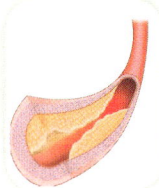

TERM	WORD ANALYSIS
thrombus THROM-bus	from Greek, for *lump, clot, or even curd of milk*

DEFINITION blood clot

NOTE: The difference between a thrombus and an embolus is twofold. A *thrombus* is a clot of blood and is stationary. An *embolus* is foreign material and is in motion. When a thrombus breaks off, it becomes a *thromboembolus*.

TERM	WORD ANALYSIS
varicose veins VAR-ih-kohs VAYNS	varicose veins swollen, twisted veins

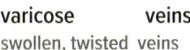

DEFINITION enlarged, dilated veins toward the surface of the skin

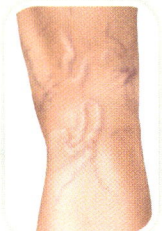

diagnostic procedures

TERM	WORD ANALYSIS
cardiac catheterization KAR-dee-ak KATH-eh-ter-ih-ZAY-shun	cardi / ac heart / pertaining to catheter / ization catheter / procedure

DEFINITION process of inserting a tube (catheter) into the heart
NOTE: The word *catheter* comes from Greek words meaning *to go inside*. By passing a tube through arteries, doctors are able to diagnose and treat heart problems without performing major surgery.

TERM	WORD ANALYSIS
echocardiogram EK-oh-KAR-dee-oh-GRAM	echo / cardio / gram echo / heart / record

DEFINITION image of the heart produced using sound waves; the same procedure as an ultrasound performed on pregnant women, but instead it is performed on a heart

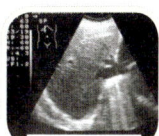

Steve Allen/Getty Images

TERM	WORD ANALYSIS
echocardiography EK-oh-KAR-dee-AW-grah-fee	echo / cardio / graphy echo / heart / writing procedure

DEFINITION use of sound waves to produce an image of the heart; the same procedure as an ultrasound performed on pregnant women, but instead it is performed on a heart

TERM	WORD ANALYSIS
electrocardiogram eh-LEK-troh-KAR-dee-oh-GRAM	electro / cardio / gram electricity / heart / record

DEFINITION record of the electrical currents of the heart

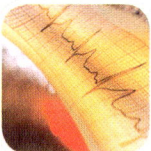

Brand X/Getty Images

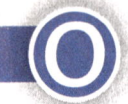

diagnostic procedures *continued*

TERM	WORD ANALYSIS	
electrocardiography eh-LEK-troh-KAR-dee-AW-grah-fee	electro / cardio / graphy electricity / heart / writing procedure	
DEFINITION procedure for recording the electrical currents of the heart		
transesophageal echocardiogram TRANZ-eh-SOF-ah-JEE-al EK-oh-KAR-dee-oh-GRAM	trans / esophag / eal through / esophagus / pertaining to	
	echo / cardio / gram echo / heart / record	
DEFINITION record of the heart using sound waves performed by inserting the transducer into the esophagus		

radiology

TERM	WORD ANALYSIS
angiogram AN-jee-oh-GRAM	angio / gram vessel / record
DEFINITION record of the blood vessels	
angiography AN-jee-AW-grah-fee	angio / graphy vessel / writing procedure
DEFINITION procedure to describe the blood vessels	
arteriogram ar-TER-ee-oh-GRAM	arterio / gram artery / record
DEFINITION record of an artery	
venogram VEE-noh-gram	veno / gram vein / record
DEFINITION record of a vein	

professional terms

TERM	WORD ANALYSIS		
blood pressure blud PRESH-ir	blood pressure		
DEFINITION the force exerted by blood on the walls of blood vessels			

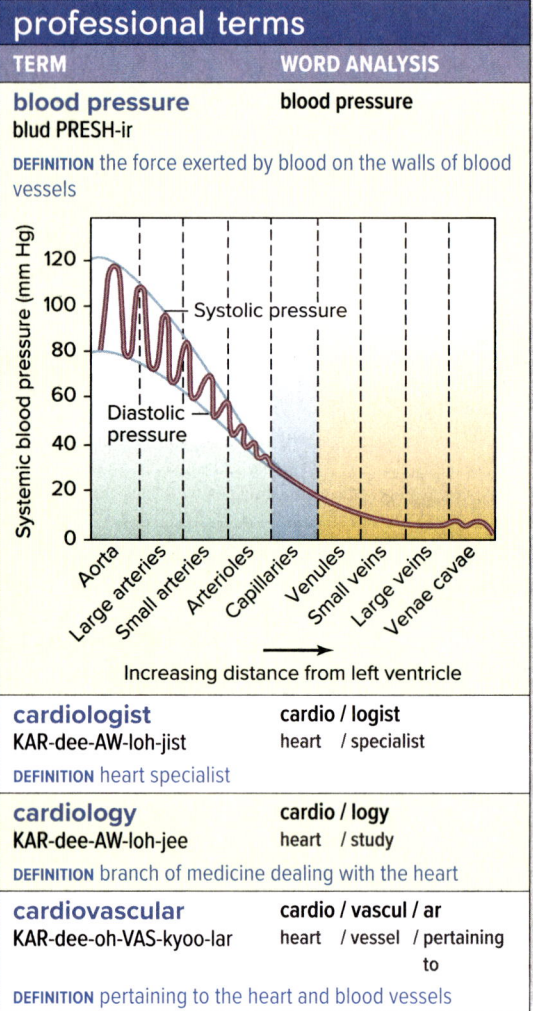

cardiologist KAR-dee-AW-loh-jist	cardio / logist heart / specialist		
DEFINITION heart specialist			
cardiology KAR-dee-AW-loh-jee	cardio / logy heart / study		
DEFINITION branch of medicine dealing with the heart			
cardiovascular KAR-dee-oh-VAS-kyoo-lar	cardio / vascul / ar heart / vessel / pertaining to		
DEFINITION pertaining to the heart and blood vessels			

PRONUNCIATION

EXERCISE 1   Indicate which syllable(s) is emphasized when pronounced.

> EXAMPLE: bronchitis bron<u>chi</u>tis

1. murmur _____

2. thrombus _____

3. embolus _____

4. venogram _____

5. ischemia _____

6. occlusion _____

7. varicose veins _____

8. aortic stenosis _____

TRANSLATION

EXERCISE 2   Break down the following words into their component parts.

> EXAMPLE: synesthesia   *syn | es | the | sia*

1. cardiology _____

2. angiography _____

3. aortic stenosis _____

4. echocardiography _____

5. electrocardiography _____

3. angiogram _____

4. arteriogram _____

5. venogram _____

6. arteriorrhexis _____

7. atherosclerosis _____

8. vena cava _____

9. echocardiogram _____

10. electrocardiogram _____

11. transesophageal echocardiogram _____

12. cardiovascular (2 roots) _____

13. coronary circulation _____

EXERCISE 3   Underline and define the word parts from this chapter in the following terms.

1. cardiologist _____

2. cardiomegaly _____

EXERCISE 4   Select the correct option for each given translation.

> EXAMPLE: hypoglycemia   *hypo over | <u>under</u>   glyc salt | <u>sugar</u>   -emia <u>blood</u> | urine condition*

1. *tachycardia* = fast/slow (*tachy*) + heart condition (*cardia*)

2. *bradycardia* = fast/slow (*brady*) + heart condition (*cardia*)

3. *arteriosclerosis* = artery/blood vessel/vein (*arterio*) + hard condition (*sclerosis*)

EXERCISE 5   Fill in the blanks.

1. *myocardium* = heart _____ tissue

2. *pericardium* = tissue _____ the heart

3. *endocardium* = tissue lining the _____ of the heart

4. *epicardium* = tissue lining the _____ of the heart

EXERCISE 6 Match the term on the left with its definition on the right.

_____ 1. murmur

_____ 2. varicose veins

_____ 3. occlusion

_____ 4. ischemia

_____ 5. embolus

_____ 6. thrombus

a. abnormal heart sound

b. blood clot; from Greek, for *lump, clot,* or even *curd of milk*

c. mass of matter present in the blood; from Greek, for *stopper,* as in the opening of a bottle

d. enlarged, dilated vein toward the surface of the skin

e. blockage of blood flow to an organ

f. closing or blockage of a passage; from Latin, for *to close off*

EXERCISE 7 Translate the following terms as literally as possible.

> EXAMPLE: **nasopharyngoscope**   *an instrument for looking at the nose and throat*

1. cardiovascular _____

2. endocardium _____

3. epicardium _____

4. myocardium _____

5. pericardium _____

6. bradycardia _____

7. tachycardia _____

8. angiography _____

9. atherosclerosis _____

10. arteriorrhexis _____

GENERATION

EXERCISE 8 Build a medical term from the information provided.

> EXAMPLE: **inflammation of the sinuses**   *sinusitis*

1. study of the heart _____

2. record of a vein (use *ven/o*) _____

3. record of the blood vessels (use *angi/o*)

_____

4. record of an artery _____

5. hardening of an artery _____

6. enlarged heart _____

7. record of the electrical currents of the heart

_____

EXERCISE 9 Multiple-choice questions. Select the correct answer(s).

1. A *transesophageal echocardiogram* is
   a. a record of the heart using sound waves performed by inserting the transducer into the esophagus
   b. an image of the heart produced using sound waves while the patient experiences increases of exercise stress
   c. a procedure to look inside blood vessels that are currently undergoing stress
   d. none of these

2. Which of the following statements about the term *echocardiogram* are true? (Select all that apply.)
   a. image of the heart produced using sound waves
   b. image of the heart produced using electrical currents

c. procedure to look inside blood vessels

d. ultrasound of the heart

3. *Blood pressure* is (select all that apply)
   a. from Latin, for *to go in a circle*
   b. the force exerted by blood on the walls of vessels
   c. the moving of blood from the heart through the vessels and back to the heart
   d. none of these

4. A blockage in a blood vessel caused by a mass of matter present in the blood is known as a(n)
   a. atherosclerosis   c. thrombus
   b. embolism   d. arteriosclerosis

5. The hardening of an artery due to buildup of plaque is known as
   a. atherosclerosis   c. thrombus
   b. embolism   d. arteriosclerosis

6. An abnormal heart sound is a
   a. cardiac anomaly   c. coronary anomaly
   b. cardiophony   d. murmur

7. Which of the following statements about the term *cardiac catheterization* are true? (Select all that apply.)
   a. It is the process of inserting a tube into the heart.
   b. Doctors are able to diagnose and treat heart problems without performing major surgery by performing this process.
   c. It comes from the root *cardio,* meaning heart, and Greek words meaning *to go inside.*
   d. None of these.

EXERCISE 10 Briefly describe the difference between each pair of terms.

1. echocardiography, electrocardiography

   _____

2. embolus, embolism

   _____

3. embolus, thrombus

   _____

4. ischemia, occlusion

   _____

9.4 Diagnosis and Pathology

Problems with the heart can begin even before birth. Patients may be born with flaws in the structure of their heart (*congenital heart defect*). Among the most common flaws are holes in the wall of the heart (*atrial septal defect* and *ventricular septal defect*).

Another type of flaw the heart can have is in its electrical system. A problem with electrical signals can cause an abnormal rhythm in the heartbeat (*arrhythmia, dysrhythmia*). Some rhythm problems are very minor and don't even require treatment. Others, such as *ventricular fibrillation,* are medical emergencies. Ventricular fibrillation occurs when the main squeezing muscle fibers of the heart do not coordinate. As a result, no blood flow occurs. Unless treated, a patient will likely die of the condition.

When the muscle fibers of the heart do not work as well as they are supposed to (*cardiomyopathy*), the heart may cease to function properly (*cardiac insufficiency*). These problems usually develop over time. Cardiomyopathies can involve muscle that is too floppy (*dilated*), too tight (*restrictive*), or too weak (*congestive*). One type involves muscle that is too thick (*hypertrophic*) and can cause sudden death while a person is playing sports. This is a major reason for physical exams prior to playing sports.

The heart is not a common site for infection, but when it does become infected, the condition is usually very serious. Infection can be inside the muscle (*myocarditis*) or along the lining of the heart and vessels (*endocarditis*).

The heart can be inflamed as a result of other illnesses as well. One site for inflammation is the thin lining on the outside of the heart (*pericarditis*), which can cause fluid to collect around the heart (*pericardial effusion*) and make it more difficult for the heart to work well.

The most common heart problem involves the blood supply to the muscle fibers of the heart. Just as the rest of the body needs blood to take in nutrients

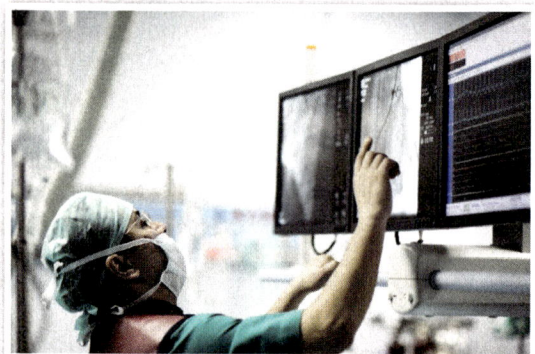

Imaging procedures are the most frequently used tools doctors use to diagnose heart issues.
UygarGeographic/Getty Images

and remove harmful waste, the heart needs it too. Coronary arteries serve this purpose. Floating fat in the blood (*cholesterol*) can accumulate and harden in the arteries of the heart. This process is called *atherosclerosis.* When the coronary arteries get blocked enough that it prevents sufficient blood flow, the heart muscle fibers do not get the oxygen they need. As a result, the muscle dies—a heart attack (*myocardial infarction*).

Common to all heart problems is the possibility of the heart failing to adequately pump the blood to the rest of the body (*congestive heart failure*). The heart's inability to pump all the blood that reaches it creates a bottleneck effect, which leads to fluid accumulation in the lungs or body. The symptoms of heart failure depend on which side of the heart is affected.

Other blood vessel problems include a blockage (*deep vein thrombosis*) or bulge (*aneurysm*) in the vessel. Vessels can also become inflamed. An inflamed vein (*phlebitis*) is usually a problem involving just one part of a single vein. Inflammation of several blood vessels (*vasculitis*) can present in many different ways, depending on the type of vessels affected.

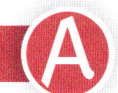

heart

TERM	WORD ANALYSIS
atrial septal defect (ASD) AY-tree-al SEP-tal DEE-fekt **DEFINITION** flaw in the septum that divides the two atria of the heart	atri / al atrium / pertaining to sept / al septum / pertaining to de / fect bad / made

Mixing blood from left (oxygenated) and right (unoxygenated) atria

Atrial septal defect

cardiac arrest KAR-dee-ak ah-REST **DEFINITION** cessation of functional circulation	cardi / ac arrest heart / pertaining to stop
cardiomyopathy KAR-dee-oh-mai-AW-pah-thee **DEFINITION** disease of the heart muscle	cardio / myo / pathy heart / muscle / disease
congenital heart defect con-JEN-ih-tal HART DEE-fekt **DEFINITION** flaw in the structure of the heart present at birth	con / genit / al together / birth / pertaining to heart de / fect heart bad / made
congestive heart failure con-JES-tiv HART FAYL-yir **DEFINITION** heart failure characterized by the heart cavity being unable to pump all the blood out of itself (*congestive*)	con / gest / ive together / bring / pertaining to heart failure
endocarditis EN-doh-kar-DAI-tis **DEFINITION** inflammation of the tissue lining the inside of the heart	endo / card / itis inside / heart / inflammation

heart *continued*

TERM	WORD ANALYSIS
myocardial infarction MAI-oh-KAR-dee-al in-FARK-shun **DEFINITION** death of heart muscle tissue NOTE: The term *infarction* originally referred to a blocked blood vessel, but it came to refer to the death of tissue resulting from the blockage.	myo / cardi / al muscle / heart / pertaining to in / farct / ion in / stuff / condition
myocardial ischemia MAI-oh-KAR-dee-al ih-SKEE-mee-ah **DEFINITION** blockage of blood to the heart muscle	myo / cardi / al muscle / heart / pertaining to isch / emia hold back / blood condition
myocarditis MAI-oh-kar-DAI-tis **DEFINITION** inflammation of the heart muscle	myo / card / itis muscle / heart / inflammation
pericarditis PER-ee-kar-DAI-tis **DEFINITION** inflammation of the tissue around the heart	peri / card / itis around / heart / inflammation
ventricular septal defect (VSD) ven-TRIK-yoo-lar SEP-tal DEE-fekt **DEFINITION** flaw in the septum that divides the two ventricles of the heart	ventricul / ar ventricle / pertaining to sept / al septum / pertaining to de / fect bad / made

circulation

TERM	WORD ANALYSIS
aneurysm AN-yir-IZ-um **DEFINITION** bulge in a blood vessel NOTE: The *an-* prefix here doesn't meet *not;* rather, it is short for *ana* and means *up* or *out.* The *not* meaning is much more common, but there are also a few important examples of the *up/out* meaning, such as *anabolic.*	an / eury / sm up / wide / condition

circulation *continued*

TERM	WORD ANALYSIS
angioma AN-jee-OH-mah	angi / oma vessel / tumor
DEFINITION blood vessel tumor	

Nau Nau/Shutterstock

TERM	WORD ANALYSIS
arteriopathy ar-TER-ee-AW-pah-thee	arterio / pathy artery / disease
DEFINITION disease of the arteries	
arteritis AR-ter-AI-tis	arter / itis artery / inflammation
DEFINITION inflammation of the arteries	
deep vein thrombosis DEEP VAYN throm-BOH-sis	deep vein deep vein thromb / osis clot / condition
DEFINITION formation of a blood clot in a vein deep in the body, most commonly the leg	

circulation *continued*

TERM	WORD ANALYSIS
hypertension HAI-per-TEN-shun	hyper / tens / ion over / stretch / condition
DEFINITION high blood pressure	
hypotension HAI-poh-TEN-shun	hypo / tens / ion under / stretch / condition
DEFINITION low blood pressure	
phlebitis fleh-BAI-tis	phleb / itis vein / inflammation
DEFINITION inflammation of the veins	
thrombophlebitis THROM-boh-fleh-BAI-tis	thrombo / phleb / itis clot / vein / inflammation
DEFINITION inflammation of vein caused by a clot	

TRANSLATION

EXERCISE 1 Break down the following words into their component parts.

> EXAMPLE: **nasopharyngoscope**
> *naso | pharyngo | scope*

1. angioma _____
2. arteritis _____
3. phlebitis _____
4. endocarditis _____
5. myocarditis _____
6. pericarditis _____
7. cardiomyopathy _____
8. myocardial ischemia _____

EXERCISE 2 Underline and define the word parts from this chapter in the following terms.

1. cardiac arrest _____
2. arteriopathy _____
3. thrombophlebitis _____
4. myocardial infarction (2 roots) _____
5. atrial septal defect (2 roots) _____
6. ventricular septal defect (2 roots) _____

EXERCISE 3 Match the term on the left with its definition on the right.

_____ 1. hypertension   a. bulge in a blood vessel

_____ 2. hypotension   b. flaw in the structure of the heart, present at birth

_____ 3. deep vein thrombosis   c. heart failure characterized by the heart cavity being unable to pump all the blood out of itself

_____ 4. congestive heart failure   d. high blood pressure

_____ 5. congenital heart defect   e. low blood pressure

_____ 6. aneurysm   f. formation of a blood clot in a vein deep in the body, most commonly the leg

EXERCISE 4 Translate the following terms as literally as possible.

> EXAMPLE: **nasopharyngoscope** *an instrument for looking at the nose and throat*

1. arteriopathy _____
2. atrial septal defect _____
3. ventricular septal defect _____

GENERATION

EXERCISE 5 Build a medical term from the information provided.

> EXAMPLE: **inflammation of the sinuses** *sinusitis*

1. inflammation of the veins (use *phleb/o*)
_____

2. blood vessel tumor (use *angi/o*)
_____

3. inflammation of the arteries
_____

4. inflammation of the heart vessels
_____

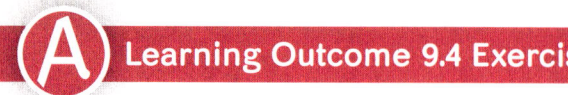
5. inflammation of the heart muscle

_____

6. disease of the heart muscle

_____

7. inflammation of the tissue lining the inside of
the heart _____

8. inflammation of the tissue around the heart

_____

9. inflammation of a vein caused by a clot

_____

EXERCISE 6 Multiple-choice questions. Select the correct
answer.

1. _Cardiac arrest_ is
   a. bulge in a blood vessel
   b. cessation of functional circulation
   c. death of heart muscle tissue
   d. fluid pouring out into the tissue around the
   heart
   e. flow of blood backward from the aorta back
   into the heart

2. An _aneurysm_ is
   a. bulge in a blood vessel
   b. cessation of functional circulation
   c. death of heart muscle tissue
   d. fluid pouring out into the tissue around the
   heart
   e. flow of blood backward from the aorta back
   into the heart

3. The formation of a blood clot in a vein deep in
the body, most commonly the leg, is known as
   a. aneurysm
   b. angioedema
   c. angioma
   d. deep vein thrombosis
   e. thrombophlebitis

EXERCISE 7 Briefly describe the difference between each pair
of terms.

1. hypertension, hypotension _____

2. congenital heart defect, congestive heart failure

_____

3. myocardial infarction, myocardial ischemia

_____

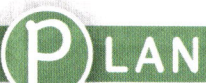

P **LAN**

9.5 Treatments and Therapies

Medications for treating the heart deal with alleviating the pain associated with low oxygen to the heart (_antianginal_) and with correcting the heart's electrical signals (_antiarrhythmics_). Medicines can also work on blood vessels. They can cause the vessels to squeeze down (_vasoconstrictor, vasopressor_), which causes blood pressure to increase, or they can cause them to dilate (_vasodilator_), which lowers the blood pressure. _Thrombolytics_ can work on both the heart and blood vessels. They work by breaking down dangerous accumulations that can develop in the heart or blood vessels.

In the past, the vast majority of procedures to physically correct heart problems used to include cutting open the patient's chest (_cardiothoracic surgery_) for direct access to the heart. While these more invasive means are now less common, they are still necessary for some types of surgeries such as making an alternate blood vessel route (_anastomosis_) for congenital heart defects. A similar procedure is a very common treatment for blocked heart vessels. In a procedure known as _coronary artery bypass graft,_ a blood vessel from another part of the body is used to make an alternate route for blood to get to the heart around

an area of blockage. This is the most common type of heart surgery. Now, less invasive techniques are often preferred. One such treatment for coronary artery disease involves passing instruments up a patient's blood vessels into the heart (*percutaneous coronary intervention*). Once the instrument is inside the coronary artery, there are several options for treatment. A balloon can be inflated to crush the buildup (*balloon angioplasty*), a mesh tube can be inserted (*stent*), or the buildup can be destroyed (*atherectomy*).

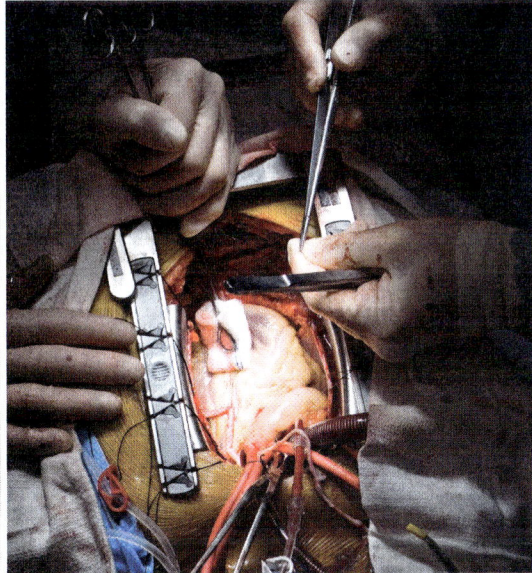

Though less-invasive techniques have been developed in recent years for a variety of heart procedures, for certain procedures—such as coronary artery bypass surgery—doctors still must employ cardiothoracic surgery.

aaM Photography, Ltd./Getty Images

pharmacology

TERM	WORD ANALYSIS			
antianginal AN-tee-AN-jih-nal	anti against	/ angin / *angina* (choke)	/ al / agent	
DEFINITION drug that prevents or relieves the symptoms of angina pectoris				
antiarrhythmic AN-tee-a-RITH-mik	anti against	/ a / no	/ rrhythm / rhythm	/ ic / agent
DEFINITION drug that opposes an irregular heartbeat				
anticoagulant AN-tee-koh-AG-yoo-lant	anti against	/ coagul / coagulation	/ ant / agent	
DEFINITION drug that opposes the coagulation of the blood				
antihypertensive AN-tee-HAI-per-TEN-siv	anti against	/ hyper / over	/ tens / stretch	/ ive / agent
DEFINITION drug that opposes high blood pressure				
thrombolytic THROM-boh-LIH-tik	thrombo clot	/ lyt / loose	/ ic / agent	
DEFINITION drug that breaks down clots				

Steve Gschmeissner/ Science Source

TERM	WORD ANALYSIS		
vasoconstrictor VAS-oh-kin-STRIK-tor	vaso vessel	/ constrict / narrowing	/ or / agent
DEFINITION drug that constricts or narrows the diameter of a blood vessel			
vasodilator VAS-oh-DAI-lay-tor	vaso vessel	/ dilat / expanding	/ or / agent
DEFINITION drug that causes the relaxation or expansion of a blood vessel			
vasopressor VAS-oh-PRES-or	vaso vessel	/ press / press	/ or / agent
DEFINITION drug that constricts or narrows the diameter of a blood vessel			

heart procedures

TERM	WORD ANALYSIS
cardiopulmonary bypass KAR-dee-oh-PUL-mon-AR-ee BAI-pas	cardio / pulmon / ary heart / lung / pertaining to **bypass**

DEFINITION procedure that temporarily circulates and oxygenates a patient's blood during the portion of heart surgery in which the heart is stopped

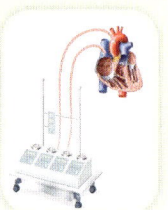

| **cardiopulmonary resuscitation (CPR)**
 KAR-dee-oh-PUL-mon-AR-ee re-SIS-ih-TAY-shun | cardio / pulmon / ary <br> heart / lung / pertaining to <br> re / suscit / ation <br> again / stir up / procedure |

DEFINITION basic life support
NOTE: Despite its name, CPR does not actually *resuscitate* an unconscious patient. Rather, through artificial breathing and chest compression, an unresponsive patient's blood circulates and is kept oxygenated until further steps can be taken.

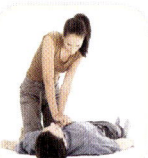

Stockbyte Platinum/ Alamy Stock Photo

| **cardioversion**
 KAR-dee-oh-VER-zhun | cardio / vers / ion <br> heart / turn / procedure |

DEFINITION returning a heart to normal rhythm

| **coronary artery bypass graft (CABG)**
 KOR-ah-NAR-ee AR-ter-ee BAI-pas GRAFT | coronary artery bypass graft |

DEFINITION borrowed piece of blood vessel used to bypass a blocked artery in the heart

heart procedures *continued*

TERM	WORD ANALYSIS
coronary artery bypass surgery KOR-ah-NAR-ee AR-ter-ee BAI-pas SIR-jir-ee	coronary artery bypass surgery

DEFINITION surgery to bypass a blocked artery in the heart

| **percutaneous coronary intervention**
 PER-koo-TAY-nee-us KOR-ah-NAR-ee IN-ter-VEN-shun | per / cutane / ous <br> through / skin / pertaining to <br> coron / ary <br> heart / pertaining to <br> intervention |

DEFINITION alternate treatment for a coronary artery that passes instruments up a patient's blood vessels into the heart

| **valvotomy**
 val-VAW-toh-mee | valvo / tomy <br> valve / incision |

DEFINITION incision into a heart valve
NOTE: Alternative spelling *valvulotomy*, using *valvulo*, is also acceptable.

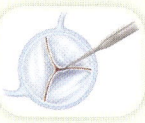

| **valvuloplasty**
 VAL-voo-loh-PLAS-tee | valvulo / plasty <br> valve / reconstruction |

DEFINITION surgical reconstruction of a heart valve

circulation procedures

TERM	WORD ANALYSIS
angioplasty AN-jee-oh-PLAS-tee	angio / plasty vessel / reconstruction

DEFINITION surgical reconstruction of a vessel

| **angiorrhaphy**
 AN-jee-OR-ah-fee | angio / rrhaphy <br> vessel / suture |

DEFINITION suture of a vessel

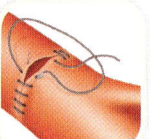

| **aortorrhaphy**
 ay-or-TOR-ah-fee | aorto / rrhaphy <br> aorta / suture |

DEFINITION suture of the aorta

9.5 Treatments and Therapies

circulation procedures *continued*	
TERM	**WORD ANALYSIS**
arteriorrhaphy ar-TER-ee-OR-ah-fee	arterio / rrhaphy artery / suture
DEFINITION suture of an artery	
atherectomy A-ther-EK-toh-mee	ather / ectomy fatty plaque / removal
DEFINITION surgical removal of fatty plaque within an artery	

circulation procedures *continued*	
TERM	**WORD ANALYSIS**
endarterectomy END-ar-ter-EK-toh-me	end / arter / ectomy inside / artery / removal
DEFINITION surgical removal of the inside of an artery	
phlebectomy fleb- EK-toh-mee	phleb / ectomy vein / removal
DEFINITION surgical removal of a vein	

Learning Outcome 9.5 Exercises

PRONUNCIATION

EXERCISE 1   Indicate which syllable(s) is emphasized when pronounced.

EXAMPLE: bronchitis bron<u>chi</u>tis

1. angioplasty (2 syllables) _____
2. valvotomy _____
3. cardioversion (2 syllables) _____
4. phlebectomy _____

TRANSLATION

EXERCISE 2   Break down the following words into their component parts.

EXAMPLE: nasopharyngoscope
naso | pharyngo | scope

1. vasodilator _____
2. angioplasty _____
3. antihypertensive _____
4. anticoagulant _____
5. thrombolytic _____
6. embolectomy _____
7. cardioversion _____

EXERCISE 3   Underline and define the word parts from this chapter in the following terms.

1. atherectomy _____
2. phlebectomy _____
3. endarterectomy _____

4. valvotomy _____   8. arteriorrhaphy _____

5. valvuloplasty _____   9. vasoconstrictor _____

6. angiorrhaphy _____   10. percutaneous coronary intervention _____

7. aortorrhaphy _____   11. cardiopulmonary bypass _____

EXERCISE 4   Match the term on the left with its definition on the right.

_____   1. coronary artery bypass surgery

a. borrowed piece of blood vessel used to bypass a blocked artery in the heart

_____   2. coronary artery bypass graft

b. drug that opposes an irregular heartbeat

_____   3. antiarrhythmic

c. drug that prevents or relieves the symptoms of angina pectoris

_____   4. cardiopulmonary resuscitation

d. alternate treatment for the coronary artery that passes instruments up a patient's blood vessels into the heart

_____   5. percutaneous coronary intervention

e. basic life support: artificial breathing and chest compression

_____   6. antianginal

f. surgery to bypass a blocked artery in the heart

EXERCISE 5   Translate the following terms as literally as possible.

> EXAMPLE: *nasopharyngoscope*   *an instrument for looking at the nose and throat*

1. valvuloplasty _____

2. angioplasty _____

3. angiorrhaphy _____

4. aortorrhaphy _____

5. arteriorrhaphy _____

6. vasoconstrictor _____

7. vasodilator _____

8. cardioversion _____

EXERCISE 6   Fill in the blanks.

1. *antihypertensive* = drug that opposes _____
_____

2. *anticoagulant* = drug that opposes _____
_____

3. *thrombolytic* = drug that _____
_____

4. *antiarrhythmic* = drug that opposes a(n)
_____

5. *antianginal* = drug that prevents or relieves the symptoms of _____

GENERATION

EXERCISE 7 Build a medical term from the information provided.

> EXAMPLE: inflammation of the sinuses *sinusitis*

1. surgical removal of a vein (use *phleb/o*)

   _____

2. incision into a heart valve

   _____

3. surgical removal of the inside of an artery

   _____

4. surgical removal of fatty plaque (within an artery) _____

EXERCISE 8 Multiple-choice questions. Select the correct answer.

1. A procedure that temporarily circulates and oxygenates a patient's blood during the portion of heart surgery in which the heart is stopped is known as
   a. anastomosis
   b. cardiopulmonary bypass
   c. cardiopulmonary resuscitation
   d. percutaneous coronary intervention
   e. none of these

2. Which of the following statements about the abbreviation *CPR* is NOT true?
   a. It is basic life support.
   b. It keeps a patient's blood circulating and oxygenated.
   c. It is a process of artificial breathing and chest compression.
   d. It resuscitates an unconscious patient.
   e. It stands for cardiopulmonary resuscitation.

EXERCISE 9 Briefly describe the difference between each pair of terms.

1. vasoconstrictor, vasodilator _____

   _____

2. coronary artery bypass graft, coronary artery bypass surgery _____

   _____

9.6 Electronic Health Records

Cardiology Admission Note

 Subjective

Chief Complaint: VSD, postop.

History of Present Illness:

Sharon Jackson is a 12-month-old female with a history of **VSD** first discovered on **echocardiogram** shortly after birth. She has been followed by cardiology. She had been **hemodynamically** stable until the past month, when her parents noticed that she had increased difficulty eating. She would sweat after eating and become **cyanotic** with exertion. Her mother followed up with Sharon's **cardiologist,** who sent her to our office for consult.

Sharon's symptoms were consistent with congestive heart failure. It was decided to surgically correct her VSD. She underwent a sternotomy and atriotomy for patch placement in the ventricular septum to correct her VSD. This was performed with cardiopulmonary bypass under the guidance of a perfusionist. Sharon tolerated the procedure well and is now being admitted for postoperative observation and care.

Review of Systems: No fever, cough, congestion, vomiting, diarrhea.

Medications: IV antibiotics.

Allergies: No known drug allergies.

Past Medical History: Noncontributory.

Past Surgical History: None.

Social History: Stays at home with mother.

Two school-aged siblings.

Family History: Noncontributory.

 Objective

Vital Signs: Temp: 99.2; Heart rate: 94; Respiratory rate: 26; Blood pressure: 94/64.

Physical Exam

General: Sedated and intubated.

Head: NCAT. Mucous membranes moist. PERRLA.

Cardiovascular: RRR with soft systolic murmur.

Respiratory: CTA.

Abdomen: Soft, nontender, nondistended.

Neurologic: Sedated.

Skin: No cyanosis, clubbing, edema.

Labs: CBC normal.

Imaging: CXR–No cardiomegaly.

ImageSource/Getty Images

 Assessment

1. Postop for VSD repair—routine postop orders and care.

2. When patient switches to PO, we will d/c IV ABx, and at discharge, she will continue antibiotics as needed for endocarditis prophylaxis.

—Miles O'Keefe, PA

EXERCISE 1   Match the term on the left with its definition on the right.

_C_   1. cardiology

_g_   2. cardiologist

_d_   3. cardiomegaly

_b_   4. echocardiogram

_h_   5. endocarditis

_e_   6. ventricular septal defect

_f_   7. congestive heart failure

_a_   8. cardiopulmonary bypass

a. procedure that temporarily circulates and oxygenates a patient's blood during a portion of heart surgery in which the heart is stopped

b. image of the heart produced using sound waves; the same procedure as an ultrasound performed on pregnant women, but instead is performed on the heart

c. branch of medicine dealing with the heart

d. enlarged heart

e. flaw in the septum that divides the two ventricles of the heart

f. heart failure characterized by the heart cavity being unable to pump all the blood out of itself

g. heart specialist

h. inflammation of the tissue lining the inside of the heart

EXERCISE 2   Fill in the blanks.

1. Using the data recorded at the patient's physical examination, fill in the following blanks.

   a. T: _____

   b. HR: _____

   c. RR: _____

   d. Cardiovascular (*give definition:* _____
   _____
   _____)

2. According to the history of present illness, Sharon's symptoms were consistent with *congestive heart failure* (give abbreviation:
   _____).

3. Sharon's sternotomy (*sterno* = sternum + *tomy* = _____) and atriotomy were performed with _____
   (a procedure that temporarily circulates and oxygenates a patient's blood during a portion of heart surgery in which the heart is stopped).

EXERCISE 3   True or false questions. Indicate true answers with a T and false answers with an F.

1. The patient is 12 years old. _F_____

2. The patient has a Hx of ventricular septal defect. _T_____

3. The patient's VSD was first discovered on EKG shortly after birth. _____

4. The patient has CHF. _T_____

5. The patient has an enlarged heart. _____

6. The patient will not need to continue her antibiotics once she is discharged. _F_____

EXERCISE 4   Multiple-choice questions. Select the correct answer(s).

1. Sharon underwent an *atriotomy.* Which of the following is an accurate breakdown of the term?

   a. *atrio* (aorta) + *tomy* (cut) = incision into the upper chamber of the heart

   b. *atrio* (aorta) + *tomy* (removal) = incision into the lower chamber of the heart

c. *atrio* (atrium) + *tomy* (cut) = incision into the lower chamber of the heart

d. *atrio* (atrium) + *tomy* (cut) = incision into the upper chamber of the heart

e. *atrio* (atrium) + *tomy* (removal) = incision into the upper chamber of the heart

2. To correct her VSD, a patch was placed on Sharon's *ventricular septum.* Select all that apply to the term *ventricular septum:*

   a. Septum comes from a Latin word meaning *partition or dividing structure* and can refer to any wall dividing two cavities.

   b. The term comes from Roman architecture where it referred to the large open area in the center of every Roman house off of which all the other rooms of the house branched out. (atrium)

   c. The ventricle is the lower portion of each side of the heart.

   d. The ventricle is the upper portion of each side of the heart.

   e. The word *ventricle* is a combination of *venter* (stomach) plus the diminutive suffix *-icle* and means *little stomach.*

3. Sharon was "*hemodynamically* stable until the past month." The root *hemo* means

   a. artery

   b. blood

   c. heart

   d. vein

   e. vessel

4. Sharon will be given antibiotic as needed for *endocarditis prophylaxis.* Which of the following is an accurate breakdown of the term?

   a. *endo* (inside) + *card* (heart) + *itis* (inflammation) + *prophylaxis* (preventive treatment)

   b. *endo* (inside) + *card* (heart) + *itis* (inflammation) + *prophylaxis* (treatment of symptoms)

   c. *endo* (outside) + *card* (heart) + *itis* (inflammation) + *prophylaxis* (treatment of symptoms)

   d. *endo* (outside) + *card* (heart) + *itis* (inflammation) + *prophylaxis* (preventive treatment)

   e. none of these

Quick Reference

glossary of roots

ROOT	DEFINITION	ROOT	DEFINITION
angi/o	vessel	phleb/o	vein
aort/o	aorta	sept/o	septum (plural, septa)
arteri/o	artery	valvul/o	valve
ather/o	fatty plaque	vas/o, vascul/o	vessel
atri/o	atrium (upper chamber)	ven/o	vein
cardi/o	heart	ventricul/o	ventricle (lower chamber)
coron/o	heart (crown)		

cardiovascular system abbreviations

ABBREVIATION	DEFINITION
A-fib	atrial fibrillation
ASD	atrial septal defect
BP	blood pressure
CABG	coronary artery bypass graft
CAD	coronary artery disease
CHF	congestive heart failure
DVT	deep vein thrombosis
ECHO	echocardiogram
EKG	electrocardiogram
HTN	hypertension
MI	myocardial infarction
MRA	magnetic resonance angiography
MVP	mitral valve prolapse
NSR	normal sinus rhythm
PCI	percutaneous coronary intervention
SCA	sudden cardiac arrest
SV	stroke volume
TEE	transesophageal echocardiogram
VSD	ventricular septal defect

The Respiratory System–Pulmonology

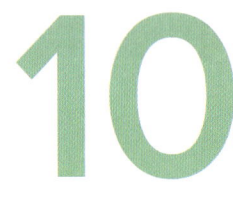

10

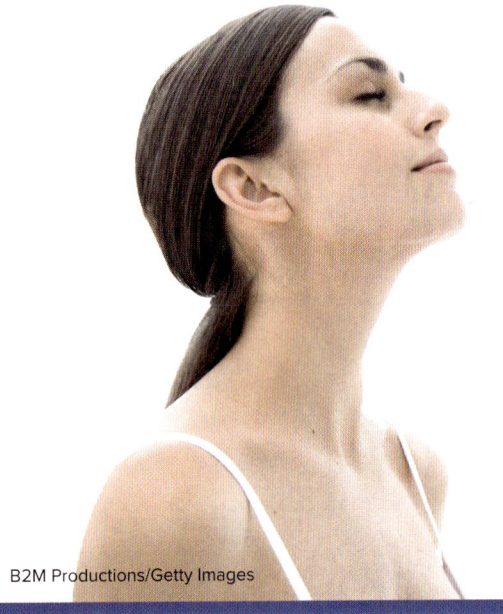

B2M Productions/Getty Images

Learning Outcomes

Upon completion of this chapter,
you will be able to:

10.1 Identify the **roots/word parts** associated with the **respiratory system.**

(S) 10.2 Translate the **Subjective** terms associated with the **respiratory system.**

(O) 10.3 Translate the **Objective** terms associated with the **respiratory system.**

(A) 10.4 Translate the **Assessment** terms associated with the **respiratory system.**

(P) 10.5 Translate the **Plan** terms associated with the **respiratory system.**

10.6 Distinguish terms associated with the **respiratory system** in the context of **electronic health records.**

Introduction and Overview of the Respiratory System

Simply put, the main job of the respiratory system is to deliver oxygen to the blood and carry carbon dioxide away from it. As we breathe in (*inhale*), we are taking in oxygen-rich air. As air passes through the respiratory tract, it is cleaned, warmed, and moistened. The air reaches its end point in the lungs, where it comes in contact with the blood. There, oxygen is exchanged for carbon dioxide. Finally, the waste air passes back out through the nose and mouth (*exhale*).

It helps to view the anatomy of the respiratory system as a tree. The mouth, nose, and throat form the tree's roots. The trachea is the tree's trunk; it leads to large branches (*bronchi*). Each branch splits into more branches (other bronchi) that further lead to twigs (*bronchioles*) and leaves (*alveoli*).

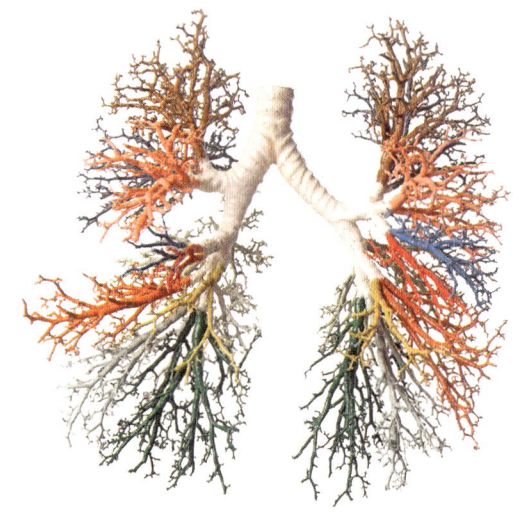

This image of the lungs shows the branching of the airways from the trachea to the bronchi, bronchioles, and down to the alveoli.

Dorling Kindersley/Getty Images

10.1 Word Parts of the Respiratory System

Upper Respiratory System

The entry point for air into the body is primarily through the nose, with some air entering through the mouth. The nose serves to warm, clean, and moisten the air. The nose consists of two nostrils (*nares*), a septum (*septum*), and tube-shaped cartilage inside the nose (*turbinates*). The nose is very vascular, which means that it contains many blood vessels, which is why the nose bleeds easily. The blood in these vessels warms the air as it enters the rest of the respiratory tract. In addition, multiple hairs line the nose and filter out dust and other particles. Finally, the nose produces mucus, which helps clean and moisten the air.

The air passes through the nose or mouth and proceeds into the throat (*pharynx*). There are three parts to the pharynx: the nasopharynx, the oropharynx, and the laryngopharynx. The laryngopharynx contains the vocal cords (*larynx*). When air passes across these cords upon exhalation, the cords vibrate at certain speeds—just like a harmonica or saxophone.

These vibrations make sounds, which we use to form speech. The air continues down the windpipe (*trachea*). The trachea is surrounded by bumpy rings of cartilage that prevent it from caving in.

---

adenoid

ROOT: *adenoid/o*

EXAMPLES: adenoidectomy, adenoiditis

NOTES: The word *adenoid* is formed by adding a suffix to the root *adeno,* which means *gland: aden/o + oid =* resembling a gland.

---

tonsil

ROOT: *tonsill/o*

EXAMPLES: tonsillectomy, tonsillitis

NOTES: The word *tonsil* comes from a Latin word meaning *almond.* The Latin word has two *l*s, but in English, one disappears.

---

nose

ROOTS: *nas/o (Latin for* nose*), rhin/o (Greek for* nose*)*

EXAMPLES: nasogastric tube, nasendoscope, rhinorrhea, rhinoplasty

NOTES: Rhinoceros is the combination of *rhino* and *ceros* (horn), which means *horn nose.*

A poet named Publius Ovidius Naso (43 BC–17 AD) lived in ancient Rome. Perhaps you know him by the much shorter name Ovid. Apparently, he or one of his ancestors had quite a prominent nose—hence the root *naso.*

---

larynx (voice box)

ROOT: *laryng/o*

EXAMPLES: laryngospasm, laryngitis

NOTES: Remember: the letter *g* is soft when followed by an *i* and hard when followed by an *o* (e.g., laryn**GO**spasm vs. laryn**JI**tis).

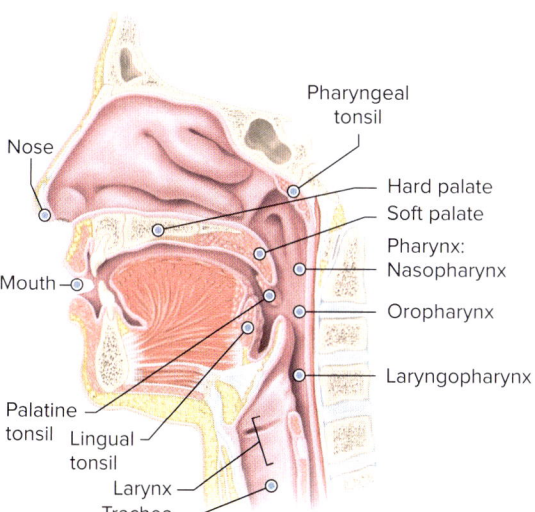

Nose

Pharyngeal tonsil

Hard palate
Soft palate
Pharynx:
Nasopharynx

Mouth

Oropharynx

Laryngopharynx

Palatine tonsil
Lingual tonsil

Larynx
Trachea

pharynx (throat)

ROOT: *pharyng/o*

EXAMPLES: pharyngitis, pharyngostenosis

NOTES: The pharynx is the pathway used by both food and air.

trachea (windpipe)

ROOT: *trache/o*

EXAMPLES: tracheotomy, tracheostomy

NOTES: From the Greek word for *rough,* because of the bumpy ridges that line the outside of the trachea.

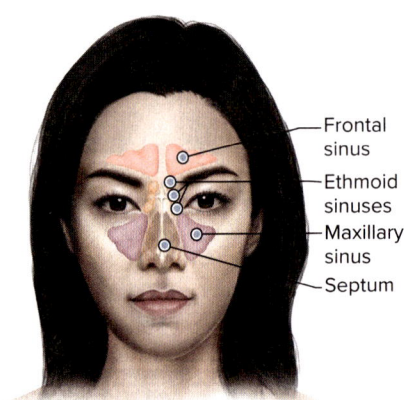

Frontal sinus
Ethmoid sinuses
Maxillary sinus
Septum

septum (plural: septa)

ROOT: *sept/o*

EXAMPLES: septectomy, septoplasty

NOTES: *Septum* comes from a Latin word meaning *partition* or *dividing structure* and can refer to any wall dividing two cavities. Of the numerous septa throughout the body, the easiest to find is the nasal septum. If you place your index fingers in each nostril and press them together, you will feel the nasal septum. If your nasal septum leans to one side, you have a deviated septum.

sinus

ROOTS: *sin/o, sinus/o*

EXAMPLES: sinusitis, sinusotomy

NOTES: From a Latin word meaning *hollow* or *cavity, sinus* refers generally to any hollow area—specifically, those in bones.

Lower Respiratory System

After passing the *trachea,* the air finally makes its way to the lungs via two main *bronchi* (right and left). As with the trachea, rings of cartilage surround the bronchi for support. The bronchi further branch into five *lobar bronchi*—three on the right and two on the left. These branches define the five *lobes* of the lung. Each lobar bronchus breaks into smaller segments (*segmental bronchi*) that further branch into smaller airways known as *bronchioles.* The bronchioles end in clusters of *alveoli,* tiny balloon-like structures surrounded by small blood vessels. At this point, oxygen passes into the blood, and carbon dioxide passes out of the blood.

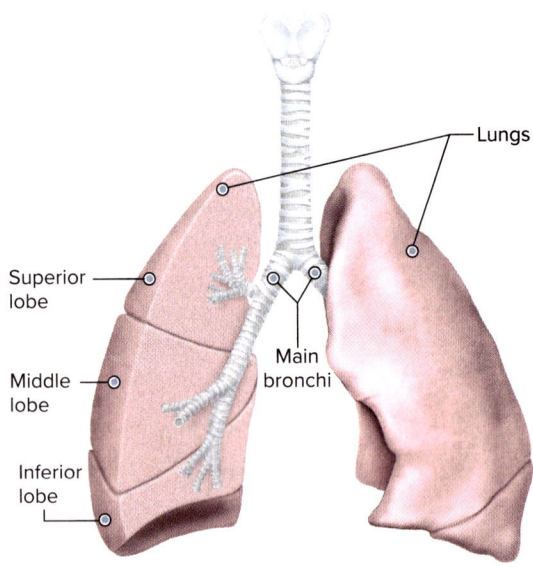

Lungs
Superior lobe
Main bronchi
Middle lobe
Inferior lobe

air or lungs

ROOTS: *pneum/o, pneumat/o, pneumon/o*

EXAMPLES: pneumomelanosis, pneumatology, pneumonia

NOTES: These roots can mean either *lung* or *air.* Context and familiarity will help in determining which to use. For instance, it makes more sense to translate *pneumothorax* as *air in the chest* rather than *lung in the chest.*

The term *pneumatic* can also be found in the construction world. It refers to any tool that moves by forcing air into it (i.e., a pneumatic drill), as opposed to hydraulic tools, which involve the use of water instead of air (i.e., a hydraulic lift).

lungs

ROOT: *pulmon/o*

EXAMPLES: pulmonologist, pulmonary

NOTES: *Pulmon/o* is listed by itself instead of with the various forms of *pneum/o* because whereas *pulmon/o* means only lung, *pneum/o* can mean both lung (as in *pneumonia*) and air (as in *pneumothorax*).

lobe

ROOT: *lob/o*

EXAMPLES: lobectomy, lobotomy

NOTES: A *lobe* is a well-defined portion of any organ. The main organs that have lobes are the lungs, brain, and liver.

What is the difference between a *lobectomy* and a *lobotomy*?

bronchus

ROOTS: *bronch/o, bronchi/o*

EXAMPLES: bronchoscope, bronchiostenosis

NOTES: The main branches from the trachea into each lung.

alveolus (air sac)

ROOT: *alveol/o*

EXAMPLES: alveolitis, alveolar

NOTES: *Alveolus* comes from a Latin word meaning *hollow* or *cavity.* The two main types are *pulmonary alveoli,* the air sacs in the lungs, and *dental alveoli,* the sockets in the jaw from which teeth emerge.

If you place your tongue on the roof of your mouth and move it forward, you will feel a bump called the *alveolar ridge* right before you get to your teeth.

chest

ROOTS: *thorac/o, pector/o (also pectus), steth/o*

EXAMPLES: thoracic, pectoralgia, pectus excavatum, stethoscope

NOTES: The root *pector/o* can also stand as a word by itself. When it does, however, the ending changes slightly, from *pectoro* to *pectus;* hence, pectus excavatum.

The term *stethoscope* literally means *an instrument for looking at the chest,* but of course, you do not look with a stethoscope—you listen.

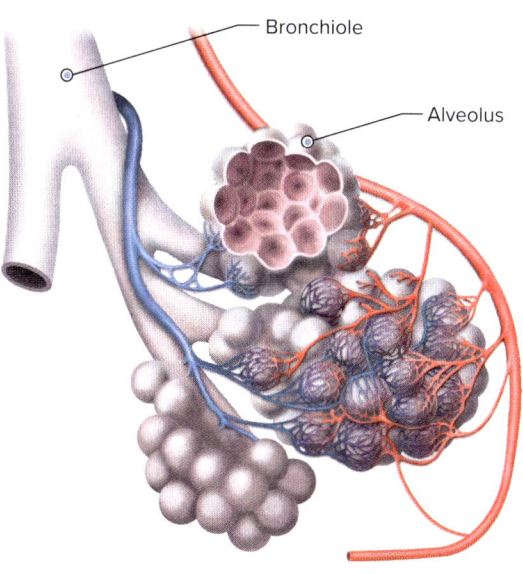

Bronchiole

Alveolus

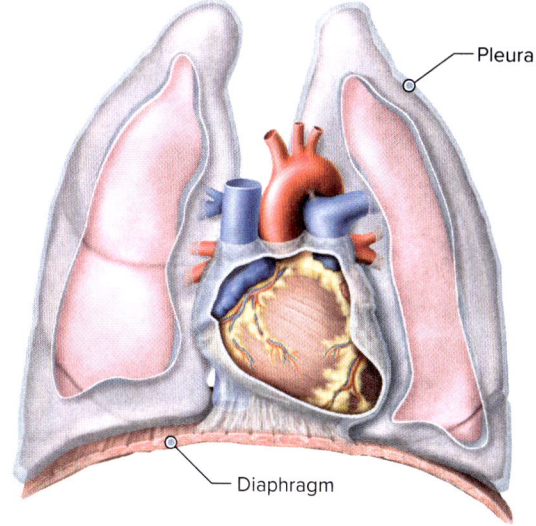

Pleura

Diaphragm

bronchiole

ROOT: *bronchiol/o*

EXAMPLES: bronchiolitis, bronchiolectasis

NOTES: The root *bronchiole* is actually formed by adding a diminutive suffix to another root: *bronch/o + iole = little bronchus,* which is a smaller subdivision of the bronchial tubes.

pleura

ROOT: *pleur/o*

EXAMPLES: pleuritis, pleurectomy

NOTES: The *pleura* is a membrane surrounding the lungs.

diaphragm

ROOT: *phren/o*

EXAMPLES: phrenospasm, phrenoplegia

NOTES: In addition to the diaphragm, *phren/o* can also refer to the brain (as in the term *schizophrenia*). The rationale comes from the ancient Greek view of the mind. The Greeks believed that the chest was the seat of emotion and reason. As that view changed and the location of the mind moved from the chest to the brain, the word for mind became applied to both regions of the body.

Process of Respiration

Although air begins its journey in the nose and mouth, the work of breathing actually starts with two sets of muscles: the muscles between the ribs (*intercostal*) and a horizontal muscle (*diaphragm*) that lies between the chest and the abdomen. When these muscles shorten (*contract*), they cause the chest to enlarge, which decreases chest (*thoracic*) pressure. As a result, air is literally sucked into the lungs.

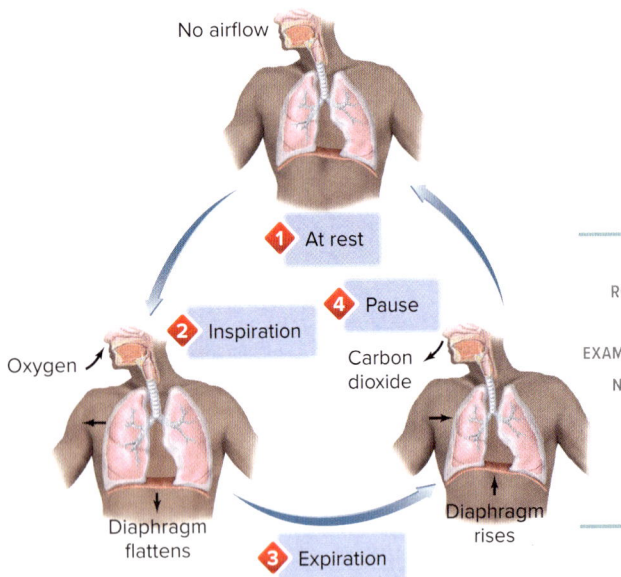

No airflow

1 At rest

4 Pause

2 Inspiration

Oxygen

Carbon dioxide

Diaphragm flattens

Diaphragm rises

3 Expiration

oxygen

ROOT: *ox/o*

EXAMPLES: hypoxia, hypoxemia

NOTES: *Hypoxia* refers to a lack of oxygen in tissue cells. *Hypoxemia* refers to lack of oxygen in the blood. If a hypoxic patient is also hypoxemic, then oxygen is not getting into the blood. If the person is not hypoxemic, then the problem lies in the transfer of oxygen from blood to tissue. Diagnosing this problem is similar to tracking a package: If a customer does not receive a package, the delivery chain could have broken down in any number of places along the way. The package might never have been sent, might not have made it on the delivery truck, or might not have been delivered to the right door.

breathing

ROOTS: *spir/o, -pnea*

EXAMPLES: spirometry, sleep apnea

NOTES: *Spir/o* also occurs in other words:

- *Perspire* translates as *to breathe through*.
- *Conspire* translates as *to breathe together*—no doubt coming from the idea that people who are *conspiring* can be thought of as being huddled together and breathing the same air.
- *Expire* also contains the *spir/o* root and means *to breathe out*. It was originally written as *exspire,* but the letter s was dropped because *x* is made up of two *k* sounds. To test this, say *expire* and *exspire*. They are rarely pronounced differently.

Note: *-pnea* is most often used as a suffix to indicate a type of breathing.

carbon dioxide

ROOTS: *capn/o (Greek for smoke), carb/o (Latin for coal)*

EXAMPLES: hypercapnia, hypocarbia

NOTES: One of the treatments for hyperventilation is to have the person breathe into a paper bag. A person who is hyperventilating has *hypocarbia* and thus needs to increase the carbon dioxide in his or her respiratory system.

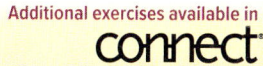
TRANSLATION

EXERCISE 1 Match the word part on the left with its definition on the right.

_____ 1. adenoid/o   a. windpipe

_____ 2. sin/o   b. tonsil

_____ 3. tonsill/o   c. sinus

_____ 4. sept/o   d. nose

_____ 5. pharyng/o   e. adenoids

_____ 6. laryng/o   f. septum

_____ 7. rhin/o   g. voice box

_____ 8. trache/o   h. pharynx

EXERCISE 4 Match the word part on the left with its definition on the right.

_F_ 1. bronch/o   a. air

_G_ 2. pleur/o   b. lung

_C_ 3. lob/o   c. lobe

_d_ 4. alveol/o   d. alveolus

_a_ 5. pneum/o   e. chest

_H_ 6. phren/o   f. bronchus

_B_ 7. pulmon/o   g. pleura

_e_ 8. thorac/o   h. diaphragm

EXERCISE 2 Translate the following word parts.

1. sinus/o _____

2. adenoid/o _____

3. pharyng/o _____

4. tonsill/o _____

5. nas/o _____

6. sept/o _____

7. trache/o _____

8. laryng/o _____

EXERCISE 5 Translate the following word parts.

1. lob/o _____

2. pleur/o _____

3. bronchiol/o _____

4. steth/o _____

5. pneumat/o _____

6. alveol/o _____

7. pneumon/o _____

8. pector/o _____

9. pulmon/o _____

10. phren/o _____

EXERCISE 3 Break down the following words into their component parts and define.

> EXAMPLE: **sinusitis** _sinus | itis_
> _inflammation of the sinuses_

1. laryngitis _____

2. tonsillitis _____

3. septectomy _____

4. nasendoscope _____

5. pharyngostenosis _____

EXERCISE 6 Break down the following words into their component parts and define.

> EXAMPLE: **sinusitis** _sinus | itis_
> _inflammation of the sinuses_

1. pneumonia _____

2. bronchitis _____

3. pleuritis _____

4. lobectomy _____

5. alveolitis _____

6. stethoscope _____

7. phrenoplegia _____

8. bronchiostenosis _____

EXERCISE 7   Translate the following word parts.

1. ox/o _____

2. carb/o _____

3. capn/o _____

4. spir/o _____

5. -pnea _____

EXERCISE 8   Match the word part on the left with its definition on the right.

_____ 1. ox/o   a. oxygen

_____ 2. capn/o   b. breathing

_____ 3. spir/o   c. carbon dioxide

GENERATION

EXERCISE 9   Identify the roots for the following definitions.

1. tonsil _____

2. adenoid _____

3. pharynx _____

4. trachea _____

5. nose _____

6. throat _____

7. voice box _____

EXERCISE 10 Build a medical term from the information provided.

1. inflammation of the throat _____

_____

2. inflammation of the sinus _____

_____

3. incision into the trachea _____

_____

4. discharge from the nose _____

_____

5. surgical removal of the tonsils _____

_____

6. creation of an opening in the trachea _____

_____

7. surgical reconstruction of the septum _____

_____

EXERCISE 11 Identify the roots for the following definitions.

1. bronchus _____

2. pleura _____

3. lobe _____

4. bronchiole _____

5. alveolus _____

6. diaphragm _____

7. lungs _____

8. chest _____

9. air or lungs _____

10. air sac _____

EXERCISE 12 Build a medical term from the information provided.

1. chest pain _____

2. the study of the lungs _____

3. instrument to look into the bronchus _____

4. involuntary contraction of the diaphragm

   _____

5. inflammation of the smaller subdivisions of the bronchus _____

EXERCISE 13 Break down the follow ing words into their component parts and define.

> EXAMPLE: **sinusitis**   *sinus | itis*
> *inflammation of the sinuses*

1. hypercapnia _____

2. hypoxemia _____

3. apnea _____

EXERCISE 14 Identify the roots for the following definitions.

1. breathing _____

2. oxygen _____

3. carbon dioxide _____

EXERCISE 15 Build a medical term from the information provided.

1. deficient oxygen _____

2. excessive carbon dioxide _____

3. instrument for measuring breathing _____

   _____

ⓈUBJECTIVE

10.2 Patient History, Problems, Complaints

The most common patient respiratory complaint is coughing. Depending on whether *sputum* is present, a cough can be described as either *productive* or *nonproductive*. A productive cough is also known as *expectoration*. Coughing blood (*hemoptysis*) is generally a more worrisome symptom.

Other respiratory symptoms include changes in the breathing patterns and pain. Descriptions of the breathing pattern reflect the speed of breathing (*tachypnea, bradypnea*), the depth of breathing (*hyperventilation, hypoventilation*), or the work involved in breathing (*orthopnea, dyspnea*). While pain is a less frequent symptom in the respiratory system than in other systems, it should never be overlooked. When chest pain happens during *inspiration* or with a cough, it is known as *pleuritic chest pain.* If pain occurs at these intervals, the pain may be distinguished as respiratory in nature.

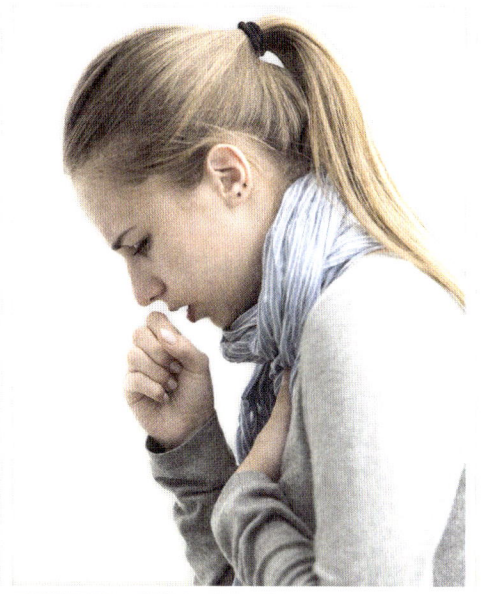

AlexRaths/Getty Images

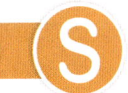

breathing processes

TERM	WORD ANALYSIS
apnea AP-nee-ah	a / pnea not / breathing
DEFINITION cessation of breathing	
bradypnea brad-ip-NEE-ah	brady / pnea slow / breathing
DEFINITION slow breathing	
dyspnea disp-NEE-ah	dys / pnea bad / breathing
DEFINITION difficulty breathing	
eupnea YOOP-nee-ah	eu / pnea good / breathing
DEFINITION good/normal breathing	
hyperpnea hai-perp-NEE-ah	hyper / pnea over / breathing
DEFINITION heavy breathing	
hypopnea hai-POP-nee-ah	hypo / pnea under / breathing
DEFINITION shallow breathing	
orthopnea or-thop-NEE-ah	ortho / pnea straight / breathing
DEFINITION able to breathe only in an upright position	
tachypnea ta-KIP-nee-ah	tachy / pnea fast / breathing
DEFINITION rapid breathing	
hyperventilation hai-per-ven-ti-LAY-shun	hyper / ventil / ation over / breathing / process
DEFINITION overbreathing; the condition of having too much air flowing into and out of the lungs; leads to hypocapnia	
hypoventilation hai-poh-ven-ti-LAY-shun	hypo / ventil / ation under / breathing / process
DEFINITION underbreathing; the condition of having too little air flowing into and out of the lungs; leads to hypercapnia	

upper respiratory

TERM	WORD ANALYSIS
epistaxis ep-ee-STAKS-is	from the Greek word epistazo, meaning *to drip out or upon*
DEFINITION a nosebleed	
rhinorrhea rai-no-REE-yah	rhino / rrhea nose / discharge
DEFINITION runny nose	

lower respiratory

TERM	WORD ANALYSIS
phrenospasm fre-no-SPAZ-um	phreno / spasm diaphragm / involuntary contraction
DEFINITION involuntary contraction of the diaphragm (also known as the hiccups)	
pleuralgia plur-AL-jah	pleur / algia pleura / pain
DEFINITION pain in the pleura	
pleurodynia plur-oh-DAI-nee-ah	pleuro / dynia pleura / pain
DEFINITION pain in the pleura	
thoracalgia thor-a-KAL-jah	thorac / algia chest / pain
DEFINITION chest pain	

discharges and secretions

TERM	WORD ANALYSIS
expectoration eks-pec-tor-A-shun	ex / pector / ation out / chest / process
DEFINITION coughing or spitting material out of the lungs	
hemoptysis heem-op-TIS-is	hemo / ptysis blood / cough
DEFINITION coughing up blood	
sputum SPYOO-tum	Latin for *spit*
DEFINITION mucus discharged from the lungs by coughing	

PRONUNCIATION

EXERCISE 1   Indicate which syllable(s) is emphasized when pronounced.

EXAMPLE: bronchitis bron<u>chi</u>tis

1. eupnea _____

2. hypopnea _____

3. dyspnea _____

4. hypoventilation _____

5. phrenospasm _____

6. hemoptysis _____

TRANSLATION

EXERCISE 2   Underline and define the word parts from this chapter in the following terms.

1. tachypnea _____

2. hypopnea _____

3. phrenospasm _____

4. pleuralgia _____

5. thoracalgia _____

6. hyperventilation _____

7. expectoration _____

EXERCISE 3   Match the term on the left with its definition on the right.

_____ 1. apnea

_____ 2. eupnea

_____ 3. dyspnea

_____ 4. orthopnea

_____ 5. hyperventilation

_____ 6. epistaxis

_____ 7. rhinorrhea

_____ 8. pleurodynia

_____ 9. hemoptysis

_____ 10. sputum

a. cessation of breathing

b. pain in the pleura

c. normal breathing

d. runny nose

e. coughing up blood

f. able to breathe only in an upright position

g. nosebleed

h. overbreathing, or too much air flowing into and out of the lungs

i. mucus discharged from the lungs by coughing

j. difficulty breathing

EXERCISE 4   Break down the following words into their component parts.

EXAMPLE: nasopharyngoscope
naso | pharyngo | scope

1. bradypnea _____

2. hyperpnea _____

3. rhinorrhea _____

4. phrenospasm _____

5. pleurodynia _____

6. thoracalgia _____

7. hypoventilation _____

8. hemoptysis _____

EXERCISE 5 Translate the following terms as literally as possible.

EXAMPLE: nasopharyngoscope *an instrument for looking at the nose and throat*

1. orthopnea _____

2. hyperpnea _____

3. hypopnea _____

4. pleuralgia _____

5. thoracalgia _____

6. hyperventilation _____

7. hypoventilation _____

GENERATION

EXERCISE 6 Build a medical term from the information provided.

EXAMPLE: inflammation of the sinuses *sinusitis*

1. not breathing _____

2. good breathing _____

3. difficulty breathing _____

4. slow breathing _____

5. fast breathing _____

6. pain in the pleura _____

7. runny nose _____

8. involuntary contraction of the diaphragm ___

_____

9. coughing up blood _____

EXERCISE 7 Multiple-choice questions. Select the correct answer.

1. *Epistaxis* comes from the Greek word meaning *to drip out or upon* and is used to indicate
   a. a nosebleed
   b. a runny nose
   c. mucus on the lungs
   d. a wet cough

2. The Latin word for *spit*, which indicates mucus discharged by the lungs, is
   a. spasm
   b. sputum
   c. mucus
   d. wet cough

3. Which of the following is NOT a term related to describing a breathing process?
   a. hyperventilation
   b. hypopnea
   c. bradypnea
   d. hemoptysis

4. Which of the following is NOT a term to describe pain in the lower respiratory system?
   a. pleuralgia
   b. rhinorrhea
   c. pleurodynia
   d. thoracalgia

5. Which term describes a patient who is coughing up blood?
   a. rhinorrhea
   b. epistaxis
   c. hemoptysis
   d. dyspnea

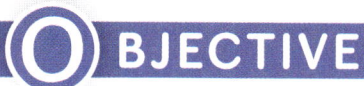

10.3 Observation and Discovery

When gathering clues about the status of a patient's respiration, a health care professional may use physical findings, labs, and specialized tests or imaging. Sights and sounds are valuable tools in the physical exam of a patient with a respiratory problem. Inspection may reveal an abnormal chest shape, a patient working harder to breathe, or a change in skin color. When listening to the patient's chest (*auscultation*), an examiner may notice changes in breathing sounds.

Lab data mainly deal with the levels of carbon dioxide and oxygen in the blood. *Capnography* and *oximetry* are fast tests that provide this information, but more specialized tests examine how well the lungs work.

Spirometry measures the strength of breathing, whereas a *ventilation–perfusion scan* measures how effectively oxygen and blood reach different parts of the lungs. Finally, it may be necessary to get a closer look to get to the root of the problem (e.g., *bronchoscopy* and *thorascopy*).

physical findings and examination methods

TERM	WORD ANALYSIS
auscultation ah-skul-TAY-shun	from the Latin word *ausculto,* meaning *to listen*
DEFINITION using a stethoscope to listen to the chest	
cyanosis sai-an-O-sis	cyan / osis blue / condition
DEFINITION a bluish color in the skin caused by insufficient oxygen	

pathology

TERM	WORD ANALYSIS
atelectasis ah-tel-EK-ta-sis	a / tel / ectasis not / complete / expansion
DEFINITION incomplete expansion	
bronchiectasis bron-key-EK-ta-sis	bronchi / ectasis bronchus / expansion
DEFINITION expansion of the bronchi	
hemothorax heem-oh-THOR-aks	hemo / thorax blood / chest
DEFINITION blood in the chest	
phrenoplegia fre-no-PLEE-jah	phreno / plegia diaphragm / paralysis
DEFINITION paralysis of the diaphragm	

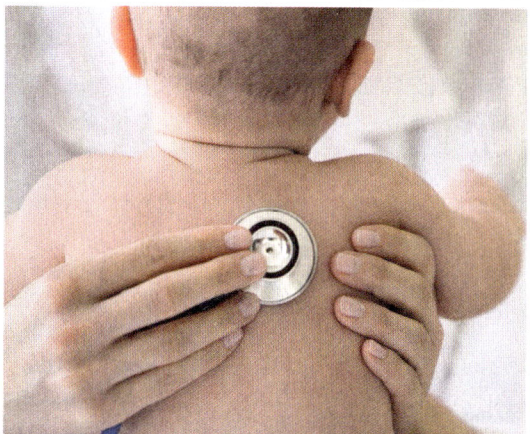

A doctor's first step in gathering data for a diagnosis is to listen to lung function using a stethoscope.

Tetra Images /Alamy

pathology *continued*

TERM	WORD ANALYSIS
pleural effusion PLUR-al ef-YOO-zhun	pleur / al pleura / pertaining to
DEFINITION fluid pouring out into the pleura NOTE: The prefix in *effusion* is actually *ex*. The *x* turns to an *f* when followed by an *f*. Why? Say *exfusion* 10 times. Most people slur *exfusion* into *effusion* because it is easier to say.	ex / fusion out / pour
pneumohemothorax new-moh-hee-moh-THOR-aks	pneumo / hemo / thorax air / blood / chest
DEFINITION air and blood in the chest	
pneumothorax new-moh-THOR-aks	pneumo / thorax air / chest
DEFINITION air in the chest	
pulmonary edema pul-mon-AIR-ee ah-DEE-ma	pulmon / ary lung / pertaining to edema swelling
DEFINITION swelling in the lungs	

laboratory data

TERM	WORD ANALYSIS
hypercapnia hai-per-CAP-nee-yah	hyper / capn / ia over / carbon / condition dioxide
DEFINITION excessive carbon dioxide	
hypercarbia hai-per-CAR-bee-yah	hyper / carb / ia over / carbon / condition dioxide
DEFINITION excessive carbon dioxide	
hypocapnia hai-poh-CAP-nee-yah	hypo / capn / ia under / carbon / condition dioxide
DEFINITION insufficient carbon dioxide	
hypocarbia hai-poh-CAR-bee-yah	hypo / carb / ia under / carbon / condition dioxide
DEFINITION insufficient carbon dioxide	
hypoxemia hai-poks-EEM-ee-yah	hyp(o) / ox / emia under / oxygen / blood condition
DEFINITION insufficient oxygen in the blood	
hypoxia hai-POKS-ee-yah	hyp(o) / ox / ia under / oxygen / condition
DEFINITION insufficient oxygen	

diagnostic procedures

TERM	WORD ANALYSIS
bronchoscopy bron-KOS-koh-pee	broncho / scopy bronchus / looking procedure
DEFINITION procedure to look inside the bronchi	

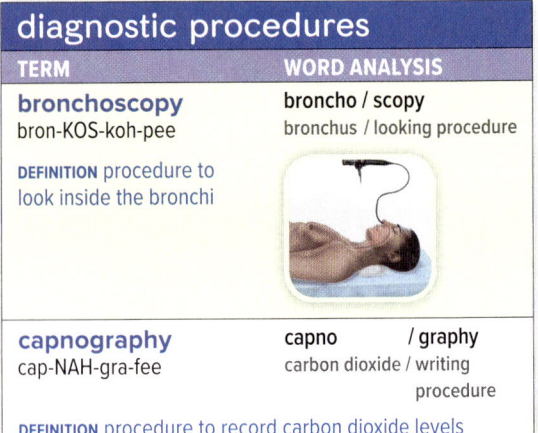

capnography cap-NAH-gra-fee	capno / graphy carbon dioxide / writing procedure
DEFINITION procedure to record carbon dioxide levels	

diagnostic procedures *continued*

TERM	WORD ANALYSIS	
capnometer cap-NOM-eh-ter	capno carbon dioxide	/ meter / instrument to measure
DEFINITION instrument to measure carbon dioxide levels		
oximetry ok-SIM-ah-tree	oxi oxygen	/ metry / measuring procedure
DEFINITION procedure to measure oxygen levels		
polysomnography po-lee-som-NAH-gra-fee	poly / somno multiple / sleep	/ graphy / writing procedure
DEFINITION recording multiple aspects of sleep		

TERM	WORD ANALYSIS	
pulmonary function testing pul-mon-AIR-ee funk-shun TES-ting	pulmon / ary lung / pertaining to function testing	
DEFINITION a group of tests used to evaluate the condition and operation of the lungs		
spirometry speer-AH-me-tree	spiro breathing	/ metry / measuring procedure
DEFINITION procedure to measure breathing		

diagnostic procedures *continued*

TERM	WORD ANALYSIS	
thoracoscopy thor-a-KOS-koh-pee	thoraco / scopy chest / looking procedure	

DEFINITION examination of the chest
NOTE: This word is sometimes shortened to *thoriscopy* to make it easier to say.

radiology

TERM	WORD ANALYSIS	
computed tomography com-PYOO-ted tom-O-grah-fee	computed tomo / graphy cut / writing procedure	
DEFINITION an imaging procedure using a computer to cut NOTE: *Cut* in this context does not mean incision but rather using a computer to view "slices" of a patient's organs.		
pulmonary angiography pul-mon-AIR-ee an-jee-AH-grah-fee	pulmon / ary lung / pertaining to angio / graphy blood vessel / writing procedure	
DEFINITION an imaging procedure for recording pulmonary blood vessel activity		
ventilation–perfusion scan ven-ti-LAY-shun–per-FYOO-shun skan	ventil / ation – breathing / process per / fusion through / pour	
DEFINITION a scan that tests whether a problem in the lungs is caused by airflow (ventilation) or blood flow (perfusion)		

Learning Outcome 10.3 Exercises

TRANSLATION

EXERCISE 1 Underline and define the word parts from this chapter in the following terms.

1. pulmonary _____

2. hypercarbia _____

3. hypocapnia _____

4. hypoxia _____

5. capnography _____

6. bronchoscopy _____

7. spirometry _____

8. thoracoscopy _____

EXERCISE 2   Match the term on the left with its definition on the right.

_____ 1. cyanosis

_____ 2. auscultation

_____ 3. atelectasis

_____ 4. pleural effusion

_____ 5. hypoxemia

_____ 6. ventilation–perfusion scan

_____ 7. computed tomography

_____ 8. pulmonary function testing

a. a scan that tests whether a problem in the lungs is caused by airflow or blood flow

b. a bluish color in the skin

c. a recording procedure using a computer to view "cuts" of a patient's organs

d. fluid pouring out into the pleura

e. deficient oxygen in the blood

f. using a stethoscope to listen to the chest

g. a group of tests used to evaluate the condition and operation of the lungs

h. incomplete expansion

EXERCISE 3   Break down the following words into their component parts.

EXAMPLE: nasopharyngoscope
naso | pharyngo | scope

1. hemothorax _____

2. phrenoplegia _____

3. capnometer _____

4. oximetry _____

5. hypercapnia _____

6. hypocarbia _____

7. pneumothorax _____

8. pneumohemothorax _____

9. thoracoscopy _____

10. bronchiectasis _____

11. polysomnography _____

12. pulmonary angiography _____

EXERCISE 4   Translate the following terms as literally as possible.

EXAMPLE: nasopharyngoscope   _an instrument for looking at the nose and throat_

1. oximetry _____

2. hypercapnia _____

3. hypocarbia _____

4. hypercarbia _____

5. hypocapnia _____

6. hypoxia _____

7. thoracoscopy _____

8. capnography _____

9. hemothorax _____

10. pneumohemothorax _____

11. bronchiectasis _____

12. polysomnography _____

13. pulmonary angiography _____

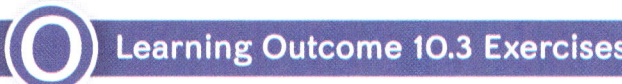

Learning Outcome 10.3 Exercises

GENERATION

EXERCISE 5 Build a medical term from the information provided.

> EXAMPLE: inflammation of the sinuses   *sinusitis*

1. swelling in the lungs _____
2. air in the chest _____
3. paralysis of the diaphragm _____
4. instrument to measure carbon dioxide levels _____
5. procedure to look inside the bronchi _____
   _____
6. procedure to measure breathing _____
   _____

EXERCISE 6 Multiple-choice questions. Select the correct answer.

1. A health care professional uses a stethoscope as part of the following procedure:
   a. auscultation   c. endoscopy
   b. polysomnography   d. capnography

2. Which of the following terms pertains to the diaphragm?
   a. pleural effusion   c. phrenoplegia
   b. pulmonary edema   d. pneumothorax

3. Which procedure measures oxygen levels?
   a. spirometry   c. bronchoscopy
   b. capnography   d. oximetry

4. The term *hemothorax* means that there is which of the following in the chest?
   a. blood   c. chyle
   b. pus   d. air

ASSESSMENT

10.4 Diagnosis and Pathology

Since the upper respiratory tract is the first line of defense, infections in this area are very common. While inflammation in these areas (*rhinitis, sinusitis, pharyngitis, laryngitis,* etc.) is not *always* caused by infection, infection is certainly the most common cause. The lower respiratory tract has its share of infections as well, with the most common being *bronchitis* and *pneumonia. Asthma* and *chronic obstructive pulmonary disorder* are long-term, noninfectious causes of illness that can be serious.

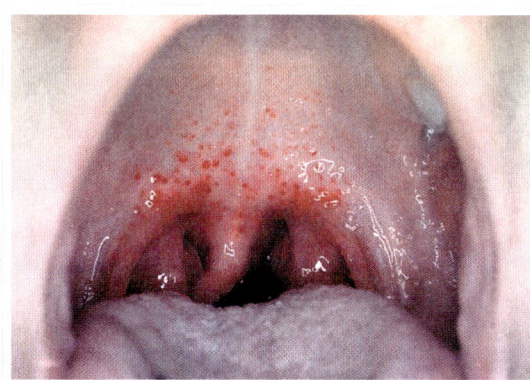

"Open up and say 'Ah'" is the way many examinations involving the respiratory system begin.
Source: Centers for Disease Control

upper respiratory pathology

TERM	WORD ANALYSIS
laryngitis la-rin-JAI-tis	laryng / itis larynx / inflammation
DEFINITION inflammation of the larynx	
laryngotracheobronchitis la-rin-go-tray-key-o-bron-KAI-tis	laryngo / tracheo / bronch / itis larynx / trachea / bronchus / inflammation
DEFINITION inflammation of the larynx, trachea, and bronchi	
rhinitis rai-NAI-tis	rhin / itis nose / inflammation
DEFINITION inflammation of the nasal passages	
pansinusitis pan-sai-nus-AI-tis	pan / sinus / itis all / sinus / inflammation
DEFINITION inflammation of all sinuses	
sinusitis sai-nus-AI-tis	sinus / itis sinus / inflammation
DEFINITION inflammation of the sinus	
sleep apnea sleep AP-nee-ah	a / pnea not / breathing
DEFINITION a condition where the patient ceases to breathe while asleep	

lower respiratory pathology

TERM	WORD ANALYSIS
asthma AZ-ma	from the Greek word for *panting* or *gasping*
DEFINITION a disease causing episodic narrowing and inflammation of the airway NOTE: The name describes the wheezing and shortness of breath that accompanies an attack.	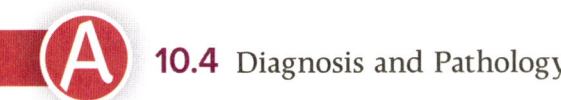 Louis-Paul St-Onge/ Getty Images
bronchiolitis bron-kee-yo-LAI-tis	bronchiol / itis bronchiole / inflammation
DEFINITION inflammation of a bronchiole	

lower respiratory pathology
continued

TERM	WORD ANALYSIS
bronchitis bron-KAI-tis	bronch / itis bronchus / inflammation
DEFINITION inflammation of the bronchi	
chronic obstructive pulmonary disease (COPD) KRON-ik ob-STRUKT-iv pul-mon-AIR-ee dih-EEZ	chron / ic time / pertaining to ob / struct / ive in the way / build / pertaining to pulmon / ary lung / pertaining to
DEFINITION a group of lung diseases characterized by the continual blockage of lung passages	
emphysema im-fi-ZEE-ma	from the Greek word *emphysan,* meaning to *inflate*
DEFINITION a disease that causes the alveoli to lose elasticity; emphysema patients can inhale but have difficulty exhaling	
pleurisy PLUR-ih-see	pleur / isy pleura / inflammation
DEFINITION another word for pleuritis	
pleuritis plur-AI-tis	pleur / itis pleura / inflammation
DEFINITION inflammation of the pleura	
pneumoconiosis new-moh-con-i-OH-sis	pneumo / coni / osis lung / dust / condition
DEFINITION a lung condition caused by dust	
pneumonia new-MOH-nee-yah	pneumon / ia lung / condition
DEFINITION a lung condition	

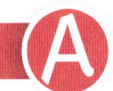

10.4 Diagnosis and Pathology

lower respiratory pathology *continued*	
TERM	**WORD ANALYSIS**
pneumonitis new-moh-NAI-tis	pneumon / itis lung / inflammation
DEFINITION inflammation of the lung	
pulmonary embolism pul-mon-AIR-ee em-bol-IZ-um	pulmon / ary lung / pertaining to embol / ism embolus / condition
DEFINITION blockage in the pulmonary blood supply	

oncology	
TERM	**WORD ANALYSIS**
bronchiogenic carcinoma bron-kee-oh-JEN-ic car-si-NO-ma	bronchio / genic bronchus / beginning in carcin / oma cancer / tumor
DEFINITION a cancerous tumor originating in the bronchi	

Learning Outcome 10.4 Exercises

TRANSLATION

EXERCISE 1 Break down the following words into their component parts.

> EXAMPLE: nasopharyngoscope
> *naso | pharyngo | scope*

1. bronchiolitis _____

2. pansinusitis _____

3. pneumoconiosis _____

4. pulmonary embolism _____

5. laryngotracheobronchitis _____

6. bronchiogenic carcinoma _____

EXERCISE 2 Underline and define the word parts from this chapter in the following terms.

1. laryngitis _____

2. rhinitis _____

3. sinusitis _____

4. bronchitis _____

5. pulmonary _____

6. pleuritis _____

_____

EXERCISE 3 Match the term on the left with its definition on the right.

_____ 1. sleep apnea   a. a disease that causes the alveoli to lose their elasticity

_____ 2. asthma   b. blockage in the pulmonary blood supply

_____ 3. emphysema   c. a lung disease caused by the continual blocking of lung passages

_____ 4. chronic obstructive pulmonary disease   d. a condition where the patient ceases to breathe while asleep

_____ 5. pleurisy   e. inflammation of the pleura

_____ 6. pulmonary embolism   f. a disease causing episodic narrowing and inflammation of the airway

EXERCISE 4 Translate the following terms as literally as possible.

> EXAMPLE: nasopharyngoscope *an instrument for looking at the nose and throat*

1. pneumonia _____

2. pleuritis _____

3. rhinitis _____

4. pansinusitis _____

5. laryngotracheobronchitis _____

6. bronchiogenic carcinoma _____

GENERATION

EXERCISE 5 Build a medical term from the information provided.

> EXAMPLE: inflammation of the sinuses *sinusitis*

1. inflammation of the larynx _____

2. inflammation of all sinuses _____

3. inflammation of the lung _____

4. inflammation of the bronchi _____

5. a lung condition caused by dust _____

EXERCISE 6 Multiple-choice questions. Select the correct answer(s).

1. The Greek word for *panting* or *gasping* is
   a. emphysema   c. pleurisy
   b. asthma   d. embolism

2. *Emphysema* comes from the Greek word meaning _____ and describes a disease that causes the alveoli to lose their elasticity.
   a. to deflate   c. to inflate
   b. to stretch   d. to loosen

3. Select the terms that pertain to the upper respiratory system.
   a. bronchitis   e. pleuritis
   b. laryngitis   f. pneumonitis
   c. laryngotracheobronchitis   g. rhinitis
   d. pansinusitis   h. sinusitis

4. Select the terms that pertain to the lower respiratory system.
   a. bronchitis   e. pleuritis
   b. laryngitis   f. pneumonitis
   c. laryngotracheobronchitis   g. rhinitis
   d. pansinusitis   h. sinusitis

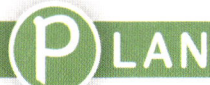

P LAN

10.5 Treatments and Therapies

Most respiratory illnesses respond to medicines. Bronchi-opening medicines (*bronchodilators*) given through an *inhaler device* or a machine (*nebulizer*) help people with asthma or chronic obstructive pulmonary disorder. Cough-stopping (*antitussive*) medicines are popular, but not necessarily very helpful.

With some illnesses, more aggressive intervention is needed. Surgeries of the upper airway are among the most common procedures. Lower airway surgeries,

such as cutting out part of the lung (*lobectomy*), are less common. Very ill patients or patients who are undergoing surgery may need to have a tube placed in the mouth and into the windpipe (*endotracheal tube*). The tube is then attached to a breathing machine.

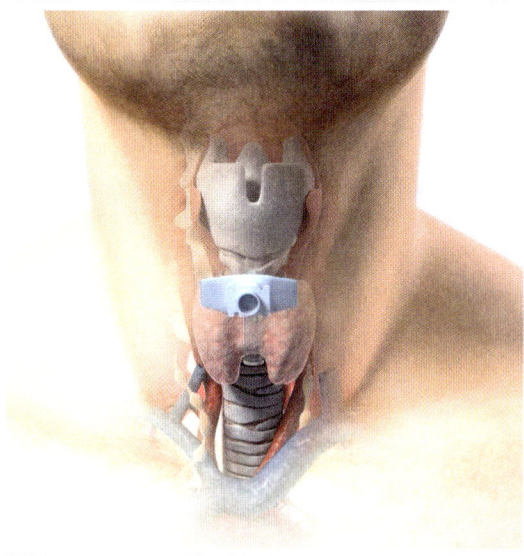

One way of bypassing a patient's obstructed airway is through a tracheostomy, creating an artificial opening in the trachea to allow air to enter the lungs easier.

MedicalRF.com

upper respiratory procedures

TERM	WORD ANALYSIS
endotracheal intubation en-doh-TRAY-kee-al in-too-BAY-shun	endo / trache / al inside / trachea / pertaining to in / tub / ation in / tube / process
DEFINITION insertion of a tube inside the trachea	
laryngectomy la-rin-JEK-toe-mee	laryng / ectomy larynx / removal
DEFINITION removal of the larynx	
tracheostomy tray-kee-AH-stoh-mee	tracheo / stomy trachea / creation of an opening
DEFINITION creation of an opening in the trachea	

upper respiratory procedures
continued

TERM	WORD ANALYSIS
tracheotomy tray-kee-AH-toe-mee	tracheo / tomy trachea / incision
DEFINITION incision into the trachea	

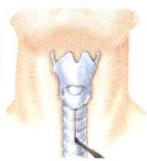

lower respiratory procedures

TERM	WORD ANALYSIS
cardiopulmonary resuscitation (CPR) kar-dee-oh-pul-mon-AIR-ee ree-sus-i-TAY-shun	cardio / pulmon / ary heart / lung / pertaining to re / suscit / ation again / awaken / process
DEFINITION method of artificially maintaining blood flow and airflow when breathing and pulse have stopped	

NOTE: *Suscit* is formed by adding the prefix *sub-* to the Latin word *cito,* which means *to move. Suscit = sub + cito = to move from beneath,* and thus *to raise* or *awaken.* The *cito* root is found in other words such as *excite, incite,* and *recite.*

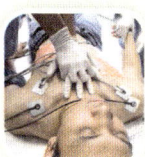

ERproductions Ltd/Blend Images LLC

lobectomy loh-BEK-toe-mee	lob / ectomy lobe / removal
DEFINITION removal of a lobe	

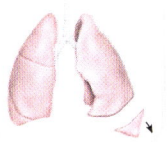

lower respiratory procedures
continued

TERM	WORD ANALYSIS
pleuropexy ploo-rah-PEK-see	**pleuro / pexy** pleura / fixation
DEFINITION reattachment of the pleura	
pneumonectomy new-mon-EK-toe-mee	**pneumon / ectomy** lung / removal
DEFINITION removal of a lung	
thoracocentesis thor-a-koh-sin-TEE-sis	**thoraco / centesis** chest / puncture
DEFINITION puncture of the chest	
thoracentesis thor-a-sin-TEE-sis	**thora [co] / centesis** chest / puncture
DEFINITION puncture of the chest NOTE: This word drops a syllable from *thoracocentesis* to make it easier to say.	
thoracostomy thor-a-KOS-toe-mee	**thoraco / stomy** chest / creation of an opening
DEFINITION creation of an opening in the chest	
thoracotomy thor-a-KAH-toe-mee	**thoraco / tomy** chest / incision
DEFINITION incision into the chest	

pharmacology

TERM	WORD ANALYSIS
antitussive an-tee-TUSS-iv	**anti / tuss / ive** against / cough / agent
DEFINITION a drug that prevents coughing	

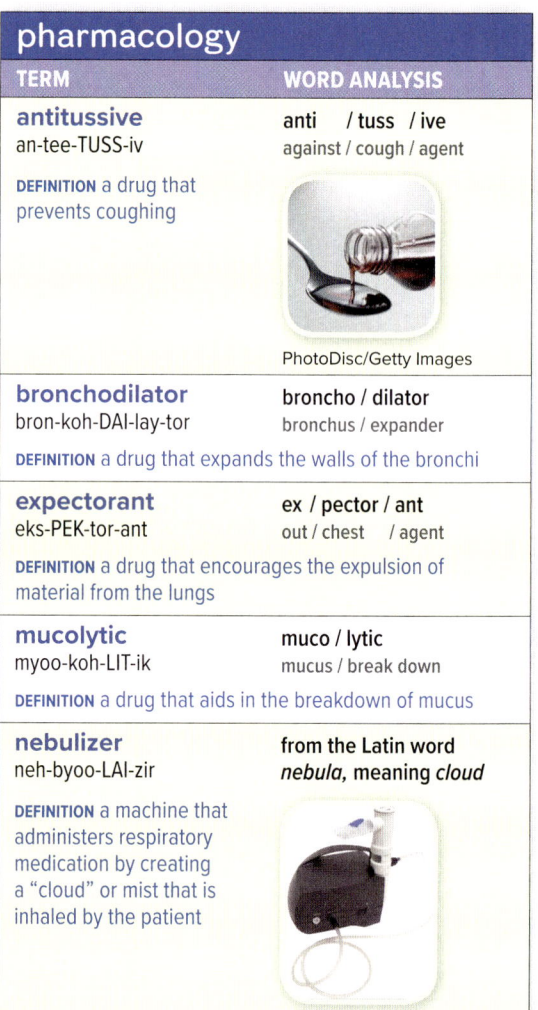

PhotoDisc/Getty Images

bronchodilator bron-koh-DAI-lay-tor	**broncho / dilator** bronchus / expander
DEFINITION a drug that expands the walls of the bronchi	
expectorant eks-PEK-tor-ant	**ex / pector / ant** out / chest / agent
DEFINITION a drug that encourages the expulsion of material from the lungs	
mucolytic myoo-koh-LIT-ik	**muco / lytic** mucus / break down
DEFINITION a drug that aids in the breakdown of mucus	
nebulizer neh-byoo-LAI-zir	from the Latin word *nebula*, meaning *cloud*
DEFINITION a machine that administers respiratory medication by creating a "cloud" or mist that is inhaled by the patient	

Stockbyte/Getty Images

PRONUNCIATION

EXERCISE 1 Indicate which syllable(s) is emphasized when pronounced.

EXAMPLE: bronchitis bron<u>chi</u>tis

1. lobectomy _____

2. antitussive _____

3. tracheostomy _____

4. thoracentesis _____

5. thoracostomy _____

TRANSLATION

EXERCISE 2 Break down the following words into their component parts.

EXAMPLE: nasopharyngoscope
naso | pharyngo | scope

1. tracheotomy _____

2. pneumonectomy _____

3. thoracostomy _____

4. tracheostomy _____

5. pleuropexy _____

6. thoracocentesis _____

7. antitussive _____

8. expectorant _____

9. mucolytic _____

EXERCISE 3 Underline and define the word parts from this chapter in the following terms.

1. laryngectomy _____

2. thoracocentesis _____

3. expectorant _____

4. endotracheal _____

EXERCISE 4 Match the term on the left with its definition on the right.

_____ 1. thoracotomy

_____ 2. nebulizer

_____ 3. thoracentesis

_____ 4. endotracheal intubation

_____ 5. cardiopulmonary resuscitation

a. insertion of a tube inside the trachea

b. a machine that administers respiratory medication by creating a "cloud" or mist that is inhaled by the patient

c. a puncture of the chest

d. a method of artificially maintaining blood flow and airflow when breathing and pulse have stopped

e. incision into the chest

EXERCISE 5 Translate the following terms as literally as possible.

EXAMPLE: nasopharyngoscope *an instrument for looking at the nose and throat*

1. antitussive _____

2. expectorant _____

3. pneumonectomy _____

4. tracheotomy _____

5. tracheostomy _____

6. thoracostomy _____

7. pleuropexy _____

8. thoracocentesis _____

9. mucolytic _____

GENERATION

EXERCISE 6 Build a medical term from the information provided.

> EXAMPLE: inflammation of the sinuses *sinusitis*

1. removal of the larynx _____

2. removal of a lobe _____

3. reattachment of the pleura _____

4. a drug that expands the walls of the bronchi

   _____

5. incision into the chest _____

6. a drug that prevents coughing _____

EXERCISE 7 Multiple-choice questions. Select the correct answer(s).

1. A *nebulizer* administers medication by creating a mist to be inhaled by a patient. It comes from the Latin word *nebula,* meaning
   a. mist
   b. smoke
   c. cloud
   d. medication

2. Select the terms that pertain to the upper respiratory system.
   a. laryngectomy   d. pneumonectomy
   b. lobectomy   e. mucolytic
   c. tracheotomy

3. Select the terms that pertain to the lower respiratory system.
   a. laryngectomy   d. pneumonectomy
   b. lobectomy   e. mucolytic
   c. tracheotomy

4. Which drug is used to break down mucus?
   a. antitussive   c. expectorant
   b. bronchodilator   d. mucolytic

10.6 Electronic Health Records

Emergency Department Visit

Chief Complaint:	**Hemoptysis**
History of Present Illness:	The patient has been brought to the emergency department by her mother. She is a 22-year-old female with **cystic fibrosis.** She has had a 1-day history of **hemoptysis.** She has been feeling tired for 5 days. Her mother says that the patient has had mild **dyspnea** and cough. The patient's last **PFTs** were much worse than normal for her. She has not had any **epistaxis,** bleeding from her gums, bloody stool, or easy bruising.
Past Medical History:	Cystic fibrosis; bronchiectasis.
Medications:	**Inhaled** antibiotic (tobramycin); **mucolytic** agent (pulmozyme); vitamins ADEK; **bronchodilator** (albuterol).
Allergies:	NKDA.
Social:	She is a nonsmoker. She is a sophomore in college and lives with her parents.
Surgical History:	None.
Physical Exam:	RR: 30; HR: 92; Temp: 102.1°F; BP: 90/57; **Pulse ox:** 89%
Gen:	Mildly **cyanotic.** In mild **respiratory distress.** Her nose and mouth are a little dry.
HEENT:	Her ear drums and ear canals are normal.
CV:	Mildly **tachycardic.** No murmur. Her pulses are a little weak.
Resp:	**Tachypneic,** shallow breaths, breath sounds are weaker than normal **bilaterally.**
GI:	Normal. Her liver and spleen are not large.
Emergency Department Course:	When she came to the **ED,** the patient was in **acute respiratory distress.** She was **intubated** with an **endotracheal tube** and placed on **SIMV.** A **CXR** verified correct placement in her trachea. She had poor circulation, so she was given **IVF** and transfused with 2 units of blood **(prbcs).** An **ABG** showed **hypoxemia** and **hypercapnia,** both of which improved on follow-up **ABG** after she was intubated. The **pulmonology** team was contacted; the team decided **bronchoscopy** would be best. The team found that she was bleeding in her **bronchi** and treated her with **endobronchial electrocautery.** Afterward, she was transferred to the **ICU** for further care.

EXERCISE 1 Fill in the blanks.

1. The patient has cystic fibrosis and a 1-day history of _____
   (coughing up blood).

2. The patient has had *dyspnea* (give definition: _____).

3. Her recent PFTs (give definition: _____)
   were significantly worse than previously.

4. Her medical history includes cystic fibrosis as well as _____
   (expansion of the bronchi).

5. Among her medications is albuterol, a *bronchodilator* (give definition: _____
   _____).

6. Her physical exam revealed that she has mild cyanosis (give definition: _____
   _____) and her breathing was rapid or _____.

7. The patient was then intubated with a tube in her _____.
   They used a bedside CXR (give definition: _____) to confirm correct
   placement.

8. ABG (give definition: _____) revealed
   hypoxemia (give definition:_____)
   and _____ (excessive carbon dioxide).

9. The pulmonologist performed a bronchoscopy (give definition: _____).

EXERCISE 2 Multiple-choice questions. Select the correct answer.

1. Which is a symptom mentioned by the patient?
   a. coughing up blood
   b. runny nose
   c. sleeplessness
   d. sore throat

2. How was the patient breathing when examined in the ED?
   a. rapidly
   b. slowly
   c. not at all
   d. heavily

3. The chart says the patient was taking shallow breaths. What is another term for that?
   a. hyperpnea
   b. hypopnea
   c. orthopnea
   d. apnea

4. Where was a tube placed in the patient?
   a. nowhere
   b. into the nose
   c. into the trachea
   d. into the nose and throat

5. What did the analysis of the patient's arterial blood gases reveal?
   a. deficient oxygen levels
   b. excessive carbon dioxide
   c. both
   d. neither

EXERCISE 3 True or false questions. Indicate true answers with a T and false answers with an F.

1. The patient has had a recent nosebleed. _____

2. The patient takes medication for constricted bronchial tubes. _____

3. The doctor noted the patient's skin had a slight blue color. _____

Quick Reference

glossary of roots

ROOT	DEFINITION	ROOT	DEFINITION
adenoid/o	adenoid	phren/o	diaphragm
bronch/o, bronchi/o	bronchus	pleur/o	pleura
bronchiol/o	bronchiole	-pnea	breathing
capn/o	carbon dioxide	pneum/o, pneumat/o, pneumon/o	air or lungs
carb/o	carbon dioxide	pulmon/o	lungs
laryng/o	larynx (voice box)	rhin/o	nose
lob/o	lobe	sept/o	septum
nas/o	nose	sin/o, sinus/o	sinus
ox/o	oxygen	spir/o	breathing
palat/o	palate	thorac/o	chest
pector/o	chest	tonsill/o	tonsil
pharyng/o	pharynx (throat)	trache/o	trachea (windpipe)

respiratory system abbreviations

ABBREVIATION	DEFINITION
ABG	arterial blood gas analysis of the gases in the blood; used to determine the effectiveness of the lungs in exchanging gases
Bx	biopsy Bx (biopsy)
COPD	chronic obstructive pulmonary disease
CPAP	continuous positive airway pressure a treatment for apnea involving keeping a patient's airways open using air pressure delivered via a face mask
CPR	cardiopulmonary resuscitation
CT	computed tomography
CTA	clear to auscultation when an examination reveals nothing abnormal about a patient's lung
CXR	chest x-ray Brand X/Getty Images
ET	endotracheal
IRDS	infant respiratory distress syndrome
LTB	laryngotracheobronchitis
MRI	magnetic resonance imaging
OSA	obstructive sleep apnea
PE	pulmonary embolism
PET	positron emission tomography
PFT	pulmonary function test
PSG	polysomnography
SOB	shortness of breath
T&A	tonsillectomy and adenoidectomy
TB	tuberculosis
URI	upper respiratory infection
V/Q	ventilation–perfusion scan

The Gastrointestinal System—Gastroenterology 11

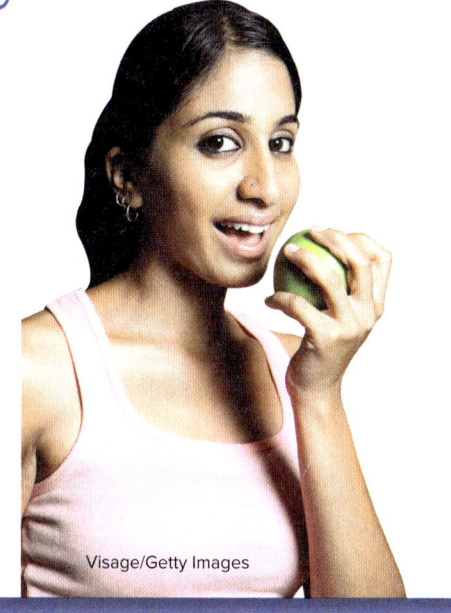

Visage/Getty Images

Learning Outcomes

Upon completion of this chapter, you will be able to:

11.1 Identify the **roots/word parts** associated with the **gastrointestinal system.**

S 11.2 Translate the **Subjective** terms associated with the **gastrointestinal system.**

O 11.3 Translate the **Objective** terms associated with the **gastrointestinal system.**

A 11.4 Translate the **Assessment** terms associated with the **gastrointestinal system.**

P 11.5 Translate the **Plan** terms associated with the **gastrointestinal system.**

11.6 Distinguish terms associated with the **gastrointestinal system** in the context of **electronic health records.**

Introduction and Overview of the Gastrointestinal System

Energy is necessary to make machines work, whether it comes from gasoline, batteries, or electricity. The body is the same way—it constantly needs energy. The gastrointestinal (GI) system is responsible for turning food into energy. As a first step, it digests the food. *Digest* comes from *di* (short for dia), meaning *through,* and *gest,* meaning *to carry. Digestion* is the process of carrying food through the body and breaking it apart into usable and unusable parts. There are three main types of usable food fuel: *protein, fat,* and *carbohydrates.* As food passes through the digestive system, the body breaks down and absorbs the usable parts and discards any unusable parts.

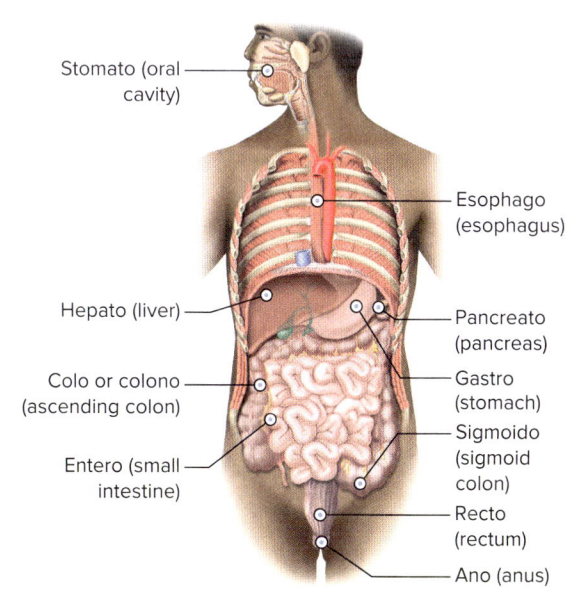

Stomato (oral cavity)

Esophago (esophagus)

Hepato (liver)

Pancreato (pancreas)

Colo or colono (ascending colon)

Gastro (stomach)

Sigmoido (sigmoid colon)

Entero (small intestine)

Recto (rectum)

Ano (anus)

The gastrointestinal system is mainly one long tube. Health care providers often talk about the system's two parts: the *upper* and *lower gastrointestinal tracts.* The upper GI tract includes the mouth, esophagus, and stomach. The lower GI tract is made up of the small and large intestines. In addition to the stomach and intestines, there are other organs that help in dealing with our nutrition. These organs are the liver, pancreas, and gallbladder.

11.1 Word Parts of the Gastrointestinal System

Upper Gastrointestinal Tract

The process of digestion begins in the mouth. When people eat, they start with chewing their food. When chewing, teeth (*dento*) tear food into smaller parts. At the same time, the salivary glands make saliva (*sialo*). The saliva helps to moisten the food to help it pass down the throat. Saliva also has chemicals that help to break the food apart.

The food is passed from the mouth down a tube (*esophago*) that leads to the stomach (*gastro*). The esophagus has two gates that keep the food moving the right way. The first gate keeps out air from the stomach, and the second gate keeps food from leaving the stomach in the wrong direction.

As we eat, food collects in the stomach. The stomach makes acid, which breaks down protein. The stomach acts almost like a blender. Through muscle contractions, the stomach mixes the food with stomach juices, including acid. This mixing process physically and chemically softens the food into a paste-like substance known as *chyme.* Food then passes through a muscle at the end of the stomach, the *pylorus,* and into the small intestine.

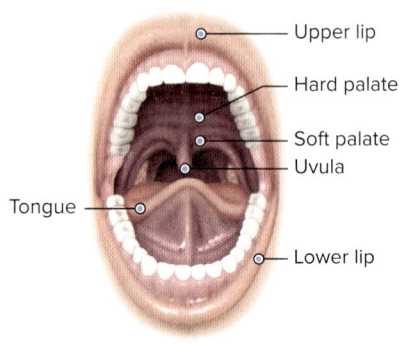

Upper lip
Hard palate
Soft palate
Uvula
Tongue
Lower lip

mouth

ROOTS: *or/o, stomat/o*

EXAMPLES: oral, stomatosis

NOTES: Most people tend to chew on the side of the mouth that corresponds to the hand with which they write. Right-handed folks use the right side of their mouth, and left-handed folks—well, you get the idea.

gums

ROOT: *gingiv/o*

EXAMPLES: gingivitis, gingivostomatitis

NOTES: This root comes from the Latin word for *gums.* Healthy gums are a pinkish-red color, but the color can vary depending on the lightness or darkness of the patient's skin.

tooth

ROOTS: *dent/o, odont/o*

EXAMPLES: dentist, odontalgia

NOTES: The enamel on the outside of the *tooth* is the hardest thing in the human body. Adult humans have 32 teeth (or they're supposed to, anyway). An opossum has 50 teeth, a mosquito has 47 teeth, and sharks have as many as 40 sets of teeth in their lifetime.

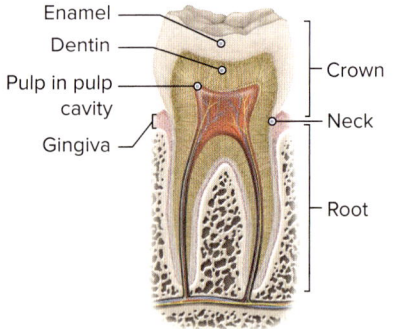

Enamel
Dentin
Pulp in pulp cavity
Gingiva
Crown
Neck
Root

tongue

ROOTS: *gloss/o, lingu/o*

EXAMPLES: glossopathy, hypoglossal, sublingual

NOTES: The strongest muscle in the human body, relative to its size, is the *tongue*. It is also the only muscle in the human body that is attached at only one end. Here's an interesting fact: Whether or not you can roll your tongue into a tube or other shapes is predetermined by your genetics.

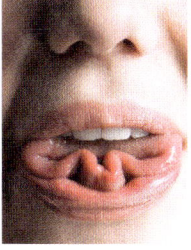

Christopher Robbins/ Getty Images

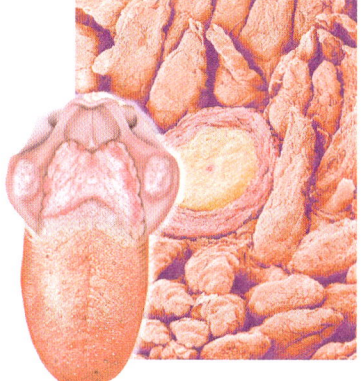

Micro Discovery/Corbis Documentary/Getty Images

stomach

ROOT: *gastr/o*

EXAMPLES: gastritis, gastropexy

NOTES: Here are two things you probably don't know about the *stomach:* It must produce a new layer of mucus every 2 weeks or it will digest itself, and when you blush, your stomach changes colors, too.

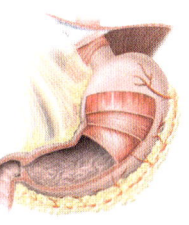

esophagus

ROOT: *esophag/o*

EXAMPLES: esophageal, esophagitis

NOTES: The *esophagus* is a tube that is about the diameter of a quarter; it connects your mouth to your stomach. The name breaks down into *eso* (carry) and *phagus* (eat) and literally means *the thing that carries what you eat,* presumably to the stomach.

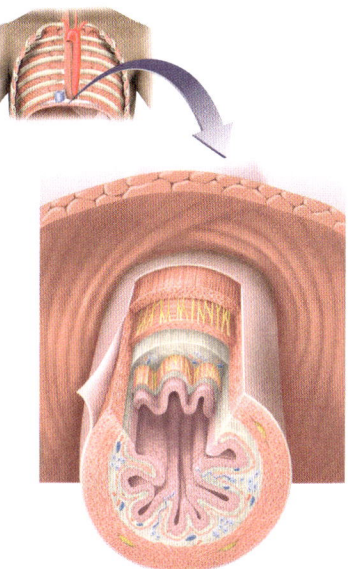

Cross section of the esophagus

Lower Gastrointestinal Tract

The lower GI tract is made up of the small and large intestines. The small intestine is the longest part of the gastrointestinal system. It is made up of three parts: the *duodenum, jejunum,* and *ileum.* Most of the chemical breakdown in the small intestine happens in its first part, the duodenum. In the duodenum, chemicals from the liver (*bile*) and the pancreas mix with the food. The food continues digestion throughout the rest of the long path of the jejunum and ileum.

From here, the food then passes into the large intestine. By this point, most of the nutrients have been absorbed. The main role of the large intestine is to absorb the water from the remaining food. The stool passes through the *ascending, transverse, descending,* and *sigmoid colon* into the *rectum,* where it waits to be excreted.

intestines

ROOT: *enter/o*

EXAMPLES: gastroenterology, dysentery

NOTES: This combining form refers to the intestines in general. It comes from a Greek word meaning *inside*. It's appropriate, because your intestines take up a great deal of space inside you. The average adult has over 20 feet of intestines.

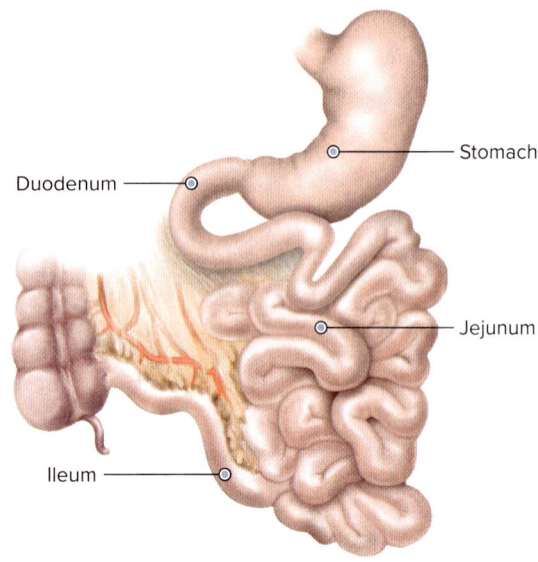

Stomach

Duodenum

Jejunum

Ileum

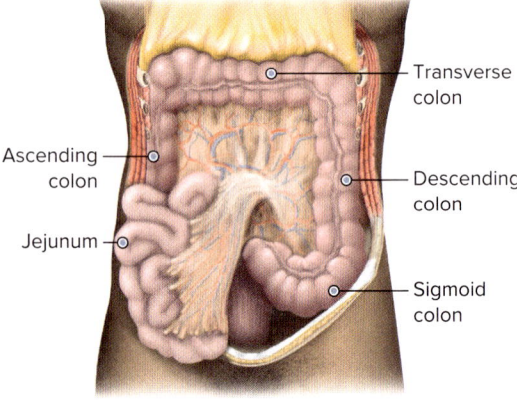

Transverse colon

Ascending colon

Descending colon

Jejunum

Sigmoid colon

duodenum

ROOT: *duoden/o*

EXAMPLES: gastroduodenoscope, duodenectomy

NOTES: The small intestine is divided into three sections: the *duodenum, jejunum,* and *ileum.* The duodenum is the first of the three sections. Its name means *twelve* and refers to the fact that its length is about the same as the width of 12 fingers.

jejunum

ROOT: *jejun/o*

EXAMPLES: jejunotomy, jejunitis

NOTES: The jejunum is the second of the small intestine's three sections. Its name means *empty* and refers to the fact that it is found empty during dissections.

ileum

ROOT: *ile/o*

EXAMPLES: ileotomy, ileitis

NOTES: The ileum is the third of the small intestine's three sections. Its name means *groin* and refers to the fact that it is located in the lower abdomen.

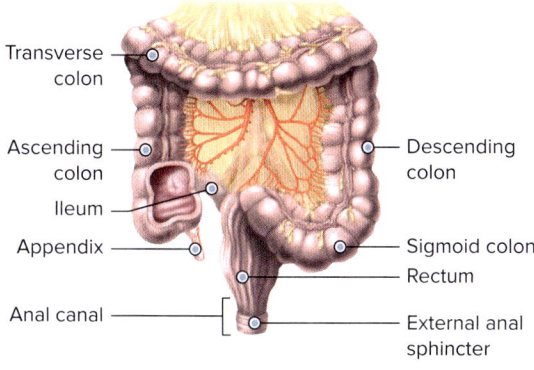

Transverse colon

Ascending colon

Ileum

Appendix

Anal canal

Descending colon

Sigmoid colon

Rectum

External anal sphincter

colon (large intestine)

ROOTS: *col/o, colon/o*

EXAMPLES: colorectal carcinoma, colitis, colonoscopy, colonectomy

NOTES: The colon starts at the bottom of the abdomen (remember, that's where the ileum ends) and is divided into three main sections: the ascending (*going up*) colon, the transverse (*going across*) colon, and the descending (*going down*) colon.

sigmoid colon

ROOT: *sigmoid/o*

EXAMPLE: sigmoidoscope

NOTES: The sigmoid colon is at the end of the colon, before the rectum begins. Its name is derived from the Greek letter *sigma* (Σ, related to the letter *s*) + *oid* (resembling). It refers to the fact it has an *s*-shaped curve.

rectum

ROOT: *rect/o*

EXAMPLES: rectoplasty, rectitis

NOTES: *Rectum* is Latin for *straight* and refers to the final portion of the colon before it arrives at the anus. Although it is straight in comparison to the rest of the intestines, the human rectum really isn't straight. It got its name from an ancient doctor named Galen, who dissected animals that really did have straight rectums.

anus

ROOT: *an/o*

EXAMPLES: anoplasty, anal fistula

NOTES: The *anus* is the sphincter or muscle at the end of the intestines that allows for the passage of feces. Its name comes from the Latin word for *ring.*

anus and rectum

ROOT: *proct/o*

EXAMPLES: proctology, proctitis

NOTES: The root *ano* refers specifically to the anus, and the root *recto* refers specifically to the rectum, but *procto* refers to both the anus and rectum.

Supporting Structures/Digestive Organs

The gastrointestinal system also includes other organs that help to break down food, including the liver and pancreas. The *liver* is the largest gland in the body. It has many roles in nutrition. It helps get rid of dangerous toxins, plays a role in energy storage, and makes a substance used to break down fat in the GI tract, called *bile.*

Bile is sent to two places: the small intestine and a storage gland called the *gallbladder.* Bile enters the small intestine by the common bile duct. Bile breaks big pieces of fat into smaller pieces of fat.

The *pancreas* is an important organ in the endocrine system. It also is part of the gastrointestinal system. The pancreas makes chemicals known as enzymes that break apart proteins, fats, and carbohydrates.

bile (gall)

ROOTS: *bil/i, chol/e*

EXAMPLES: biligenesis, cholelith

NOTES: *Bile,* which is sometimes called *gall,* is a substance produced in the liver that is required for the body to digest food.

saliva

ROOT: *sial/o*

EXAMPLE: sialoadenitis

NOTES: The average human produces between 1 and 3 pints of saliva a day. In addition to beginning the process of digestion, saliva is necessary to taste food. You cannot taste food until it is mixed with saliva.

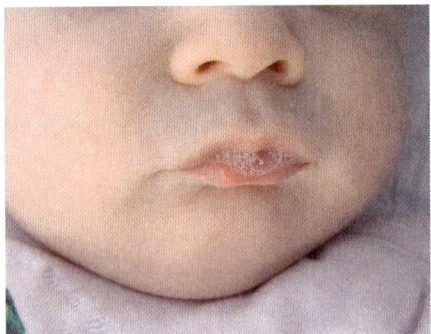

fotolinchen/Getty Images

The gastrointestinal organs are located in the part of the body known as the *abdomen* and are surrounded by a membrane that keeps everything in place. This membrane is called the *peritoneum*. It has more specific nerve fibers than the organs it surrounds. If infection or inflammation spreads to the peritoneum, the pain is usually more specific in its nature. This is very helpful when examining a patient with gastrointestinal pain.

abdomen

ROOTS: *abdomin/o, celi/o, lapar/o*

EXAMPLES: abdominocentesis, celiopathy, laparoscope

NOTES: Laparoscopic surgery is a way to perform surgery on the *abdomen* without making lengthy incisions. In fact, it is so minimally invasive that it is sometimes referred to as *Band-Aid* or *keyhole* surgery because the incisions are so small. One unique aspect of this procedure, though, is that in order to have enough room to work, surgeons must fill the abdomen with air, or blow it up like a balloon.

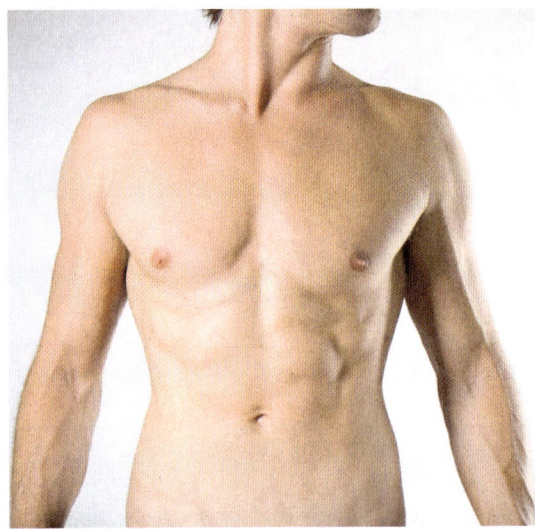

Juice Images/Alamy Stock Photo

bladder

ROOT: *cyst/o*

EXAMPLES: cholecystogram, cholecystectomy

NOTES: Once bile is produced in the liver, some of it is stored in the *gallbladder,* a small organ about the size of a pear that's located under the liver. While it is being stored, the bile becomes more concentrated in order to increase its potency. It is stored until the body needs it to help digest fatty foods.

duct

ROOT: *doch/o*

EXAMPLE: choledocholithiasis

NOTES: Okay, this is tricky. Bile leaves the liver through numerous bile *ducts*. The name for these, though, uses the root *cholangio,* for *bile vessels.* All of these little ducts eventually unite to form the *common bile duct,* a single tube that empties into the small intestine. The root *choledocho* means *bile duct* but refers to only this main duct.

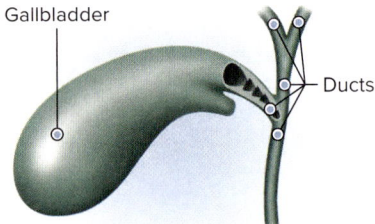

Gallbladder

Ducts

liver

ROOTS: *hepat/o, hepatic/o*

EXAMPLES: hepatitis, hepaticotomy

NOTES: The *liver,* which is located on the right side of your abdomen just below your rib cage, is the largest organ in the human body (except the skin); it can filter more than a liter of blood every minute.

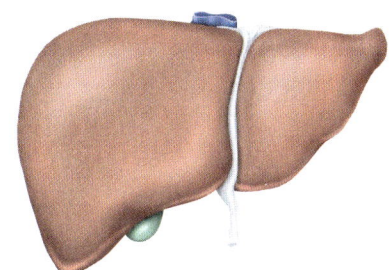

Anterior view

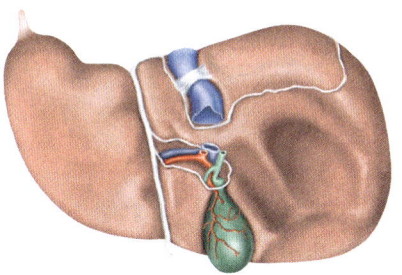

Posterior view

pancreas

ROOT: *pancreat/o*

EXAMPLES: pancreatitis, pancreatolith

NOTES: The term *pancreas* comes from two Greek words: *pan* (*all*) and *kreas* (*flesh*). People debate the reason why, but some think it is because of the organ's fleshy consistency. If you are in a restaurant and are tempted to order *sweetbreads,* be careful. It's a term used by chefs to mean *cooked pancreas.*

peritoneum

ROOT: *peritone/o*

EXAMPLE: peritoneotomy

NOTES: The peritoneum is a membrane that lines the abdominal cavity and covers most of the abdominal organs. The name comes from *peri* (*around*) and *teneo* (*stretch*) and refers to the fact that it appears to be *stretched around* the abdominal organs.

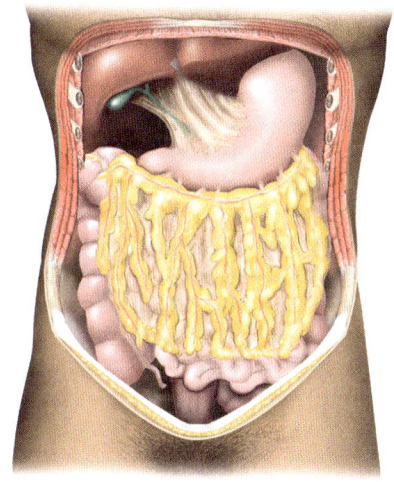

TRANSLATION

EXERCISE 1 Match the root on the left with its definition on the right. Some definitions will be used more than once.

_____ 1. dent/o

_____ 2. esophag/o

_____ 3. gingiv/o

_____ 4. lingu/o

_____ 5. or/o

_____ 6. gastr/o

_____ 7. odont/o

_____ 8. gloss/o

_____ 9. stomat/o

a. esophagus

b. gums

c. mouth

d. stomach

e. tongue

f. tooth

EXERCISE 2 Translate the following roots.

1. dent/o _____

2. esophag/o _____

3. gingiv/o _____

4. lingu/o _____

5. or/o _____

6. gastr/o _____

7. odont/o _____

8. gloss/o _____

9. stomat/o _____

EXERCISE 3 Underline and define the roots from this chapter in the following terms.

1. dentistry _____

2. orthodontics _____

3. esophageal carcinoma _____

4. gingival hyperplasia _____

5. nasogastric tube _____

6. glossorrhaphy _____

7. stomatomycosis _____

8. stomatogastric (2 roots) _____

9. esophagogastroplasty (2 roots) _____

EXERCISE 4 Break down the following words into their component parts and translate.

EXAMPLE: **sinusitis** _sinus | itis_
inflammation of the sinuses

1. dentalgia _____

2. odontalgia _____

3. stomatoplasty _____

4. esophagalgia _____

5. gastralgia _____

6. gastroplasty _____

7. gingivoplasty _____

8. glossoplasty _____

EXERCISE 5 Match the root on the left with its definition on the right.

_____ 1. proct/o

_____ 2. enter/o

_____ 3. an/o

_____ 4. rect/o

_____ 5. ile/o

_____ 6. jejun/o

_____ 7. duoden/o

_____ 8. col/o

_____ 9. sigmoid/o

a. sphincter or muscle at the end of the intestines that allows for the passage of feces; its name comes from the Latin word for *ring*

b. anus and rectum

c. end of the colon before it enters the rectum; its name is derived from the Greek letter *sigma* (Σ, related to the letter *s*) + *oid* (resembling), and it refers to the fact it has an *s*-shaped curve

d. first of three sections of the small intestine; the name means *twelve* and refers to the fact that its length is about the same as the width of 12 fingers

e. intestines

f. Latin for *straight* and refers to the final portion of the colon, before it arrives at the anus

g. starts at the bottom of the abdomen and is divided into three main sections: the ascending, the transverse, and the descending

h. the second of three sections of the small intestine, its name means *empty,* a reference to the fact that it is found empty during dissections

i. the third of three sections of the small intestine, its name means *groin,* a reference to the fact that it is located in the lower abdomen

EXERCISE 6 Translate the following roots.

1. proct/o _____

2. an/o _____

3. rect/o _____

4. colon/o _____

5. enter/o _____

6. col/o _____

7. jejun/o _____

8. duoden/o _____

9. ile/o _____

10. sigmoid/o _____

4. jejunostomy _____

5. sigmoidoscopy _____

6. rectopexy _____

7. enterorrhaphy _____

8. proctoptosis _____

9. colorectal carcinoma (2 roots) _____

10. anosigmoidoscopy (2 roots) _____

11. gastroduodenostomy (2 roots) _____

12. gastroenterostomy (2 roots) _____

EXERCISE 8 Break down the following words into their component parts and translate.

EXAMPLE: sinusitis   *sinus | itis*
                         inflammation of the sinuses

EXERCISE 7 Underline and define the roots from this chapter in the following terms.

1. anal fistula _____

2. colovaginal fistula _____

3. colostomy _____

1. rectalgia _____

2. anoplasty _____

3. proctology _____

Learning Outcome 11.1 Exercises

4. colectomy _____   7. ileotomy _____

5. duodenectomy _____   8. jejunotomy _____

6. enterectomy _____   9. sigmoidoscope _____

EXERCISE 9 Match the root on the left with its definition on the right. Some definitions will be used more than once.

_____ 1. pancreat/o

_____ 2. abdomin/o

_____ 3. lapar/o

_____ 4. sial/o

_____ 5. bil/i

_____ 6. chol/e

_____ 7. hepat/o

_____ 8. cyst/o

_____ 9. choledoch/o

_____ 10. cholangi/o

_____ 11. peritone/o

_____ 12. celi/o

a. membrane that lines the abdominal cavity and covers most of the abdominal organs; the name comes from *peri* (*around*) and *teneo* (*stretch*) and refers to the fact that it appears to be *stretched around* the abdominal organs

b. a substance produced in the liver and required for the body to digest food

c. abdomen

d. begins the process of digestion; required to taste food

e. bladder

f. located on the right side of your abdomen just below your rib cage, this, the largest organ in the human body (except the skin), can filter over a liter of blood every minute

g. main bile duct

h. pancreas

i. bile vessels through which bile leaves the liver

EXERCISE 10 Translate the following roots.

1. abdomin/o _____

2. pancreat/o _____

3. bil/i _____

4. peritone/o _____

5. celi/o _____

6. chol/e _____

7. hepatic/o _____

8. hepat/o _____

9. lapar/o _____

10. doch/o _____

11. cyst/o _____

12. sial/o _____

EXERCISE 11 Underline and define the roots *from this chapter* in the following terms.

1. abdominocentesis _____

2. biligenesis _____

3. celiomyositis _____

4. cholelithotripsy _____

5. peritoneoscopy _____

6. laparoscopic surgery _____

7. sialolithiasis _____

8. hepatomalacia _____

9. pancreatolithiasis _____

10. cholecystectomy (2 roots) _____

11. choledocholithiasis (2 roots) _____

12. hepaticogastrostomy (2 roots) _____

13. laparoenterostomy (2 roots) _____

14. cholangiopancreatography (2 roots) _____

EXERCISE 12 Break down the following words into their component parts and translate.

> EXAMPLE: **sinusitis**   *sinus | itis*
> *inflammation of the sinuses*

1. cholelith _____

2. celiotomy _____

3. cholelithotomy _____

4. cholecystalgia _____

5. choledochotomy _____

6. sialolith _____

7. abdominoplasty _____

8. hepaticotomy _____

9. laparotomy _____

10. pancreatolith _____

11. peritonitis _____

12. sialolithotomy _____

GENERATION

EXERCISE 13 Identify the roots for the following definitions.

1. esophagus _____

2. gums _____

3. stomach _____

4. tooth (2 roots) _____

5. tongue (2 roots) _____

6. mouth (2 roots) _____

EXERCISE 14 Build a medical term from the information provided.

> EXAMPLE: **inflammation of the sinuses**   *sinusitis*

1. inflammation of the mouth (use *stomat/o*)

   _____

2. inflammation of the esophagus _____

3. inflammation of the stomach _____

4. inflammation of the gums _____

5. tooth specialist (use *dent/o*) _____

6. straight teeth specialist (use *odont/o*) _____

   _____

7. inflammation of the gums and tongue (use *gloss/o*) _____

8. around tooth inflammation (use *odont/o*)

   _____

EXERCISE 15 Identify the roots for the following definitions.

1. anus _____

2. rectum _____

3. anus and rectum _____

4. ileum _____

5. jejunum _____

6. duodenum _____

7. intestines _____

8. colon (2 roots) _____

9. sigmoid colon _____

EXERCISE 16 Build a medical term from the information provided.

> EXAMPLE: **inflammation of the sinuses**   *sinusitis*

1. inflammation of the colon (use *col/o*) _____

   _____

2. inflammation of the duodenum _____

   _____

3. inflammation of the ileum _____

   _____

4. inflammation of the jejunum _____

_____

5. inflammation of the rectum _____

_____

6. surgical reconstruction of the anus _____

_____

7. instrument to look into the sigmoid colon

_____

8. inflammation of the anus and rectum (use *proct/o*) _____

9. inflammation of the ileum and colon (use *col/o*) _____

10. inflammation of the jejunum and ileum

_____

11. inflammation of the stomach, intestines, and colon (use *col/o*) _____

EXERCISE 17 Identify the roots for the following definitions.

1. peritoneum _____

2. pancreas _____

3. bladder _____

4. duct _____

5. saliva _____

6. liver (2 roots) _____

7. bile (2 roots) _____

8. abdomen (3 roots) _____

EXERCISE 18 Build a medical term from the information provided.

> EXAMPLE: inflammation of the sinuses *sinusitis*

1. inflammation of the liver (use *hepat/o*)

_____

2. inflammation of the pancreas _____

3. inflammation of the peritoneum _____

_____

4. inflammation of the bile bladder (use *chol/e*)

_____

5. incision into the bile duct (use *chol/e*)

_____

6. incision into the abdomen (use *lapar/o*)

_____

7. surgical reconstruction of the abdomen (use *abdomin/o*) _____

8. disease of the abdomen (use *celi/o*) _____

_____

EXERCISE 19 Multiple-choice questions. Select the correct answer(s).

1. Select all of the roots below that pertain to the supporting structures/digestive organs.
   a. abdomin/o   g. gingiv/o
   b. chol/e   h. hepatic/o
   c. colon/o   i. pancreat/o
   d. enter/o   j. proct/o
   e. esophag/o   k. sial/o
   f. gastr/o   l. stomat/o

2. Select all of the roots below that pertain to the lower GI tract.
   a. abdomin/o   g. gingiv/o
   b. chol/e   h. hepatic/o
   c. colon/o   i. pancreat/o
   d. enter/o   j. proct/o
   e. esophag/o   k. sial/o
   f. gastr/o   l. stomat/o

3. Select all of the roots below that pertain to the upper GI tract.
   a. abdomin/o   g. gingiv/o
   b. chol/e   h. hepatic/o
   c. colon/o   i. pancreat/o
   d. enter/o   j. proct/o
   e. esophag/o   k. sial/o
   f. gastr/o   l. stomat/o

11.2 Patient History, Problems, Complaints

Gastrointestinal complaints are a very common reason for patient visits to a health care provider. Problems of the upper gastrointestinal tract differ a bit from problems of the lower gastrointestinal tract. Pain in the upper GI tract is much more common than in the lower GI tract.

A patient may have pain in his or her mouth (*stomatodynia*). This is common with inflammation of the mouth (*stomatitis*), which may include ulcers. Esophageal pain (*esophalgia*) is very common in patients who have acid reflux disease, in which stomach acid comes up the wrong way from the stomach. Stomach pain (*gastralgia*) can be from a hole in the lining of the stomach or from inflammation.

The other common type of upper GI complaint is change in function. A patient may have discomfort with eating (*dyspepsia*); this may either be pain or general nausea. If nausea becomes severe, the body may vomit (*emesis*) the stomach's contents.

Symptoms of the lower GI tract generally relate to problems with how food moves through the tract. If food moves too fast, less of the water in it is absorbed into the body, and stools may become very watery (*diarrhea*). If food moves too slowly, the stool may become hard, causing constipation. If food doesn't move at all, there may be a blockage (*obstruction*). If the obstruction blocks even gas from passing, it's known as *obstipation*.

The supporting organs of the digestive system can cause pain as well. Gallbladder pain (*cholecystalgia*) is among the more common GI complaints in adult patients. It can be caused by blockage, infection, or both. Pancreatic pain is usually very severe and often requires strong pain medicine for relief. While diseases of the liver can also cause pain, they more often first present as yellow discoloration of the eyes and skin (*jaundice*). This is due to an accumulation of *bilirubin*.

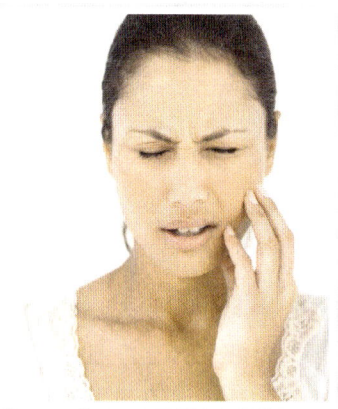

It might not seem like it, but dentalgia, or tooth pain, can be a sign of a gastroenterology problem as well as a dentistry problem.
Stockbyte/Getty Images

upper gastro tract

TERM	WORD ANALYSIS
aphagia ah-FAY-jah	a / phag / ia no / eat / condition
DEFINITION inability to eat	
dentalgia den-TAL-jah	dent / algia tooth / pain
DEFINITION tooth pain	
	Karin Dreyer/Blend Images LLC
dyspepsia dis-PEP-see-ah	dys / peps / ia bad / digestion / condition
DEFINITION bad digestion	
gastralgia gas-TRAL-jah	gastr / algia stomach / pain
DEFINITION stomach pain	

upper gastro tract *continued*

TERM	WORD ANALYSIS
gastrodynia GAS-troh-DIH-nee-ah	gastro / dynia stomach / pain
DEFINITION stomach pain	
gingivostomatitis JIN-jih-voh-STOH-mah-TAI-tis	gingivo / stomat / itis gum / mouth / inflammation
DEFINITION inflammation of the mouth and gums	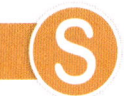
hematemesis HEM-at-EM-eh-sis	hemat / emesis blood / vomiting
DEFINITION vomiting blood	
hyperemesis HAI-per-EM-eh-sis	hyper / emesis over / vomiting
DEFINITION excessive vomiting	
odontalgia OH-dawn-TAL-jah	odont / algia tooth / pain
DEFINITION tooth pain	
odontodynia oh-DAWN-toh-DAI-nee-ah	odonto / dynia tooth / pain
DEFINITION tooth pain	
stomatitis STOH-mah-TAI-tis	stomat / itis mouth / inflammation
DEFINITION inflammation of the mouth	

lower gastro tract

TERM	WORD ANALYSIS
diarrhea DAI-ah-REE-ah	dia / rrhea through / discharge
DEFINITION passing of fluid or unformed feces	
dysentery DIS-en-TER-ee	dys / enter / y bad / intestine / condition
DEFINITION another name for diarrhea	
hemorrhoid HEM-oh-ROID	from a Greek word referring to veins likely to discharge blood
DEFINITION inflammation of the veins surrounding the anus	

supporting organs

TERM	WORD ANALYSIS
icterus IK-ter-us	from Greek, for *jaundice*
DEFINITION another name for jaundice NOTE: This word has its origins in the name of a bird with a yellow breast; it was once believed that seeing the bird would cure jaundice.	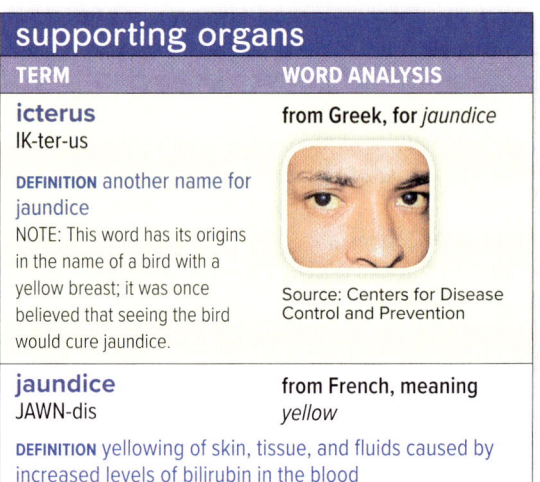 Source: Centers for Disease Control and Prevention
jaundice JAWN-dis	from French, meaning *yellow*
DEFINITION yellowing of skin, tissue, and fluids caused by increased levels of bilirubin in the blood	

PRONUNCIATION

EXERCISE 1   Indicate which syllable(s) is emphasized when pronounced.

> EXAMPLE: bronchitis bron**chi**tis

1. aphagia _____

2. jaundice _____

3. icterus _____

4. dentalgia _____

5. gastralgia _____

6. dyspepsia _____

TRANSLATION

EXERCISE 2   Break down the following words into their component parts.

> EXAMPLE: nasopharyngoscope
> *naso | pharyngo | scope*

1. stomatitis _____

2. gastrodynia _____

3. odontodynia _____

4. hematemesis _____

5. hyperemesis _____

6. dyspepsia _____

7. gingivostomatitis _____

EXERCISE 3   Underline and define the roots from this chapter in the following terms.

1. dentalgia _____

2. odontalgia _____

3. gastralgia _____

4. dysentery _____

5. gingivostomatitis (2 roots) _____

EXERCISE 4   Fill in the blanks.

1. *gastralgia* = pain in the _____

2. *dentalgia* = pain in the _____

3. *odontalgia* = pain in the _____

EXERCISE 5   Match the term on the left with its definition on the right.

_____ 1. diarrhea   a. inability to eat

_____ 2. hemorrhoid   b. bad digestion

_____ 3. dyspepsia   c. passing of fluid or unformed feces

_____ 4. jaundice   d. inflammation of the veins surrounding the anus

_____ 5. aphagia   e. yellowing of the skin, tissue, and fluids caused by increased levels of bilirubin in the blood

EXERCISE 6   Translate the following terms as literally as possible.

> EXAMPLE: nasopharyngoscope   *an instrument for looking at the nose and throat*

1. odontodynia _____

2. dyspepsia _____

3. hematemesis _____

4. hyperemesis _____

5. aphagia _____

GENERATION

EXERCISE 7 Build a medical term from the information provided.

EXAMPLE: inflammation of the sinuses *sinusitis*

1. inflammation of the mouth (use *stomat/o*)

   _____

2. inflammation of the mouth and gums (use *stomat/o*) _____

3. stomach pain (use *-dynia*) _____

4. bad intestine condition _____

EXERCISE 8 Multiple-choice questions. Select the correct answer(s).

1. Select all of the terms below that pertain to the lower GI tract.
   a. dentalgia
   b. diarrhea
   c. hematemesis
   d. hemorrhoid
   e. stomatitis

2. Select all of the terms below that pertain to the upper GI tract.
   a. dentalgia
   b. diarrhea
   c. hematemesis
   d. hemorrhoid
   e. stomatitis

3. Which of the terms below literally means *through excessive discharge* and is the passing of fluid or unformed feces?
   a. diarrhea
   b. dysentery
   c. hemorrhoid
   d. icterus

4. Which of the definitions below is the correct definition of the term *hemorrhoid?*
   a. inflammation of the skin surrounding the anus
   b. inflammation of the skin surrounding the rectum
   c. inflammation of the veins surrounding the anus
   d. inflammation of the veins surrounding the rectum
   e. none of these

O BJECTIVE

11.3 Observation and Discovery

The first component to examining a patient with gastrointestinal complaints is visual inspection. Color changes, such as jaundice, can indicate problems with the GI system. Another visual finding could be a very large, fluid-filled abdomen (*ascites*). This is usually associated with serious liver problems.

After visually inspecting the patient, the next step is to touch, or *palpate,* the abdomen. During abdominal palpation, an examiner may notice masses, pain, or tensing of the abdominal muscles in response to pain, which is known as *guarding.*

It is important to know where a patient has tenderness during the exam. The abdomen is divided into different regions to help distinguish the types of problems a patient may have. One specific goal of palpation is locating the liver's edge. An enlarged liver (*hepatomegaly*) can be a sign of disease.

Many laboratory tests for the digestive system involve examining the waste product of the digestion—that is, the stool. Some tests look for nutrients that have not been broken down or absorbed correctly. For example, fat in the stool

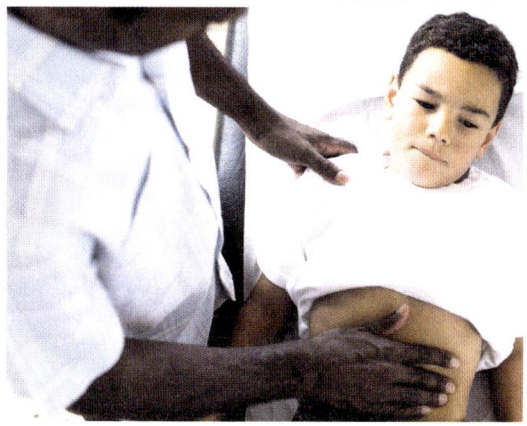

A doctor pressing on a patient's abdomen during a physical exam is checking for hepatomegaly.

Ian Hooton/Science Source

(*steatorrhea*) indicates disease. Other tests look for blood (*fecal occult blood test*) or pus in the stool, and still others look for bacteria (*stool culture*) in the stool.

A few blood tests specifically relate to the GI system. These tests involve the chemicals that organs make to break down food (*enzymes*) and include liver enzymes and pancreatic enzymes.

As with all parts of the body, images can be very helpful in diagnosing disease. X-rays, CT scans, and ultrasounds are all very common ways of assessing the abdomen and GI structures. Because the GI system is one long tube, visual inspection with a camera is also possible (*endoscopy*). Common examples include camera inspection of the entire colon (*colonoscopy*) or just the end part (*sigmoidoscopy*), as well as inspection of the esophagus, stomach, and duodenum (*esophagogastroduodenoscopy*). There are also more specialized tests that examine vessels and ducts. One common example studies the release of bile from the gallbladder (*cholangiogram*).

upper gastro tract

TERM	WORD ANALYSIS
gingivitis JIN-jih-VAI-tis	gingiv / itis gum / inflammation
DEFINITION inflammation of the gums	
stomatogastric stoh-MAT-oh-GAS-trik	stomato / gastr / ic mouth / stomach / pertaining to
DEFINITION pertaining to the mouth and stomach	
stomatosis STOH-mah-TOH-sis	stomat / osis mouth / condition
DEFINITION mouth condition	

Source: CDC/Minnesota Department of Health, R.N. Barr Library; Librarians Melissa Rethlefsen and Marie Jones

lower gastro tract

TERM	WORD ANALYSIS
flatus FLAH-tus	from Latin, for *to blow*
DEFINITION medical term for passing gas	
hernia HER-nee-ah	from Latin, for *rupture*
DEFINITION rupture or protusion of an organ through the wall that normally contains it	

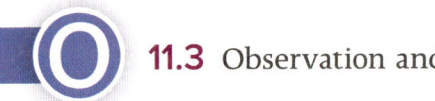

supporting organs

TERM	WORD ANALYSIS
ascites ah-SAI-teez	from the Greek word *askos,* referring to a bag made from the skin of a goat that was used to hold wine
DEFINITION retention of fluid in the peritoneum NOTE: The name comes from the patient's resemblance to an askos.	
cholelith KOH-lay-lith	chole / lith bile / stone
DEFINITION gallstone; literally, *a stone in the bile*	
hepatomegaly heh-PAT-oh-MEG-ah-lee	hepato / megaly liver / enlargement
DEFINITION enlargement of the liver 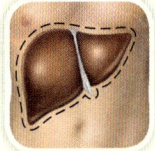	
pancreatolith pan-kree-AT-oh-lith	pancreato / lith pancreas / stone
DEFINITION stone in the pancreas	
sialolith sai-AL-oh-lith	sialo / lith saliva / stone
DEFINITION stone in the saliva	

diagnostic procedures

TERM	WORD ANALYSIS
colonoscopy COH-lon-AW-skoh-pee	colono / scopy colon / looking procedure
DEFINITION procedure for looking at the colon 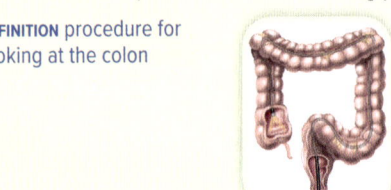	

diagnostic procedures *continued*

TERM	WORD ANALYSIS
endoscopy en-DAW-skoh-pee	endo / scopy inside / looking procedure
DEFINITION procedure of looking inside 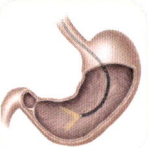	
esophagoscopy eh-SAW-fah-GAW-skoh-pee	esophago / scopy esophagus / looking procedure
DEFINITION procedure for looking inside the esophagus	
esophagogastro-duodenoscopy eh-SAW-fah-goh-GAS-stroh-DOO-aw-den-AW-skoh-pee	esophago / gastro / esophagus / stomach **duodeno / scopy** duodenum / looking procedure
DEFINITION procedure for looking inside the esophagus, stomach, and duodenum	
fecal occult blood test (FOBT) FEE-kal ah-KULT blud test	fec / al feces / pertaining to **occult blood test** hidden
DEFINITION test of feces to discover blood not visibly apparent	
gastroscopy gas-TRAW-skoh-pee	gastro / scopy stomach / looking procedure
DEFINITION procedure for looking at the stomach	
laparoscope LAP-ar-oh-skohp	laparo / scope abdomen / instrument to look
DEFINITION instrument for looking inside the abdomen 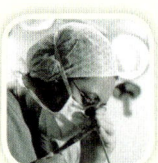	

Corbis/VCG/Getty Images

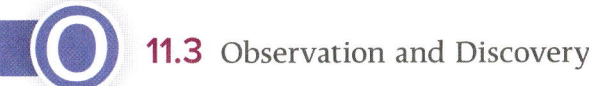

diagnostic procedures *continued*

TERM	WORD ANALYSIS
laparoscopy LAP-ar-AW-skoh-pee	laparo / scopy abdomen / looking procedure
DEFINITION procedure for looking inside the abdomen	
nasogastric tube (NGT) NAY-soh-GAS-trik TOOB	naso / gastr / ic nose / stomach / pertaining to **tube**
DEFINITION tube inserted through the nose into the stomach	

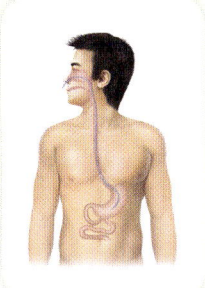

TERM	WORD ANALYSIS
proctoscope PRAWK-toh-skohp	procto / scope anus/rectum / instrument to look
DEFINITION instrument for looking at the anus and rectum	
proctoscopy prawk-TAW-skoh-pee	procto / scopy anus/rectum / looking procedure
DEFINITION procedure for looking at the anus and rectum	
sigmoidoscopy sig-moy-DAW-skoh-pee	sigmoido / scopy sigmoid / looking procedure
DEFINITION procedure for looking at the sigmoid colon	

radiology

TERM	WORD ANALYSIS
cholangiogram koh-LAN-jee-oh-gram	cholangio / gram bile vessels / record
DEFINITION record of the bile vessels (ducts)	
cholangiography koh-LAN-jee-AW-grah-fee	cholangio / graphy bile vessels / writing procedure
DEFINITION procedure for mapping the bile vessels (ducts)	
cholangiopan-creatography koh-LAN-jee-oh-PAN-kree-ah-TAW-grah-fee	cholangio / pancreato bile vessels / pancreas / graphy / writing procedure
DEFINITION procedure for mapping the bile vessels (ducts) and pancreas	
pancreatography PAN-kree-ah-TAW-graw-FEE	pancreato / graphy pancreas / writing procedure
DEFINITION procedure for mapping the pancreas	

professional terms

TERM	WORD ANALYSIS
bariatrics BAR-ee-ah-triks	bar / iatr / ics heavy / treatment / pertain- ing to
DEFINITION branch of medicine dealing with weight issues NOTE: In weather forecasts, the atmospheric pressure is called *barometric pressure*.	
gastroenterologist GAS-troh-EN-ter-AW-loh-jist	gastro / entero / logist stomach / intestines / specialist
DEFINITION specialist in the stomach and intestines	
gastroenterology GAS-troh-EN-ter-AW-loh-jee	gastro / entero / logy stomach / intestines / study
DEFINITION study of the stomach and intestines	

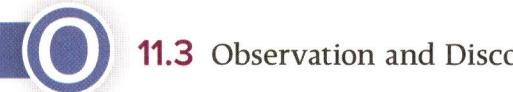

professional terms *continued*	
TERM	**WORD ANALYSIS**
orthodontics or-thoh-DAWN-tiks	orth / odont / ics straight / teeth / pertaining to
DEFINITION branch of medicine dealing with the straightening of teeth	

Keith Brofsky/Getty Images

professional terms *continued*	
TERM	**WORD ANALYSIS**
orthodontist or-thoh-DAWN-tist	orth / odont / ist straight / teeth / specialist
DEFINITION specialist in straightening teeth	
proctologist prok-TAW-loh-jist	procto / logist anus/rectum / specialist
DEFINITION specialist in the anus, rectum, and colon	
proctology prok-TAW-loh-jee	procto / logy anus/rectum / study
DEFINITION branch of medicine dealing with the anus, rectum, and colon	

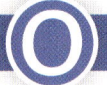

Learning Outcome 11.3 Exercises

TRANSLATION

EXERCISE 1 Break down the following words into their component parts.

> EXAMPLE: nasopharyngoscope
> *naso | pharyngo | scope*

1. laparoscope _____
2. proctoscope _____
3. endoscopy _____
4. proctology _____
5. pancreatolith _____
6. hepatomegaly _____
7. nasogastric tube _____
8. gastroenterology _____
9. orthodontics _____
10. cholangiogram _____
11. cholangiography _____
12. cholangiopancreatography _____

EXERCISE 2 Underline and define the roots from this chapter in the following terms.

1. orthodontist _____
2. proctologist _____
3. gingivitis _____
4. stomatosis _____
5. cholelith _____
6. sialolith _____
7. pancreatography _____
8. colonoscopy _____
9. esophagoscopy _____
10. gastroscopy _____
11. laparoscopy _____
12. proctoscopy _____
13. sigmoidoscopy _____
14. stomatogastric (2 roots) _____
15. gastroenterologist (2 roots) _____
16. esophagogastroduodenoscopy (3 roots)

_____

EXERCISE 3   Match the term on the left with its definition on the right.

_____ 1. hernia

_____ 2. fecal occult blood test

_____ 3. bariatrics

_____ 4. flatus

_____ 5. ascites

a. branch of medicine dealing with weight issues

b. medical term for passing gas; from the Latin word meaning *to blow*

c. retention of fluid in the peritoneum

d. rupture or protrusion of an organ through the wall that normally contains it

e. test of feces to discover blood not visibly apparent

EXERCISE 4   Fill in the blanks.

1. *proctologist* = specialist in _____

2. *orthodontist* = specialist in _____

3. *gastroenterologist* = specialist in _____

4. *colonoscopy* = procedure for looking at the

_____

5. *gastroscopy* = procedure for looking at the

_____

6. *esophagoscopy* = procedure for looking at the

_____

7. *proctoscopy* = procedure for looking at the

_____

8. *laparoscopy* = procedure for looking at the

_____

9. *sigmoidoscopy* = procedure for looking at the

_____

10. *esophagogastroduodenoscopy* = procedure for looking at the _____

EXERCISE 5   Translate the following terms as literally as possible.

> EXAMPLE: nasopharyngoscope
> *an instrument for looking at the nose and throat*

1. pancreatography _____

2. stomatosis _____

3. stomatogastric _____

4. nasogastric tube _____

5. orthodontics _____

6. cholangiopancreatography _____

GENERATION

EXERCISE 6   Build a medical term from the information provided.

> EXAMPLE: inflammation of the sinuses   *sinusitis*

1. enlargement of the liver _____

2. inflammation of the gums _____

3. stone in the pancreas _____

4. stone in the saliva _____

5. gall (bile) stone _____

6. instrument for looking inside the abdomen

_____

7. instrument for looking at the anus and rectum

_____

8. study of the stomach and intestines _____

9. study of the anus, rectum, and colon _____

EXERCISE 7 Multiple-choice questions. Select the correct answer(s).

1. A person with *ascites* has fluid retention in which part of the GI system?
   a. esophagus
   b. ileum
   c. mouth
   d. peritoneum
   e. sigmoid colon

2. An FOBT tests the feces for what?
   a. allergies
   b. bile
   c. blood
   d. sugar
   e. undigested materials

3. *Bariatrics* is a
   a. branch of medicine dealing with the anus, rectum, and colon
   b. branch of medicine dealing with digestive disorders
   c. branch of medicine dealing with intestinal issues
   d. branch of medicine dealing with weight issues
   e. none of these

4. Which of the terms below comes from the Latin word meaning *to blow?*
   a. ascites
   b. bariatrics
   c. flatus
   d. hernia

5. Which of the terms below comes from the Latin word meaning *to rupture?*
   a. ascites
   b. bariatrics
   c. flatus
   d. hernia

EXERCISE 8 Briefly describe the difference between the pair of terms.

1. cholangiogram, cholangiography _____

⒜SSESSMENT

11.4 Diagnosis and Pathology

GI problems include infection or inflammation, change in function, and problems in the GI tract's structure. Infection of the GI tract is perhaps the most common GI problem seen in the office setting. *Acute gastroenteritis* is infection of the entire tract; it presents with vomiting and/or diarrhea. Most cases are caused by a virus and require no treatment. However, food poisoning can possibly lead to life-threatening illness.

Less-common infections include infection of the liver (*hepatitis*) or pancreas (*pancreatitis*). Infectious hepatitis is generally caused by a virus and presents with pain, jaundice, and/or vomiting. The chief symptom of pancreatitis is intense pain. Inflammation of GI organs can also be caused by inherited disorders such as *ulcerative colitis* or acquired due to stress or reaction to a medication, such as stomach inflammation (*gastritis*).

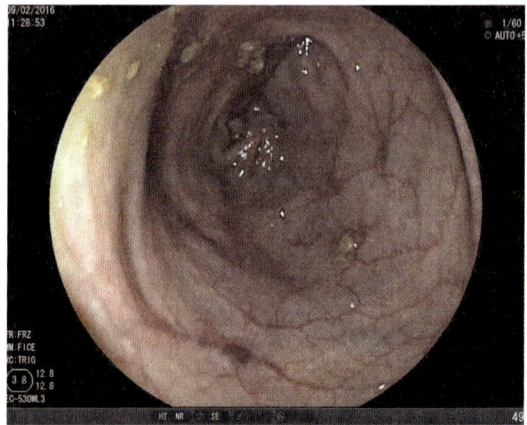

Endoscopes are invaluable tools in diagnosing problems in the digestive tract.

whitetherock photo/Shutterstock

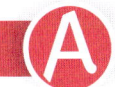

When the GI tract isn't working the way it should, food might travel in the wrong direction. For instance, when food passes from the stomach back up the esophagus (*gastroesophageal reflux*), the result can be a painful burning sensation. While medicine often helps, this problem can become severe enough to require surgery.

When the intestines do not work properly (*enteropathy*), food will often pass through without being completely digested or absorbed. Another functional GI problem occurs when a blockage exists in the tract. This can be caused by an overgrown structure in the body, such as the muscle valve at the end of the stomach (*pyloric stenosis*), or it can be caused by the development of stones over time as with gallstones (*cholelithiasis*). This blockage frequently leads to infection of the gallbladder (*cholecystitis*).

lower gastro tract

TERM	WORD ANALYSIS
colitis coh-LAI-tis	col / itis colon / inflammation
DEFINITION inflammation of the colon	
duodenitis doo-AH-den-AI-tis	duoden / itis duodenum / inflammation
DEFINITION inflammation of the duodenum	
fistula FIS-tyoo-la	from Latin, for *pipe*
DEFINITION any abnormal passageway in the body that shouldn't be there	

upper gastro tract

TERM	WORD ANALYSIS
esophagitis eh-SAWF-ah-JAI-tis	esophag / itis esophagus / inflammation
DEFINITION inflammation of the esophagus	
gastritis gas-TRAI-tis	gastr / itis stomach / inflammation
DEFINITION inflammation of the stomach	
gastroenteritis GAS-troh-EN-ter-AI-tis	gastro / enter / itis stomach / intestine / inflammation
DEFINITION inflammation of the stomach and intestines	
gastroesophageal reflux disease (GERD) GAS-troh-eh-SOF-ah-JEE-al REE-fluks dih-ZEEZ	gastro / esophag / eal stomach / esophagus / pertaining to re / flux back / flow
DEFINITION disease in which acid comes up from the stomach and damages the esophagus	

oncology

TERM	WORD ANALYSIS
colorectal carcinoma COH-loh-REK-tal KAR-sih-NOH-mah	colo / rect / al colon / rectum / pertaining to carcin / oma cancer / tumor
DEFINITION cancerous tumor of the colon or rectum	

supporting organs

TERM	WORD ANALYSIS
cholangitis KOH-lan-JAI-tis	cholang / itis bile vessels / inflammation
DEFINITION inflammation of the bile vessels (ducts)	
cholecystitis KOH-lay-sis-TAI-tis	chole / cyst / itis bile / bladder / inflammation
DEFINITION inflammation of the bile (gall) bladder	
choledocholithiasis koh-lay-DOH-koh-lith-AI-ah-sis	chole / docho / lith / iasis bile / duct / stone / presence
DEFINITION presence of a stone in the (common) bile duct	

supporting organs *continued*

TERM	WORD ANALYSIS
cholelithiasis KOH-lay-lih-THAI-ah-sis	chole / lith / iasis bile / stone / presence
DEFINITION presence of a gallstone	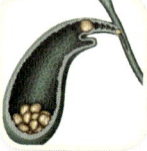
cirrhosis sir-OH-sis	from the Greek word *cirrho,* for *yellow*
DEFINITION liver disease named for the change of color in the liver NOTE: The standard Greek root for yellow is *xantho.* This word uses a much rarer root for *yellow.*	
hepatitis HEH-pah-TAI-tis	hepat / itis liver / inflammation
DEFINITION inflammation of the liver	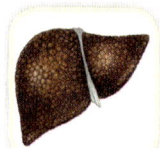

supporting organs *continued*

TERM	WORD ANALYSIS
laparocele LAP-ar-oh-seel	laparo / cele abdomen / hernia
DEFINITION abdominal hernia	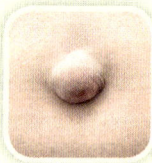 Miriam Doerr Martin Frommherz/Shutterstock
pancreatitis PAN-kree-ah-TAI-tis	pancreat / itis pancreas / inflammation
DEFINITION inflammation of the pancreas	
pancreatolithiasis PAN-kree-AH-toh-lih-THAI-ah-sis	pancreato / lith / iasis pancreas / stone / presence
DEFINITION presence of a stone in the pancreas	
peritonitis PER-ih-toh-NAI-tis	periton / itis peritoneum / inflammation
DEFINITION inflammation of the peritoneum	
sialoadenitis sai-AL-oh-AD-en-AI-tis	sialo / aden / itis saliva / gland / inflammation
DEFINITION inflammation of the salivary glands	
sialolithiasis sai-AL-oh-lih-THAI-ah-sis	sialo / lith / iasis saliva / stone / presence
DEFINITION presence of salivary stones	

A **Learning Outcome 11.4 Exercises**

TRANSLATION

EXERCISE 1 Break down the following words into their component parts.

> EXAMPLE: **nasopharyngoscope**
> *naso | pharyngo | scope*

1. gastritis _____
2. colitis _____
3. esophagitis _____
4. cholangitis _____
5. sialoadenitis _____
6. sialolithiasis _____
7. cholelithiasis _____
8. pancreatolithiasis _____
9. choledocholithiasis _____

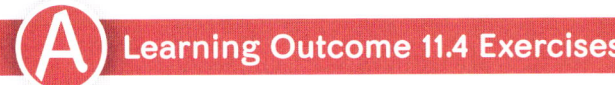

EXERCISE 2 Underline and define the roots from this chapter in the following terms.

1. pancreatitis _____
2. peritonitis _____
3. duodenitis _____
4. hepatitis _____
5. cholangitis _____
6. laparocele _____
7. sialoadenitis _____
8. gastroesophageal reflux disease (2 roots)

   _____

9. gastroenteritis (2 roots) _____
10. colorectal carcinoma (2 roots) _____
11. cholecystitis (2 roots) _____
12. choledochocele (2 roots) _____
13. gastroenterocolitis (3 roots) _____

EXERCISE 3 Match the term on the left with its definition on the right.

_____ 1. cirrhosis   a. abdominal hernia

_____ 2. fistula   b. liver disease named for the change in color in the liver

_____ 3. esophagitis   c. presence of salivary stones

_____ 4. laparocele   d. any abnormal passageway in the body that shouldn't be there

_____ 5. sialolithiasis   e. inflammation of the esophagus

_____ 6. cholelithiasis   f. presence of a gallstone

EXERCISE 4 Translate the following terms as literally as possible.

EXAMPLE: nasopharyngoscope *an instrument for looking at the nose and throat*

1. laparocele _____
2. cholangitis _____
3. colorectal carcinoma _____
4. choledocholithiasis _____

GENERATION

EXERCISE 5 Build a medical term from the information provided.

EXAMPLE: inflammation of the sinuses *sinusitis*

1. inflammation of the esophagus _____
2. inflammation of the pancreas _____
3. inflammation of the colon _____
4. inflammation of the duodenum _____
5. inflammation of the peritoneum _____
6. inflammation of the stomach _____
7. inflammation of the liver _____
8. inflammation of the stomach and intestines

   _____

9. inflammation of the bile (gall) bladder _____

   _____

10. inflammation of the salivary glands _____

    _____

EXERCISE 6 Multiple-choice questions. Select the correct answer(s).

1. A person suffering from *cirrhosis* has (select all that apply)
   a. a liver disease   d. liver cancer
   b. a purple liver   e. liver inflammation
   c. a yellow liver

2. GERD is
   a. a disease in which acid comes up from the intestines and damages the esophagus
   b. a disease in which acid comes up from the intestines and damages the stomach
   c. a disease in which acid comes up from the stomach and damages the esophagus
   d. a disease in which acid comes up from the stomach and damages the intestines
   e. none of these

3. An abnormal passageway (one that shouldn't be there) in the body is called a
    a. carcinoma   d. laparocele
    b. cirrhosis   e. stenosis
    c. fistula

EXERCISE 7 Briefly describe the difference between each pair of terms.

1. cholelithiasis, pancreatolithiasis _____

2. sialoadenitis, sialolithiasis _____

P **LAN**

11.5 Treatments and Therapies

Medicines that are utilized to help patients with GI problems generally treat issues with stomach acid and the movement of food through their GI tracts. Patients with gastroesophageal reflux and ulcers may need medicine to decrease levels of stomach acid (*antacids*). Medicines also help with food movement, including medicine to stop vomiting (*antiemetics*) or medicine to help accelerate the movement of food or aid with constipation (*cathartics*).

Nonmedication methods are also commonly used to treat GI problems. Among the most common treatments is keeping the patient from eating or drinking anything (*NPO*), which helps the GI tract rest. Another form of assistance includes inserting a tube into part of the GI tract. The most common tube is the nasogastric tube (*NGT*). This tube can either send food into the stomach, bypassing the throat, or it can be used to suck out (*aspirate*) the contents of the stomach. A tube can also be passed through the anus into the colon to administer fluid (*enema*) to help flush out stool that is stuck there.

There are two types of surgical approaches when operating on the gastrointestinal system: cutting a patient open (*laparotomy*) and inserting a camera and instruments through small holes (*laparoscopic*). The most common type of surgery involves removing part of the GI tract. When a section of the GI tract is removed, the remaining ends need to be reconnected (*anastomosis*). Occasionally, one end is attached to an opening to the outside of the body (*ostomy*), and the part past this is left disconnected. Usually,

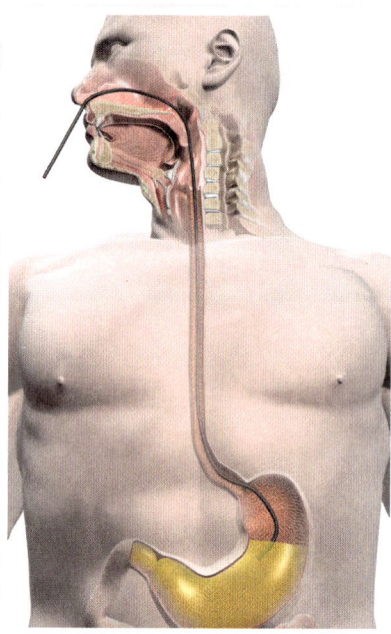

A nasogastric tube can either send food into the stomach, bypassing the throat, or can suck out (aspirate) the contents of the stomach.
3D4Medical/Science Source

this is a temporary procedure to give time for the GI tract to heal. The most common of all gastrointestinal surgeries is removal of the appendix (*appendectomy*). The appendix is a small extension off the large intestine with little to no function. If blocked, it can become infected and possibly rupture.

pharmacology

TERM	WORD ANALYSIS
antacid ant-AS-id	ant / acid against / acid
DEFINITION agent that neutralizes acid	

McGraw-Hill Education /Jill Braaten

TERM	WORD ANALYSIS
antiemetic AN-tee-EE-met-ik	anti / emet / ic against / vomiting / pertaining to
DEFINITION agent that prevents or relieves nausea or vomiting	

Helen Sessions/Alamy Stock Photo

TERM	WORD ANALYSIS
cathartic kah-THAR-tik	cathart / ic cleansing / pertaining to
DEFINITION agent that produces bowel movement	

upper gastro tract

TERM	WORD ANALYSIS
gastrectomy gas-TREK-toh-mee	gastr / ectomy stomach / removal
DEFINITION surgical removal of the stomach	
gastroduo-denostomy GAS-troh-doo-AH-den-AW-stoh-mee	gastro / duodeno / stomy stomach / duodenum / opening
DEFINITION creation of an opening between the stomach and the duodenum	

upper gastro tract *continued*

TERM	WORD ANALYSIS
glossorrhaphy glaws-OR-ah-fee	glosso / rrhaphy tongue / suture
DEFINITION suture of the tongue	
odontectomy oh-dawn-TEK-toh-mee	odont / ectomy tooth / removal
DEFINITION surgical removal of a tooth	

lower gastro tract

TERM	WORD ANALYSIS
anastomosis ah-NAS-toh-MOH-sis	ana / stom / osis up/out / mouth / condition
DEFINITION creation of an opening; a surgical procedure connecting two previously unconnected hollow tubes NOTE: The prefix *ana-* here means *out* or *up* instead of *no* or *not*. This is the same type of usage as in the word *aneurysm*.	
colostomy koh-LAW-stoh-mee	colo / stomy colon / opening
DEFINITION creation of an opening in the colon	

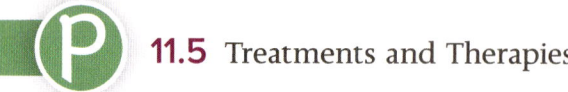

lower gastro tract *continued*

TERM	WORD ANALYSIS
duodenectomy doo-AW-den-EK-toh-mee	dudoden / ectomy duodenum / removal
DEFINITION surgical removal of the duodenum	
hemorrhoidectomy HEM-oh-roi-DEK-toh-mee	hemorrhoid / ectomy hemorrhoid / removal
DEFINITION surgical removal of hemorrhoids	
herniorrhaphy her-nee-OR-ah-fee	hernio / rrhaphy hernia / suture
DEFINITION suture of a hernia	
ileostomy IH-lee-AW-stoh-mee	ileo / stomy ileum / opening
DEFINITION creation of an opening in the ileum	

supporting organs

TERM	WORD ANALYSIS
abdominocentesis ab-DAW-min-oh-sin-TEE-sis	abdomino / centesis abdomen / puncture
DEFINITION puncture of the abdomen (usually for the purpose of withdrawing fluid)	

Stockbyte/Getty Images

TERM	WORD ANALYSIS
cholecystectomy KOH-lay-sis-TEK-toh-me	chole / cyst / ectomy bile / bladder / removal
DEFINITION surgical removal of the bile (gall) bladder	
choledocho-lithectomy KOH-lay-DOH-koh-lih-THEK-toh-mee	chole / docho / lith / ectomy bile / duct / stone / removal
DEFINITION surgical removal of a stone from the (common) bile duct	

supporting organs *continued*

TERM	WORD ANALYSIS
cholelithotripsy KOH-lay-lih-THOH-trip-see	chole / litho / tripsy bile / stone / wear down procedure
DEFINITION crushing of bile (gall) stones	
laparoscopic surgery LAP-ar-oh-SKAW-pik SIR-jir-ee	laparo / scop / ic abdomen / device to look / pertaining to **surgery**
DEFINITION the use of a laparoscope to perform minimally invasive surgery	
pancreatectomy PAN-kree-ah-TEK-toh-mee	pancreat / ectomy pancreas / removal
DEFINITION surgical removal of the pancreas	
pancreato-lithectomy PAN-kree-at-oh-lih-THECK-toh-mee	pancreato / lith / ectomy pancreas / stone / removal
DEFINITION surgical removal of stones in the pancreas	
sialoadenectomy sai-AL-oh-AD-en-EK-toh-mee	sialo / aden / ectomy saliva / gland / removal
DEFINITION surgical removal of a salivary gland	

PRONUNCIATION

EXERCISE 1 Indicate which syllable(s) is emphasized when pronounced.

EXAMPLE: bronchitis bron<u>chi</u>tis

1. antacid _____
2. cathartic _____
3. colostomy _____
4. gastrectomy _____
5. odontectomy _____
6. glossorrhaphy _____
7. herniorrhaphy _____

TRANSLATION

EXERCISE 2 Break down the following words into their component parts.

EXAMPLE: nasopharyngoscope
naso | pharyngo | scope

1. ileostomy _____
2. colostomy _____
3. glossorrhaphy _____
4. herniorrhaphy _____
5. hemorrhoidectomy _____
6. pancreatolithectomy _____
7. gastroduodenostomy _____
8. cholelithotripsy _____
9. anastomosis _____

EXERCISE 3 Underline and define the roots from this chapter in the following terms.

1. gastrectomy _____
2. odontectomy _____
3. duodenectomy _____
4. pancreatectomy _____
5. sialoadenectomy _____
6. abdominocentesis _____
7. laparoscopic surgery _____
8. cholecystectomy (2 roots) _____
9. choledocholithectomy (2 roots) _____

EXERCISE 4 Match the term on the left with its definition on the right.

_____ 1. antacid
_____ 2. antiemetic
_____ 3. cathartic
_____ 4. abdominocentesis
_____ 5. herniorrhaphy
_____ 6. colostomy
_____ 7. pancreatectomy
_____ 8. ileostomy

a. surgical removal of the pancreas
b. agent that prevents or relieves nausea or vomiting
c. creation of an opening in the ileum
d. agent that produces bowel movements
e. creation of an opening in the colon
f. agent that neutralizes acid
g. puncture of the abdomen
h. suture of a hernia

EXERCISE 5 Translate the following terms as literally as possible.

> EXAMPLE: nasopharyngoscope *an instrument for looking at the nose and throat*

1. herniorrhaphy _____
2. glossorrhaphy _____
3. duodenectomy _____
4. hemorrhoidectomy _____
5. abdominocentesis _____
6. laparoscopic surgery _____

EXERCISE 6 Fill in the blanks.

1. *colostomy* = creation of an opening in the
   _____

2. *ileostomy* = creation of an opening in the
   _____

3. *gastroduodenostomy* = creation of an opening
   between _____ and _____

GENERATION

EXERCISE 7 Build a medical term from the information provided.

> EXAMPLE: inflammation of the sinuses *sinusitis*

1. surgical removal of the stomach _____
2. surgical removal of the duodenum _____
3. surgical removal of the bile (gall) bladder
   _____
4. surgical removal of hemorrhoids _____

EXERCISE 8 Multiple-choice questions. Select the correct answer(s).

1. Select all of the terms below that pertain to the upper GI tract.
   a. cholecystectomy   d. enterectomy
   b. choledocholithectomy   e. gastrectomy
   c. duodenectomy   f. odontectomy

2. Select all of the terms below that pertain to the lower GI tract.
   a. cholecystectomy   d. enterectomy
   b. choledocholithectomy   e. gastrectomy
   c. duodenectomy   f. odontectomy

3. Select all of the terms below that pertain to the supporting organs for the GI system.
   a. cholecystectomy   d. enterectomy
   b. choledocholithectomy   e. gastrectomy
   c. duodenectomy   f. odontectomy

EXERCISE 9 Briefly describe the difference between each pair of terms.

1. sialoadenectomy, odontectomy _____
2. pancreatectomy, pancreatolithectomy _____
3. cholecystectomy, choledocholithectomy _____
4. antacid, antiemetic _____

11.6 Electronic Health Records

Clinic Note

S	**Subjective**	Mr. Robert Luno presents to our clinic with a 2-month history of intermittent post-prandial gastralgia and dyspepsia. It has become more and more frequent. He also reports occasional emesis as well, but denies hematemesis and cholemesis. He denies diarrhea and constipation.
O	**Objective**	Temp: 98.6; HR: 64; RR: 16; BP: 120/80. General: Overweight, middle-aged man in no apparent distress. HEENT: PERRLA. No conjunctival injection. No scleral icterus. Mucous membranes moist and pink. TMs normal. CV: RRR without murmur. Resp: CTA. Good air entry. Abd: Soft, nontender, nondistended. No HSM. Normative bowel sounds.
A	**Assessment**	I suspect Mr. Luno is suffering from gastroesophageal reflux. Other possibilities include gastritis, cholelithiasis, and PUD.
P	**Plan**	I will begin a trial of antacid therapy along with recommended dietary adjustments. If he does not respond to treatment in 1 month, I will schedule him for an EGD. —Constance Stiles, NP

Purestock/Getty Images

EXERCISE 1 Match the term on the left with its definition on the right.

_____ 1. antacid

_____ 2. diarrhea

_____ 3. gastritis

_____ 4. dypepsia

_____ 5. hematemesis

_____ 6. cholelithiasis

_____ 7. gastroesophageal reflux

_____ 8. esophagogastroduodenoscopy

a. agent that neutralizes acid

b. bad digestion

c. disease in which acid comes up from the stomach and damages the esophagus

d. inflammation of the stomach

e. passing of fluid or unformed feces

f. procedure for looking inside the esophagus, stomach, and duodenum

g. presence of a gallstone

h. vomiting blood

EXERCISE 2 Fill in the blanks.

1. Using the data recorded in the patient's clinic note, fill in the following blanks.
   a. The patient's temperature: _____
   b. The patient's heart rate: _____
   c. The patient's respiratory rate: _____
   d. The patient's blood pressure: _____

2. Mr. Luno presents to the clinic with a 2-month history of intermittent _gastralgia_ (give definition: _____) and _dyspepsia_ (give definition: _____).

3. He occasionally vomits, but has not vomited _____ (_hematemesis_) or vomited _____ (_cholemesis_).

EXERCISE 3 True or false questions. Indicate true answers with a T and false answers with an F.

1. The medical professional suspects the patient has GERD. _____

2. The patient has stomach pain and poor digestion. _____

3. The patient has vomited both blood and bile. _____

4. The patient has difficulty passing feces. _____

5. The patient may have a gallstone. _____

6. The patient may have peptic ulcer disease. _____

EXERCISE 4 Multiple-choice questions. Select the correct answer.

1. Which of the following symptoms did Mr. Luno report to the medical professional?
   a. cholemesis
   b. constipation
   c. diarrhea
   d. gastralgia
   e. hematemesis

2. Which of the following is NOT a possible diagnosis?
   a. cholelithiasis
   b. gastritis
   c. gastroesophageal reflux disease
   d. hepatosplenomegaly
   e. peptic ulcer disease

3. Which is the correct definition for the abbreviation *EGD?*
   a. epigastricduodenectomy
   b. epigastrodynia
   c. esophagogastroduodenoscopy
   d. esophagogastrodynia
   e. none of these

Quick Reference

glossary of roots

ROOT	DEFINITION	ROOT	DEFINITION
abdomin/o	abdomen	hepat/o	liver
an/o	anus	hepatic/o	liver
bil/i	bile (gall)	ile/o	ileum
celi/o	abdomen	jejun/o	jejunum
chol/e	bile (gall)	lapar/o	abdomen
col/o	colon (large intestine)	lingu/o	tongue
colon/o	colon (large intestine)	odont/o	tooth
cyst/o	bladder	or/o	mouth
dent/o	tooth	pancreat/o	pancreas
doch/o	duct	peritone/o	peritoneum
duoden/o	duodenum	proct/o	anus and rectum
enter/o	intestines	rect/o	rectum
esophag/o	esophagus	sial/o	saliva
gastr/o	stomach	sigmoid/o	sigmoid colon
gingiv/o	gums	stomat/o	mouth
gloss/o	tongue		

gastrointestinal system abbreviations

ABBREVIATIONS	DEFINITION
BE	barium enema
BM	bowel movement
EGD	esophagogastroduodenoscopy
ERCP	endoscopic retrograde cholangiopancreatography
EUS	endoscopic ultrasound
FOBT	fecal occult blood test
GB	gallbladder
GERD	gastroesophageal reflux disease
GI	gastrointestinal
LFT	liver function test
LLQ	left lower quadrant
LUQ	left upper quadrant
N&V	nausea and vomiting
NGT	nasogastric tube
NPO	nothing by mouth (*nil per os*)
PEG	percutaneous endoscopic gastrostomy
PUD	peptic ulcer disease
RLQ	right lower quadrant
RUQ	right upper quadrant
UGI	upper gastrointestinal

The Urinary and Male Reproductive Systems—Urology

12

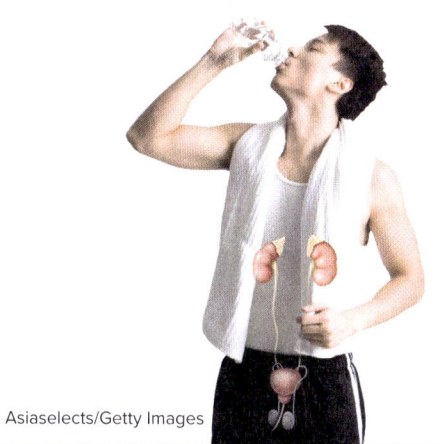

Asiaselects/Getty Images

Learning Outcomes

Upon completion of this chapter, you will be able to:

12.1 Identify the **roots/word parts** associated with the **urinary system.**

12.2 Identify the **roots/word parts** associated with the **male reproductive system.**

(S) 12.3 Translate the **Subjective** terms associated with the **urinary and male reproductive systems.**

(O) 12.4 Translate the **Objective** terms associated with the **urinary and male reproductive systems.**

(A) 12.5 Translate the **Assessment** terms associated with the **urinary and male reproductive systems.**

(P) 12.6 Translate the **Plan** terms associated with the **urinary and male reproductive systems.**

12.7 Distinguish terms associated with the **urinary and male reproductive systems** in the context of **electronic health records.**

Introduction and Overview of the Urinary and Male Reproductive Systems

So far, we have addressed body systems that are identical in men and women. What separates the sexes, of course, is their reproductive systems. Both men and women produce half the blueprints for new life, which are found in *sperm* and *eggs.* The reproductive systems are responsible for making these code carriers and for helping to bring the two together.

In medicine, the male and female reproductive systems are cared for by different specialties. The next two chapters deal with those specialties. This chapter deals with the specialty of *urology.* Since the male reproductive system shares structures with the urinary system, urology deals with both the urinary tract and the male reproductive system. The next chapter deals with the specialty of *obstetrics* and *gynecology,* which focuses specifically on the female reproductive system.

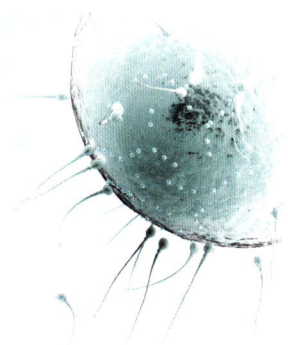

Sperm attempting to fertilize an egg.
MedicalRF.com/Getty Images

12.1 Word Parts of the Urinary System

Many homes and businesses have aquariums. People enjoy watching fish swim peacefully around in the water. In fact, some studies have shown that watching fish in an aquarium can lower a person's blood pressure.

While the fish are the main attraction, a great deal of hard work goes into keeping the water in their tank just right. The water must be cleaned and maintained with a balance of chemicals to keep a safe and clean environment for the fish to live in. Otherwise, the water becomes unsuitable for life.

The kidneys, the unsung heroes of the body, perform a similar function for the blood. The cells of the body are in constant contact with the blood, just as fish are always in contact with the water in an aquarium. Cells require just the right balance of pH, minerals, water, and sugar, and the kidneys monitor and regulate these levels. If they did not perform their job, blood would soon become toxic.

The basic working unit of the kidney is called the *nephron.* There are more than 2 million nephrons in a single kidney. Blood passes through the kidneys into a cluster of small blood vessels known as the *glomerulus.* Here, the blood is filtered, with water and nutrients being forced into the surrounding

capsule around the glomerulus. This filtered liquid (filtrate) then flows through a series of small tubes.

These tubes flow next to blood vessels. As the filtrate passes through this series of tubes, much of the water and nutrients in it are reabsorbed back into the bloodstream. At the same time, the remaining unfiltered waste is forced into the last part of the tubes.

These tubes containing waste dump into a basin known as the *renal pelvis.* Long vessels from each kidney, called *ureters,* drain these collecting areas into the *bladder,* a large holding bag for urine. When the bladder becomes full, a signal is sent to the muscle that is holding the urine in the bladder. When this muscle relaxes, the urine empties out of the body through the *urethra.*

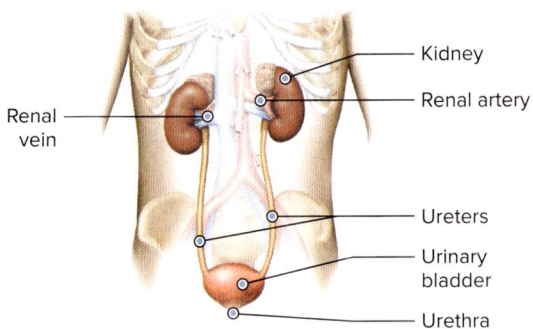

glomerulus (plural: glomeruli)

ROOT: *glomerul/o*

EXAMPLES: glomerulopathy, glomerulonephritis

NOTES: *Glomerulus* comes from a Latin word meaning *little ball* and refers to the little balls of blood vessels inside the kidney. These serve as the primary place for filtering the blood to form urine.

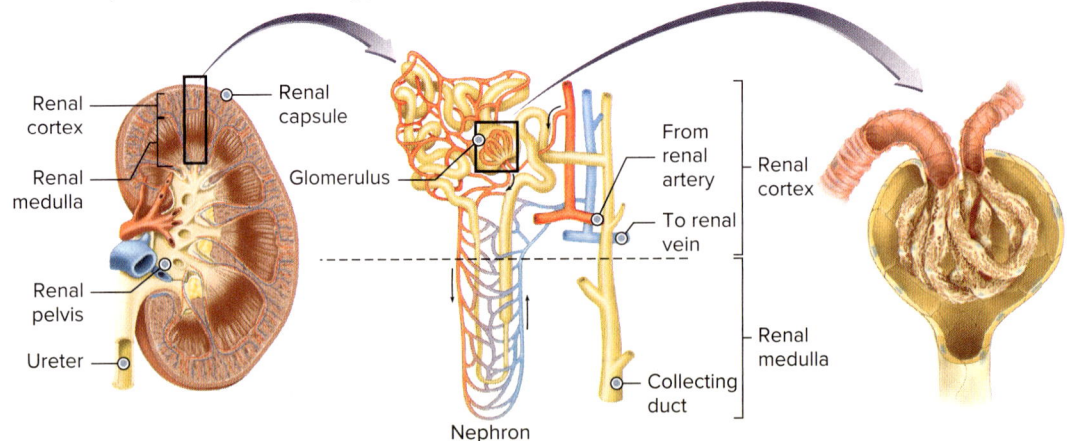

kidney

ROOTS: *nephr/o, ren/o*

EXAMPLES: nephrology, nephritis, renal failure

NOTES: Kidneys perform the necessary task of filtering the blood—at a rate of 200 quarts per day. If you lose or donate a kidney, your remaining kidney can adjust and perform the work of two by increasing the amount it filters and by increasing in size. If you are born with only one kidney, your kidney may grow to be the size of two normal kidneys.

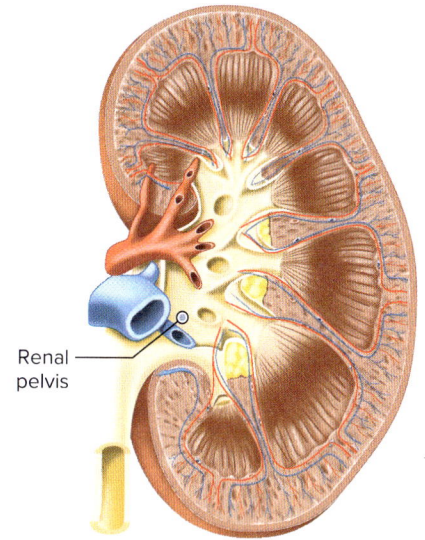

Renal pelvis

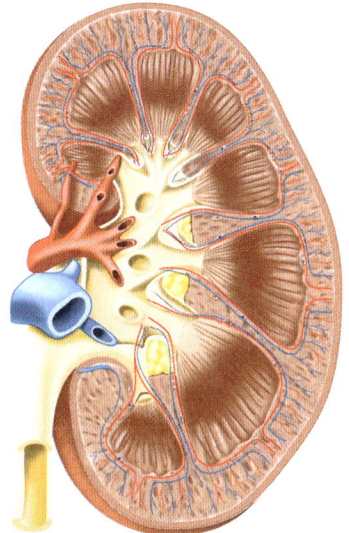

renal pelvis

ROOT: *pyel/o*

EXAMPLES: pyelonephritis, pyelitis

NOTES: *Pyelo* is a root meaning *pelvis.* There are two things that the word *pelvis* can apply to: the *skeletal pelvis,* which is where your legs and your spine attach to one another; and the *renal pelvis,* which is a series of tubes that funnel urine out of the kidneys and into the ureters and on to the bladder. *Pyelo* is used most commonly for the renal pelvis.

urine

ROOTS: *ur/o, urin/o*

EXAMPLES: urology, hematuria

NOTES: Healthy urine is completely sterile and contains ammonia molecules. This latter fact led the ancient Romans to use urine in two odd ways: to wash clothes (in fact, Romans set up large urinals outside laundries to gather urine free of charge) and to whiten teeth. It served both functions really well . . . but *gross.*

tunedin123/123RF

stone

ROOT: *lith/o*

EXAMPLES: lithiasis, lithotripsy

NOTES: Kidney stones aren't "stones"; instead, they are accumulations of mineral salts and calcium. To make sure people don't mistakenly think they are little rocks, health care professionals sometimes translate *litho* as *calculus,* a Latin word meaning—you guessed it—*little rocks.*

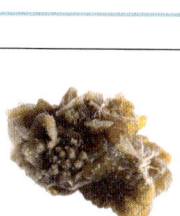

Jonathan Kirn/Getty Images

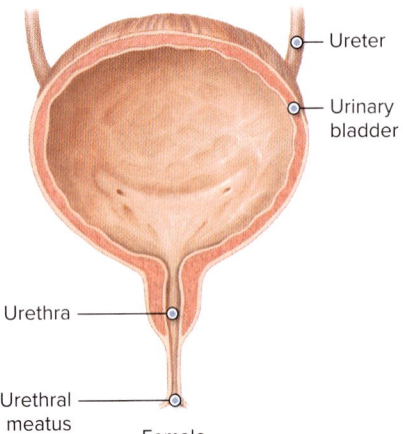

Ureter

Urinary bladder

Urethra

Urethral meatus

Female

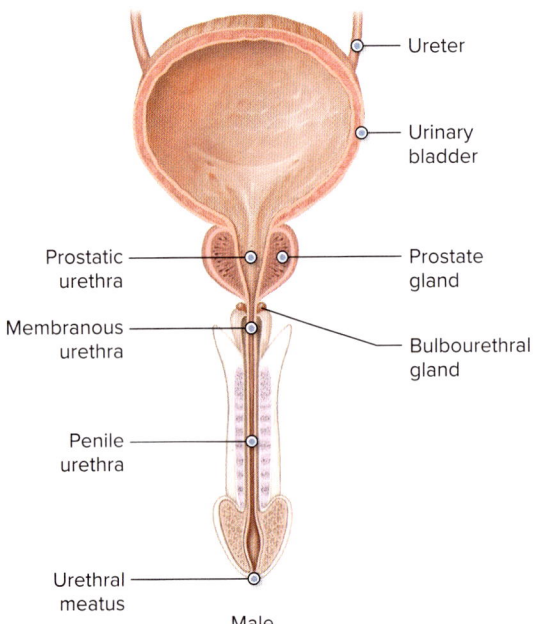

Ureter

Urinary bladder

Prostatic urethra

Prostate gland

Membranous urethra

Bulbourethral gland

Penile urethra

Urethral meatus

Male

bladder

ROOTS: *cyst/o, vesic/o*

EXAMPLES: cystotomy, cystitis, vesiculotomy, vesiculitis

NOTES: When completely full, the urinary bladder is roughly the size of a softball and can hold about 18 ounces of liquid. But it rarely reaches capacity. When the bladder is only about a quarter full, most people can't "hold it" anymore and feel an urgent need to urinate.

urethra

ROOT: *urethr/o*

EXAMPLES: urethrostenosis, urethritis

NOTES: The length of the urethra differs depending on sex. The average male urethra is about 8 inches long, and the average female urethra is 1.5 to 2 inches long. This difference is sometimes mentioned as the reason why kidney stones are more painful for men than women; in fact, some say that the pain of kidney stones is the closest men can come to the pain of giving birth. Others argue that men are just big babies. You be the judge.

ureter

ROOT: *ureter/o*

EXAMPLES: ureterocele, ureterectomy

NOTES: *Ureters* are the thick-walled tubes about 10 inches in length that carry urine from the kidneys to the bladder. Don't confuse ureters with the *urethra,* a tube that runs from the bladder to the outside world. You have two ureters, but only one urethra.

Learning Outcome 12.1 Exercises

TRANSLATION

EXERCISE 1 Translate the following roots.

1. ureter/o _____

2. urethr/o _____

3. urin/o _____

4. lith/o _____

5. nephr/o _____

EXERCISE 2   Match the root on the left with its definition on the right. Some definitions will be used more than once.

_____ 1. cyst/o

_____ 2. vesic/o

_____ 3. ur/o

_____ 4. pyel/o

_____ 5. glomerul/o

_____ 6. ren/o

_____ 7. ureter/o

a. bladder

b. from Latin, for *little ball;* refers to little balls of blood vessels inside the kidney that serve as the primary place for filtering the blood to form urine

c. organ that filters the blood

d. series of tubes that funnel urine out of the kidneys and into the ureter and on to the bladder

e. thick-walled tubes about 10 inches in length that carry urine from the kidneys to the bladder

f. urine

EXERCISE 3   Underline and define the roots from this chapter in the following terms.

1. glucosuria _____

2. renal angiography _____

3. pyelogram _____

4. vesicocele _____

5. laparonephrectomy _____

6. cystolithectomy (2 roots) _____

7. nephroureterectomy (2 roots) _____

EXERCISE 4   Fill in the blanks.

1. *ureteralgia:* pain in the _____

2. *urethroplasty:* surgical reconstruction of the

_____

3. *nephralgia:* pain in the _____

4. *lithectomy:* removal of a(n) _____

5. *glomerulopathy:* disease of the _____

6. *cystalgia:* pain in the _____

7. *uropathy:* disease of the _____

EXERCISE 5   Break down the following words into their component parts and translate.

EXAMPLE: sinusitis   *sinus | itis*
                         inflammation of the sinuses

1. ureteroplasty _____

2. urethrectomy _____

3. nephrologist _____

4. renal failure _____

5. pyeloplasty _____

6. vesicotomy _____

7. nephrolithotomy _____

GENERATION

EXERCISE 6   Identify the roots for the following definitions.

1. ureter _____

2. urethra _____

3. glomerulus _____

4. stone _____

5. renal pelvis _____

6. urine (2 roots) _____

7. bladder (2 roots) _____

8. kidney (2 roots) _____

EXERCISE 7   Build a medical term from the information provided.

EXAMPLE: inflammation of the sinuses   *sinusitis*

1. inflammation of the bladder (use *cyst/o*)

_____

2. inflammation of the ureter   _____

_____

3. inflammation of the renal pelvis   _____

_____

4. inflammation of a stone in the kidney (use *nephr/o*)   _____

5. inflammation of the glomerulus and kidney (use *nephr/o*)   _____

6. inflammation of the renal pelvis and bladder (use *cyst/o*)   _____

7. inflammation of the bladder and ureter (use *cyst/o*)   _____

8. inflammation of the ureter and renal pelvis

_____

12.2 Word Parts of the Male Reproductive System

The male reproductive system shares structures with the urinary system. For this reason, *urologists* deal with both urinary tract problems and male genital problems. The male reproductive system is made up of the *testicles,* the *epididymis,* the *seminiferous tubules,* the *prostate gland,* and the *penis.*

The structures of the male genital system can be divided by their function into three categories: those that make and store *sperm,* those that make special carrier fluid for sperm, and the outer parts. The first category makes and stores sperm. Each sperm carries half of the blueprint for a human life (23 chromosomes). The organ that makes these blueprint carriers is called a *gonad.* The male gonads are the *testicles,* and the female gonads are the *ovaries.*

In addition to making sperm, the testicles also produce *testosterone,* the male hormone that causes male character traits such as muscle growth and facial hair. While sperm cells are made in the testicles, they are stored in the *epididymis.* During sexual intercourse, the sperm cells travel out of the epididymis via ducts called the *vas deferens.* Sperm cells mix with a carrier fluid known as *semen.*

The majority of this fluid is made in the *seminal vesicles* and the prostate gland. At climax, the semen is ejected out of the body (*ejaculation*) through the penis.

The third category of structures is the visible parts of the male reproductive system: the penis and the *scrotum.* These are also known as the male *genitals.* The penis is the organ for directing urine and sperm outside the body, and the scrotum is the external sac that holds the testicles in place outside the body.

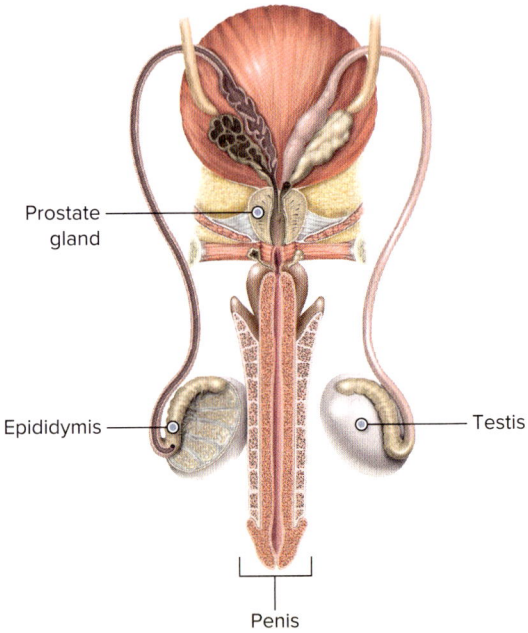

Prostate gland

Epididymis

Testis

Penis

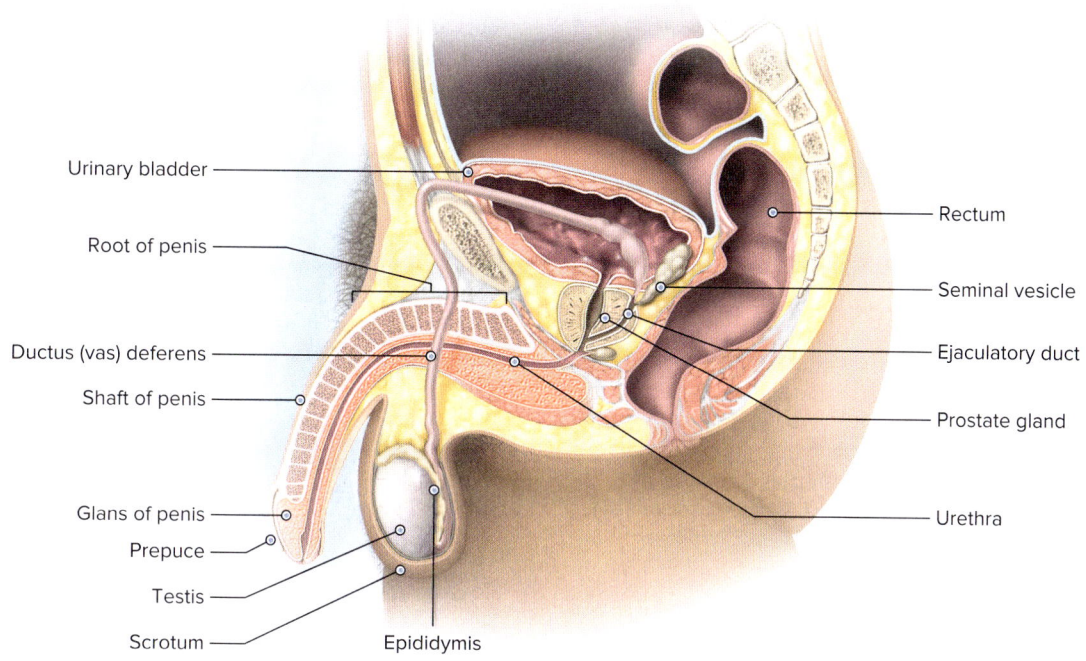

Urinary bladder

Root of penis

Ductus (vas) deferens

Shaft of penis

Glans of penis

Prepuce

Testis

Scrotum

Epididymis

Rectum

Seminal vesicle

Ejaculatory duct

Prostate gland

Urethra

penis

ROOT: *balan/o*

EXAMPLES: balanorrhea, balanitis

NOTES: The root *balano* comes from a Greek word meaning *acorn;* this is an allusion to the shape of the tip of the penis. It was also the word the Greeks used to refer to a deadbolt lock on a door.

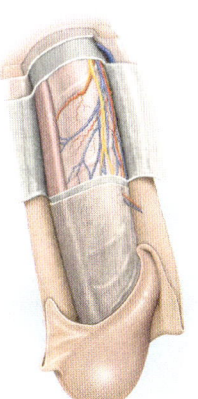

Enigma/Alamy Stock Photo

epididymis

ROOT: *epididym/o*

EXAMPLES: epididymotomy, epididymectomy

NOTES: The *epididymis,* an oblong organ that sits on top of each testicle, is the place where sperm cells complete their final level of development and are stored. Interestingly, the root *didymis* means *twins,* so the name of this organ is literally *upon the twins.*

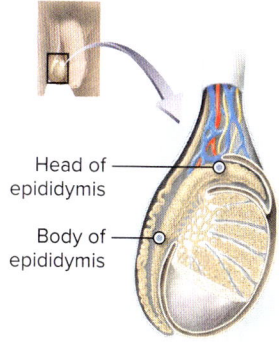

Head of epididymis

Body of epididymis

testicle

ROOTS: *orch/o, orchi/o, orchid/o, test/o, testicul/o*

EXAMPLES: orchitis, orchiopexy, anorchidism, testitis

NOTES: You likely noticed right away that one of the main roots for *testicle* is similar to the word *orchid*. Believe or not, the flower is named for the organ, and not the other way around. The plant was called an *orchid* because some believed that its roots looked like a pair of testicles.

prostate

ROOT: *prostat/o*

EXAMPLES: prostatitis, prostatomegaly

NOTES: The *prostate* is an organ in the male reproductive tract that surrounds the urethra. The name *prostate* breaks down into *pro (before)* and *state (stand)* and literally translates to mean *the one that stands before or in front of*. It was so named because of its position in front of the urinary bladder.

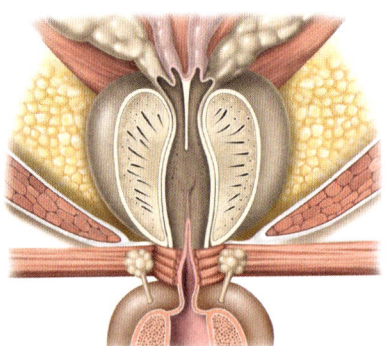

sperm

ROOTS: *sperm/o, spermat/o, sperm/i*

EXAMPLES: aspermia, spermicide, spermatocele

NOTES: *Sperm* (from Greek, for *seed*) is produced in the testicles. It takes roughly 10 weeks to produce a single sperm. Sperm can sit in the epididymis for as long as 2 weeks before being ejaculated. These sperm can survive in the female reproductive tract for as long as 5 days. Because the male's sperm determines the sex of a baby, sperm can be either male or female. Male sperm are faster swimmers, but weaker. Female sperm are slower, but stronger.

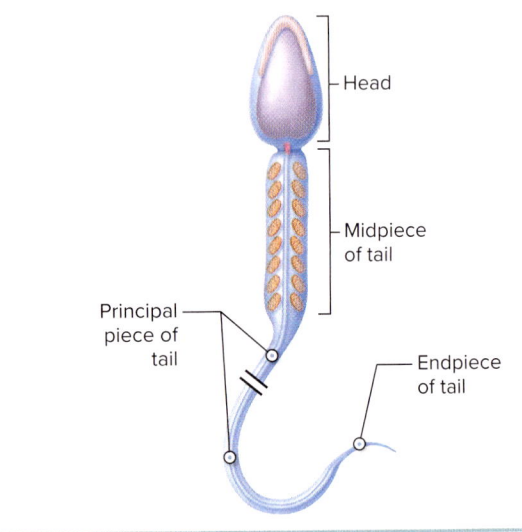

Learning Outcome 12.2 Exercises

TRANSLATION

EXERCISE 1   Translate the following roots.

1. prostat/o _____

2. test/o _____

3. spermat/o _____

4. epididym/o _____

5. orchid/o _____

6. orch/o _____

7. balan/o _____

EXERCISE 2   Match the root on the left with its definition on the right. Some definitions will be used more than once.

_____ 1. test/o

_____ 2. prostat/o

_____ 3. sperm/o

_____ 4. balan/o

_____ 5. orchi/o

_____ 6. epididym/o

a. organ in the male reproductive tract surrounding the urethra; the name literally translates into *the one that stands before or in front of*

b. from Greek, for *acorn,* an allusion to the shape of its tip

c. from Greek, for *seed;* produced in the testicles

d. organ that sits on top of each testicle; the place where sperm cells complete their final level of development and are stored

e. testicle

EXERCISE 3   Underline and define the roots from this chapter in the following terms.

1. spermicide _____

2. testicular carcinoma _____

3. epididymectomy _____

4. balanorrhea _____

5. anorchidism _____

6. prostatovesiculectomy (2 roots) _____

EXERCISE 4   Break down the words into their component parts and translate.

| EXAMPLE: | sinusitis | *sinus | itis* |
| | | *inflammation of the sinuses* |

1. epididymotomy _____

2. orchidectomy _____

3. orchiodynia _____

4. prostatectomy _____

5. aspermia _____

GENERATION

EXERCISE 5   Identify the roots for the following definitions.

1. prostate _____

2. epididymis _____

3. penis _____

4. sperm (3 roots) _____

5. testicle (5 roots) _____

EXERCISE 6   Fill in the blanks.

1. *testitis:* inflammation of the _____

2. *prostatorrhea:* discharge from the _____

3. *spermatogenesis:* creation of _____

4. *orchitis:* inflammation of the _____

5. *balanoplasty:* surgical reconstruction of the _____

6. *epididymo-orchitis:* inflammation of the _____ and _____

EXERCISE 7   Build a medical term from the information provided.

1. inflammation of the testicle (use *orchid/o*) _____

2. inflammation of a testicle (use *test/o*) _____

3. inflammation of the prostate _____

4. inflammation of the epididymis _____

5. inflammation of the penis _____

6. inflammation of the prostate and bladder (use *cyst/o*) _____

7. inflammation of the testicle (use *orch/o*) and epididymis _____

12.3 Patient History, Problems, Complaints

Patients with urinary system problems frequently seek medical care with one of two types of problems: pain or problems with urinating. Pain is a very common symptom of infections of the urinary system.

Pain with urination (*dysuria*) is the most common symptom of an infection in the urinary tract. A simple urinary tract infection also may cause pain in the bladder (*cystalgia*). If the infection spreads to the kidney(s), the patient may have kidney pain (*nephralgia*). Severe kidney pain that comes in waves (*renal colic*) is a very good indicator of a kidney stone. The urethra is also a common source of pain (*urethralgia*) when infected or irritated by chemicals. Difficulty with urination may present with inability to hold urine in (*incontinence, enuresis*). Patients may also urinate too frequently (*polyuria*) or not enough (*oliguria*). Complete lack of urination (*anuria*) is a serious symptom that represents either a blockage or kidney failure. A patient's urine itself may be a concern, as he or she may notice blood (*hematuria*) or pus (*pyuria*) in the urine.

Male patients may have special genitourinary issues that are unique to them. When genital pain is a concern, the testicle (*orchialgia, orchiodynia*) is the most common site. Male patients may also have problems with erections. They can be painful and prolonged (*priapism*) or may not last long enough for sexual intercourse (*impotence*). Finally, a male patient may have concerns with penile discharge (*balanorrhea, urethrorrhea*). This is often an indicator of a sexually transmitted infection.

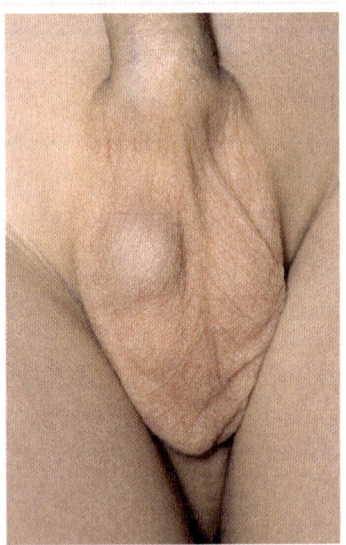

Though a patient might notice only one testicle, usually a medical exam is required to determine whether the missing testicle is not there (*anorchidism*) or is hidden (*cryptorchidism*).

Dr. P. Marazzi/Science Source

urinary tract

TERM	WORD ANALYSIS		
anuria an-YUR-ee-ah	an / ur / ia no / urine / condition		
DEFINITION lack of urination			
cystalgia sis-TAL-jah	cyst / algia bladder / pain		
DEFINITION pain in the bladder			
cystodynia SIS-toh-DAI-nee-ah	cysto / dynia bladder / pain		
DEFINITION pain in the bladder			
dysuria dis-YUR-ee-ah	dys / ur / ia bad / urine / condition		
DEFINITION painful urination			
enuresis EN-yur-EE-sis	from Greek, for *to urinate*		
DEFINITION involutary urination			
hematuria HEE-mah-TUR-ee-ah	hemat / ur / ia blood / urine / condition		
DEFINITION bloody urination			
incontinence in-CON-tih-nentz	in / con / tinence not / together / hold		
DEFINITION inability to control urination			

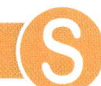
urinary tract *continued*

TERM	WORD ANALYSIS
oliguria aw-lih-GYIR-ee-ah	olig / ur / ia few / urine / condition
DEFINITION low urine output	
polydipsia PAW-lee-DIP-see-ah	poly / dips / ia many / thirst / condition
DEFINITION excessive thirst	
polyuria PAW-lee-YUR-ee-ah	poly / ur / ia many / urine / condition
DEFINITION excessive urination	
pyuria pai-YUR-ee-ah	py / ur / ia pus / urine / condition
DEFINITION pus in the urine	
urethrodynia yoo-REE-throh-DAI-nee-ah	urethro / dynia urethra / pain
DEFINITION pain in the urethra	
urethrorrhea yoo-REE-throh-REE-ah	urethro / rrhea urethra / discharge
DEFINITION discharge from the urethra	
urodynia YUR-oh-DAI-nee-ah	uro / dynia urine / pain
DEFINITION painful urination	

male genitalia

TERM	WORD ANALYSIS
balanorrhea BAL-ah-noh-REE-ah	balano / rrhea penis / discharge
DEFINITION discharge from the penis	
orchialgia OR-kee-AL-jah	orchi / algia testicle / pain
DEFINITION testicle pain	
orchichorea OR-kee-kor-EE-ah	orchi / chorea testicle / dance
DEFINITION involuntary jerking movement of the testicles	
orchidoptosis OR-kih-dop-TOH-sis	orchido / ptosis testicle / drooping condition
DEFINITION downward displacement of a testicle	
orchiodynia OR-kee-oh-DAI-nee-ah	orchio / dynia testicle / pain
DEFINITION testicle pain	
priapism PREE-ap-izm	from ancient Greek minor fertility god named Priapus, who is always shown with a large and permanently erect penis
DEFINITION persistent and painful erection	

TRANSLATION

EXERCISE 1 Break down the following words into their component parts.

EXAMPLE: nasopharyngoscope
naso | pharyngo | scope

1. anuria _____
2. dysuria _____
3. cystodynia _____
4. orchiodynia _____
5. incontinence _____

EXERCISE 2 Underline and define the root from this chapter in the following terms.

1. urethrorrhea _____
2. orchichorea _____
3. balanorrhea _____
4. orchidoptosis _____
5. enuresis _____

EXERCISE 3 Fill in the blanks.

1. *cystalgia:* pain in the _____
2. *orchialgia:* pain in the _____
3. *urethrodynia:* pain in the _____
4. *urodynia:* pain in _____
5. *polydipsia:* excessive _____
6. *polyuria:* excessive _____

EXERCISE 4 Translate the following terms as literally as possible.

EXAMPLE: nasopharyngoscope   *an instrument for looking at the nose and throat*

1. cystalgia _____
2. hematuria _____
3. oliguria _____
4. pyuria _____
5. orchialgia _____
6. orchichorea _____

EXERCISE 5 Match the term on the left with its definition on the right.

_____ 1. incontinence

_____ 2. hematuria

_____ 3. pyuria

_____ 4. oliguria

_____ 5. cystodynia

_____ 6. priapism

a. bloody urination

b. inability to control urination

c. low urine output

d. pain in the bladder

e. persistent and painful erection

f. pus in the urine

GENERATION

EXERCISE 6 Build a medical term from the information provided.

> EXAMPLE: inflammation of the sinuses
> *sinusitis*

1. discharge from the urethra _____
2. discharge from the penis _____
3. downward displacement of a testicle

_____

EXERCISE 7 Briefly describe the difference between each pair of terms.

1. urethrodynia, urodynia _____
2. anuria, dysuria _____
3. polydipsia, polyuria _____
4. orchiodynia, priapism _____

OBJECTIVE

12.4 Observation and Discovery

When evaluating a patient with urinary concerns, the examiner will first need to determine whether the patient is alert and oriented. Kidney failure can cause confusion and delirium and may also cause swelling (*edema*) in the feet.

The abdominal exam may uncover pain in the lower abdomen (*suprapubic tenderness*), which may be an indication of inflammation of the bladder. Pain when pushing on the lower back (*costovertebral angle*) can warn of kidney infection.

When examining male patients, the examiner will inspect the head of the penis. Does the foreskin pull back normally, or is it stuck (*phimosis*)? The exam also includes visualizing the hole through which the urine comes out (*urethral meatus*). The hole may be too small (*meatal stenosis*) or in the wrong position (*hypospadias*).

A testicular exam includes ensuring that both testes are present in the scrotum. If one is absent, it could mean that the patient is missing a testicle (*anorchid*) or that the testicle is hidden (*cryptorchid*).

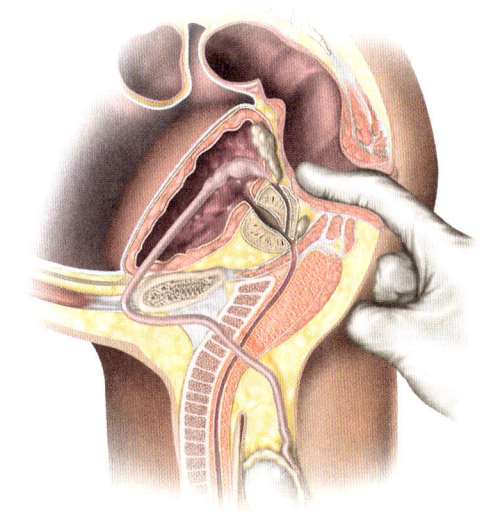

The principal way to examine the prostate is with a digital rectal exam (DRE).

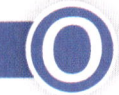

Palpation of the testicles may reveal a mass, which could be fluid (*hydrocele*), misplaced intestines (*hernia*), or a tumor.

The last part of a urologist's physical exam is the insertion of a finger in the patient's anus to feel his prostate (*digital rectal exam*). While unpleasant, this exam is very important in detecting an enlarged prostate.

Not surprisingly, laboratory testing for urinary problems focuses mostly on testing the urine directly (*urinalysis*). A routine urinalysis reveals a lot about a patient. For example, how concentrated the urine is reveals how well hydrated the patient is.

Urinalysis can also show things that are in the urine that don't belong there. Protein in the urine (*proteinuria*) is always abnormal. One specific protein that may show up in the urine is albumin (*albuminuria*). Protein spilling into the urine is a sign that the kidneys are not functioning properly. The presence of sugar (*glucosuria/glycosuria*) is also always abnormal; usually, sugar in the urine indicates that the patient has diabetes. If the patient's diabetes is severe or if he or she is dehydrated, the urine may include a by-product of fat breakdown called *ketones* (*ketonuria*). This can also happen in fasting states. Blood in the urine (*hematuria*) may not have been noticed by the patient but can

be seen with lab testing. This type of hematuria is called *microscopic hematuria* (as opposed to *gross hematuria,* which can be seen by the naked eye).

When a patient's kidneys do not work properly, there may be some abnormalities in his or her blood work, too. The patient's blood may have high potassium (*hyperkalemia*) or low sodium (*hyponatremia*) levels. Also, the blood may have an overaccumulation of a waste product known as *blood urea nitrogen* (*BUN*). When the BUN is too high, the condition is called *azotemia.*

There are also a few laboratory tests related to genital function. The main male-specific lab test in the field of urology is *sperm count,* a test of how many sperm cells are present in a patient's *semen.* This test can help detect low sperm counts (*oligospermia*) in an infertile male or confirm that there is no sperm (*azoospermia/aspermia*) in the semen of a patient who has undergone surgery to become sterile.

Sometimes, it may be necessary to examine parts of the urinary tract either with images or a camera to get a clearer understanding of the problem. *Ultrasound* offers the least invasive way of looking at many parts of the urinary system. A renal ultrasound, or *nephrosonography,* is a very common test that can help determine if the kidneys are filled with fluid (*hydronephrosis*). This is often a good indicator of an anatomical problem of the urinary tract. A bladder ultrasound can be helpful to show if a patient is retaining urine.

Among the most common types of images of the urinary tract is an *intravenous pyelogram.* In this test, the patient receives an intravenous injection of a special dye and then undergoes a CT scan of the urinary tract. This test can be very useful in showing kidney stones (*nephrolithiasis*) or problems with the anatomy of the urinary tract. For example, the CT may show that the patient's ureter is narrowing (*ureterostenosis*) or that the ureter has developed a pouch (*ureterocele*). Some patients are allergic to the special dye used in the intravenous pyelogram. In such a case, it may be necessary to insert a special camera into the bladder (*cystoscope*) or ureter (*ureteroscope*).

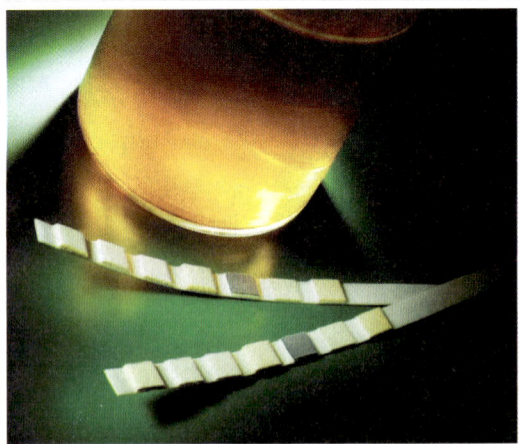

Test strips help in analyzing urine samples.
Brand X/Getty Images

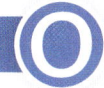

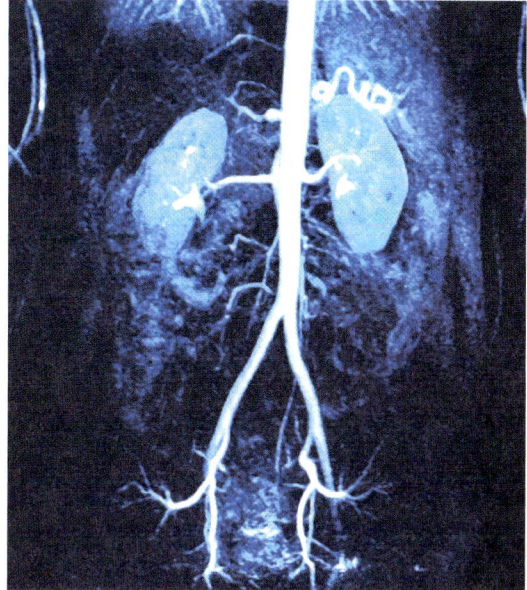

An image of the abdomen with the kidneys and bladder prominent.

Miriam Maslo/SPL/Getty Images

At times, a physician may want to watch the flow of urine (*urodynamic testing*). The most common of these types of tests involves putting dye in the patient's bladder and watching the direction of the urine as the patient urinates (*voiding cystourethrogram*).

urinary tract

TERM	WORD ANALYSIS		
albuminuria al-byoo-mih-NUR-ee-ah	albumin / protein	ur / urine	ia / condition
DEFINITION protein in the urine			
azoturia AZ-oh-TUR-ee-ah	azot / nitrogen	ur / urine	ia / condition
DEFINITION excess nitrogen in the urine			
NOTE: The *azot* root comes from the two roots *a* (not) and *zo* (living). It was applied to nitrogen because things cannot live in it.			

urinary tract *continued*

TERM	WORD ANALYSIS		
cystorrhexis SIS-toh-REK-sis	cysto / bladder	rrhexis / rupture	
DEFINITION rupture of the bladder			
dipsogenic DIP-soh-JIN-ik	dipso / thirst	genic / creating	
DEFINITION creating thirst			
glycosuria GLAI-koh-shur-EE-ah	glycos / sugar	ur / urine	ia / condition
DEFINITION sugar in the urine			
nephroptosis nef-rop-TOH-sis	nephro / kidney	ptosis / drooping condition	
DEFINITION downward displacement of a kidney			
nephrosis neh-FROH-sis	nephr / kidney	osis / condition	
DEFINITION kidney condition			
uremia ur-EE-mee-ah	ur / urine	emia / blood condition	
DEFINITION urine in the blood			
urethrostenosis yoo-REE-throh-steh-NOH-sis	urethro / urethra	sten / narrowing	osis / condition
DEFINITION narrrowing of the urethra			

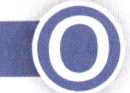

diagnostic procedures

TERM	WORD ANALYSIS
cystoscopy sis-TAWS-koh-pee	cysto / scopy bladder / looking procedure
DEFINITION process for examining the bladder	
nephroscopy ne-FRAW-skoh-pee	nephro / scopy kidney / looking procedure
DEFINITION procedure for examining a kidney	
urethroscopy yoo-ree-THRAW-skoh-pee	urethro / scopy urethra / looking procedure
DEFINITION process of examining the urethra	
urinalysis (UA) YUR-ih-NAL-ih-sis **DEFINITION** analysis of the urine NOTE: The *-in* sound at the end of *urine* combines with an *an-* sound at the beginning of *analysis* to make a single sound.	*urinalysis* is actually a shortened form of *urine analysis*

radiology

TERM	WORD ANALYSIS
nephrosonography NEF-roh-soh-NAW-grah-fee	nephro / sono / graphy kidney / sound / writing procedure
DEFINITION procedure for imaging a kidney using sound waves	
pyelogram PAI-el-oh-GRAM	pyelo / gram pelvis / record
DEFINITION image of the renal pelvis	
renal angiography REE-nal AN-jee-AW-grah-fee	ren / al kidney / pertaining to angio / graphy vessel / writing procedure
DEFINITION process of imaging a kidney blood vessel	
renal arteriogram REE-nal ar-TER-ee-oh-GRAM	ren / al kidney / pertaining to arterio / gram artery / record
DEFINITION image of a kidney artery	

radiology *continued*

TERM	WORD ANALYSIS
retrograde pyelogram REH-troh-grayd PAI-el-oh-GRAM	retro / grade backward / walk pyelo / gram pelvis / record
DEFINITION image of the renal pelvis produced by injecting a contrast dye from the bladder to the kidney NOTE: The term *retrograde* is used because the contrast goes in the opposite direction of normal urine flow.	
ultrasonography UL-trah- soh-NAW-grah-fee	ultra / sono / graphy high / sound / writing procedure
DEFINITION imaging procedure using high-frequency sound waves	
voiding cystourethrogram (VCUG) VOI-ding SIS-toh-yoo-REE-throh-GRAM	voiding urinating cysto / urethro / gram bladder / urethra / record
DEFINITION imaging procedure of the bladder and urethra produced during urination	
transrectal ultrasonography TRANZ-REK-tal UL-trah-soh-NAW-grah-fee	trans / rect / al through / rectum / pertaining to ultra / sono / graphy high / sound / writing procedure
DEFINITION procedure using a probe inserted into the rectum using high-frequency sound waves to scan through the rectum to nearby tissue (most commonly, the prostate)	

professional terms

TERM	WORD ANALYSIS
blood urea nitrogen (BUN) blud yoo-REE-ah NAI-troh-jun	blood urea nitrogen
DEFINITION nitrogen in the blood in the form of urea; it is the product of the breakdown of amino acids for energy NOTE: The level of urea in the blood can be an indicator of kidney function.	

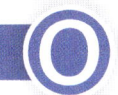

professional terms *continued*

TERM	WORD ANALYSIS	
diuresis DAI-yur-EE-sis	di	/ uresis
	through	/ urination
DEFINITION excessive urination NOTE: The prefix for this word is actually *dia*, but when the next word part starts with a vowel (as does *uresis*), the *dia* shortens to *di*.		
nephrologist neh-FRAW-loh-jist	nephro	/ logist
	kidney	/ specialist
DEFINITION specialist in the kidneys		
nephrology neh-FRAW-loh-jee	nephro	/ logy
	kidney	/ study
DEFINITION study of the kidneys		
urologist yur-AW-loh-jist	uro	/ logist
	urine	/ specialist
DEFINITION specialist in the urinary tract		

Rick Brady/McGraw-Hill Education

TERM	WORD ANALYSIS	
urology yur-AW-loh-jee	uro	/ logy
	urine	/ study
DEFINITION study of the urinary tract		

male genitalia

TERM	WORD ANALYSIS	
anorchidism an-OR-kih-DIZ-um	an / orchid	/ ism
	no / testicle	/ condition
DEFINITION lack of a testicle		

male genitalia *continued*

TERM	WORD ANALYSIS	
aspermia ay-SPER-mee-ah	a / sperm	/ ia
	no / sperm	/ condition
DEFINITION condition characterized by lack of sperm		
cryptorchidism krip-TOR-kih-DIZ-um	crypt / orchid	/ ism
	hidden / testicle	/ condition
DEFINITION hidden testicle		
hydrocele HAI-droh-SEEL	hydro	/ cele
	water	/ hernia
DEFINITION fluid-filled mass in a testicle		
hypospadias HAI-poh-SPAY-dee-as	from Greek, for *to tear underneath*	
DEFINITION birth defect in which the opening of the urethra is on the underside, instead of the end, of the penis		
phimosis fih-MOH-sis	from Greek, for *muzzle*	
DEFINITION contraction of the foreskin of the penis, preventing it from being retracted		
prostatomegaly PROS-ta-toh-MEH-gah-lee	prostato / megaly	
	prostate / enlargement	
DEFINITION abnormal enlargement of the prostate		

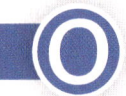

12.4 Observation and Discovery

diagnostic procedures

TERM	WORD ANALYSIS
digital rectal exam (DRE) DIJ-ih-tal REK-tal ek-ZAM	**digit** / al finger / pertaining to **rect** / al rectum / pertaining to **exam**
DEFINITION examination of the prostate using a finger inserted into the rectum	

professional terms

TERM	WORD ANALYSIS
gonads GOH-nadz	**gon** / ads creation / pair
DEFINITION pair of organs used for sexual reproduction; in males, they are the testicles, and in females, they are the ovaries	
spermatogenesis sper-MAT-oh-JIN-eh-sis	**spermato** / genesis sperm / creation
DEFINITION creation of sperm	

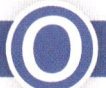

Learning Outcome 12.4 Exercises

PRONUNCIATION

EXERCISE 1 Indicate which syllable(s) is emphasized when pronounced.

> EXAMPLE: bronchitis bron<u>chi</u>tis

1. gonads _____
2. uremia _____
3. aspermia _____
4. nephroptosis _____
5. cryptorchidism _____
6. urology _____
7. urologist _____
8. nephrology _____
9. nephrologist _____
10. cystoscopy _____
11. nephroscopy _____

TRANSLATION

EXERCISE 2 Break down the following words into their component parts.

> EXAMPLE: nasopharyngoscope
> *naso | pharyngo | scope*

1. urology _____
2. nephrology _____
3. hydrocele _____
4. pyelogram _____
5. nephrosis _____
6. prostatomegaly _____
7. albuminuria _____
8. dipsogenic _____
9. aspermia _____
10. nephrosonography _____

11. ultrasonography _____
12. anorchidism _____

EXERCISE 3 Underline and define the roots from this chapter in the following terms.

1. urinalysis _____
2. nephrologist _____
3. urologist _____
4. nephroptosis _____
5. cystorrhexis _____
6. urethrostenosis _____
7. azoturia _____
8. retrograde pyelogram _____
9. diuresis _____
10. cryptorchidism _____

EXERCISE 4 Match the term on the left with its definition on the right.

_____ 1. gonads

_____ 2. blood urea nitrogen

_____ 3. digital rectal exam

_____ 4. transrectal ultrasonography

_____ 5. hypospadias

_____ 6. phimosis

a. birth defect in which the opening of the urethra is on the underside, instead of the end, of the penis

b. contraction of the foreskin of the penis, preventing it from being retracted

c. procedure using a probe inserted into the rectum using high-frequency sound waves to scan through the rectum to nearby tissue (most commonly, the prostate)

d. exam of the prostate using a finger inserted into the rectum

e. nitrogen in the blood in the form of urea; can be an indicator of kidney function

f. pair of organs used for sexual reproduction (testicles in males; ovaries in females)

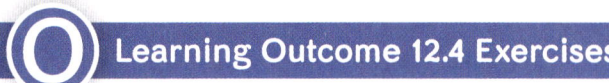

EXERCISE 5 Underline the correct option for each given translation.

> EXAMPLE: hypoglycemia   *hypo (over/<u>under</u>)*
> *pharyngo (salt/<u>sugar</u>) -emia (<u>blood</u>/urine condition)*

1. *albuminuria = albumin* protein/nitrogen + *uria* urine/blood condition

2. *glycosuria = glycos* sugar/potassium + *uria* urine/blood condition

EXERCISE 6 Fill in the blanks.

1. *urethroscopy:* process for examining the

   _____

2. *cystoscopy:* process for examining the

   _____

3. *nephroscopy:* process for examining the

   _____

4. *renal angiography:* process of imaging a(n)

   _____

EXERCISE 7 Translate the following terms as literally as possible.

> EXAMPLE: nasopharyngoscope   *an instrument for looking at the nose and throat*

1. nephrology _____

2. cystoscopy _____

3. pyelogram _____

4. spermatogenesis _____

5. urinalysis _____

6. cryptorchidism _____

7. cystorrhexis _____

8. uremia _____

9. anorchidism _____

10. dipsogenic _____

GENERATION

EXERCISE 8 Build a medical term from the information provided.

> EXAMPLE: inflammation of the sinuses   *sinusitis*

1. kidney condition (use *nephr/o*) _____

   _____

2. process of imaging a kidney blood vessel (use *ren/o*) _____

3. procedure for examining a kidney _____

   _____

4. specialist in the kidneys _____

   _____

5. abnormal enlargement of the prostate

   _____

6. downward displacement of a kidney

   _____

7. low sodium in the blood _____

   _____

8. imaging procedure using high-frequency sound waves _____

   _____

9. procedure for imaging a kidney using sound waves _____

   _____

EXERCISE 9 Multiple-choice questions. Select the correct answer(s).

1. Which of the choices below are true of the term *blood urea nitrogen?*
   a. abbreviated BUN
   b. nitrogen in the blood in the form of urea
   c. product of the breakdown of amino acids for energy
   d. level of urea in the blood can be an indicator of kidney function
   e. all of these

2. The medical term for *excessive urination* is
   a. diuresis   c. voiding
   b. uremia   d. glycosuria

3. A *hydrocele* is a fluid-filled mass in the
   a. bladder   d. testicle
   b. kidney   e. none of these
   c. prostate

4. The *digital rectal exam* and the *transrectal ultrasonography* are both procedures for examining the
   a. bladder   c. testicle
   b. kidney   d. none of these
   c. prostate

5. Which of the statements below are true of the term *retrograde pyelogram* (select all that apply)?
   a. image of the kidney
   b. image of the renal pelvis
   c. image produced by injecting a contrast dye from the bladder to the kidney
   d. image produced by injecting a contrast dye from the bladder to the urethra
   e. literally means *backward walk pelvis record*

6. Which of the statements below are true of the term *hypospadias* (select all that apply)?
   a. birth defect
   b. from Greek, for *to tear underneath*
   c. literally means *over sperm*
   d. opening of the urethra is on the end of the penis
   e. opening of the urethra is on the underside of the penis

EXERCISE 10 Briefly describe the difference between each pair of terms.

1. urologist, urology _____

2. urethrorrhea, urethrostenosis _____

   _____

3. albuminuria, azoturia _____

   _____

(A)SSESSMENT

12.5 Diagnosis and Pathology

Just like all the other body systems, the urinary system can have problems with its anatomy, infection, tumors, and blood supply. On a large scale, the vessels in patients' urinary tracts can have abnormal pouches (for example, *cystoceles*). These pouches can be harmless or cause a blockage of urine. In the case of the ureter (*ureterocele*), this pouching intrudes into the bladder. Patients may also have large cysts in the kidneys (*polycystic kidney disease*). These don't cause blockage, but they can prevent the kidneys from working correctly.

On a microscopic level, the kidneys can have all manner of problems. These general kidney problems (*nephropathy*) fall into two general types with (*nephritis*) or without (*nephrosis*) inflammation. Often, the difference is seen in a urinalysis. Nephritis will most often cause white blood cells and red blood cells to show up in the urine. Both types of diseases can be severe enough to lead to kidney failure. Kidney failure is marked by the kidney's inability to filter waste out of the blood. If this problem is not fixed, the patient will die.

The urinary tract is vulnerable to infection. Urinary tract infections (UTIs) are often divided into lower urinary tract and upper urinary tract infections, depending on whether the kidneys are involved. Lower urinary tract infections generally refer to infections of the bladder (*cystitis*). They are much more common in females than in males, and they are also frequently seen in patients whose urine flows back toward the kidneys from the bladder (*vesicoureteral reflux*).

When infection spreads to the kidneys (*pyelonephritis*), it generally becomes more severe. A patient with pyelonephritis may have back pain and, high fever, and may appear very ill. Another common infection of the urinary tract involves just the urethra (*urethritis*). The usual cause is *gonorrhea,* a sexually transmitted infection.

Tumors of the urinary tract are most common in the larger structures of the tract: the kidney (*nephroma*) or bladder (*cystoma*). The most usual presenting symptom is blood in the urine. By far, the most common cancer of the kidney is *renal cell carcinoma*. Often, there are few early warning symptoms for this cancer.

Kidneys need a constant supply of blood. Poor blood supply to the kidneys (*renal ischemia*) is usually caused by cholesterol deposits in the arteries. Another cause is narrowing of the arteries that lead to the kidney (*renal artery stenosis*). When the blood supply to the kidneys is low, the kidneys release signals to the rest of the body to increase the blood's pressure (*renovascular hypertension*). Any time a patient's high blood pressure doesn't respond to

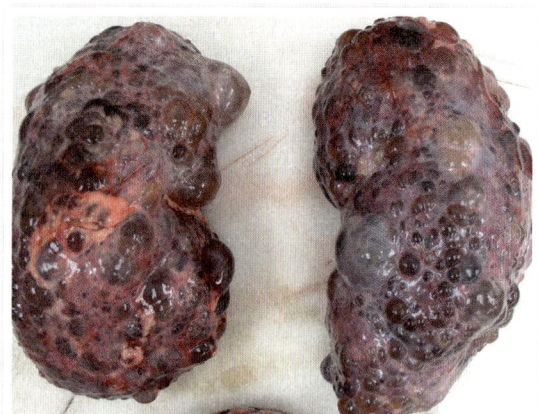
A pair of kidneys with polycystic kidney disease.

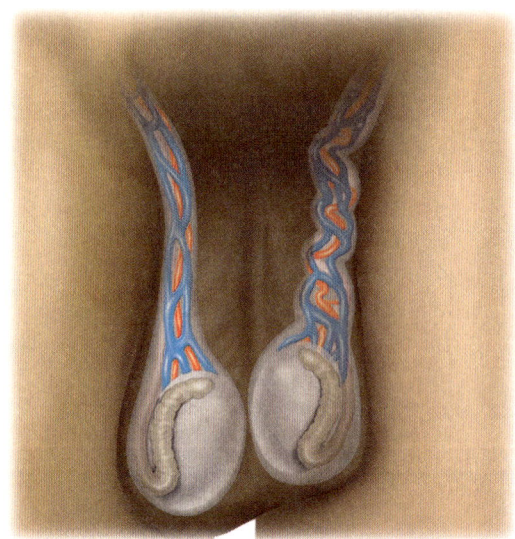
Testicular torsion—when a testicle becomes twisted—is considered a medical emergency.

typical medical management, a renal cause should be considered.

Male patients can have specific problems with their genitourinary systems. The prostate gland is a common cause of problems in older men. The prostate gland may become enlarged (*benign prostate hypertrophy*), infected (*prostatitis*), or cancerous. Prostate symptoms include pain and the blocked flow of

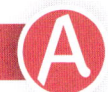

urine, leading to a weak urine stream or difficulty starting a urine stream at all.

The testicles can cause problems in any age group. *Testicular carcinoma* is the most common form of cancer in young adult men. It usually presents as a painful lump on the testicle. The testicle can also become infected (*orchitis*), a problem usually associated with the mumps.

Since testicles hang from the body, it is possible for one of them to become twisted (*testicular torsion*). This can cut off the blood supply to the testicle and is considered a medical emergency. Concerns in other parts of the reproductive system include infection of the epididymis (*epididymitis*) and swelling of the veins in the scrotum (*varicocele*).

urinary tract

TERM	WORD ANALYSIS
cystocele SIS-toh-seel	cysto / cele bladder / hernia
DEFINITION hernia of the bladder	
glomerulonephritis gloh-MER-yoo-loh-neh-FRAI-tis	glomerulo / nephr / itis glomerulus / kidney / inflammation
DEFINITION inflammation of the kidneys involving primarily the glomeruli	
hydronephrosis HAI-droh-neh-FROH-sis	hydro / nephr / osis water / kidney / condition
DEFINITION kidney condition caused by the obstruction of urine flow	

urinary tract *continued*

TERM	WORD ANALYSIS
nephritis neh-FRAI-tis	nephr / itis kidney / inflammation
DEFINITION inflammation of the kidney	
nephrolithiasis NEH-froh-lih-THAI-ah-sis	nephro / lith / iasis kidney / stone / presence
DEFINITION presence of stones in the kidney	
nephromalacia NEH-froh-mah-LAY-shah	nephro / malacia kidney / softening
DEFINITION abnormal softening of a kidney	
nephromegaly NEH-froh-MEG-ah-lee	nephro / megaly kidney / enlargement
DEFINITION abnormal enlargement of a kidney	
nephropathy neh-FRAW-pah-thee	nephro / pathy kidney / disease
DEFINITION any kidney disease	

urinary tract *continued*

TERM	WORD ANALYSIS
nephroptosis NEH-frop-TOH-sis	nephro / ptosis kidney / drooping condition
DEFINITION downward displacement of a kidney	

polycystic kidney disease (PKD) PAW-lee-SIS-tik KID-nee dih-ZEEZ	poly / cyst / ic many / cysts / pertaining to kidney disease
DEFINITION disease characterized by the formation of many fluid-filled cysts in the kidneys	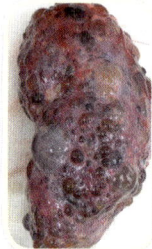

pyelitis PAI-el-AI-tis	pyel / itis pelvis / inflammation
DEFINITION inflammation of the renal pelvis	

pyelonephritis PAI-el-oh-neh-FRAI-tis	pyelo / nephr / itis pelvis / kidney / inflammation
DEFINITION inflammation of the kidney and renal pelvis	

pyelopathy PAI-el-AW-pah-thee	pyelo / pathy pelvis / disease
DEFINITION disease of the renal pelvis	

renal failure REE-nal FAY-el-yur	ren / al failure kidney / pertaining to failure
DEFINITION kidney failure	

stress urinary incontinence (SUI) stress YUR-ih-NAR-ee in-CON-tih-nentz	stress urin / ary stress urine / pertaining to in / con / tinence not / together / holding
DEFINITION loss of bladder control caused by the application of external pressure NOTE: This is the medical term for loss of bladder control due to excessive laughing, a hard cough, or similar motion.	

ureteritis yoo-REE-ter-AI-tis	ureter / itis ureter / inflammation
DEFINITION inflammation of a ureter	

ureteropyelo-nephritis yoo-REE-ter-oh-PAI-el-oh-neh-FRAI-tis	uretero / pyelo / nephr / itis ureter / pelvis / kidney / inflammation
DEFINITION inflammation of a kidney, renal pelvis, and ureter	

urethritis yoo-ree-THRAI-tis	urethr / itis urethra / inflammation
DEFINITION inflammation of the urethra	

urethrocystitis yoo-REE-throh-sis-TAI-tis	urethro / cyst / itis urethra / bladder / inflammation
DEFINITION inflammation of the urethra and bladder	

urinary tract infection (UTI) YUR-ih-NAR-ee trakt in-FEK-shun	urinary tract infection
DEFINITION infection of the urinary tract	

oncology

TERM	WORD ANALYSIS
renal cell carcinoma REE-nal SELL KAR-sih-NOH-mah	ren / al kidney / pertaining to cell carcin / oma cell cancer / tumor
DEFINITION cancer of the kidneys	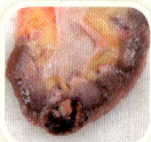

testicular carcinoma tes-TIK-yoo-lar KAR-sih-NOH-mah	testicul / ar testicle / pertaining to carcin / oma cancer / tumor
DEFINITION testicular cancer	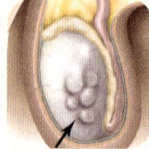

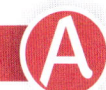

male genitalia

TERM	WORD ANALYSIS
balanitis bal-ah-NAI-tis	balan / itis penis / inflammation
DEFINITION inflammation of the penis	
benign prostate hyperplasia (BPH) beh-NAIN PROS-tayt HAI-per-PLAY-zhah	benign prostate friendly prostate hyper / plas / ia over / formation / condition
DEFINITION noncancerous overdevelopment of the prostate, also known as *enlarged prostate*	
orchiditis OR-kih-DAI-tis	orchid / itis testicle / inflammation
DEFINITION inflammation of the testicles	
orchitis or-KAI-tis	orch / itis testicle / inflammation
DEFINITION inflammation of the testicles	
prostatitis PRAWS-tah-TAI-tis	prostat / itis prostate / inflammation
DEFINITION inflammation of the prostate	

male genitalia *continued*

TERM	WORD ANALYSIS
testitis tes-TAI-tis	test / itis testicle / inflammation
DEFINITION inflammation of a testicle	
varicocele VAR-ih-koh-SEEL	varico / cele twisted / tumor
DEFINITION overexpansion of the blood vessels of the testicles, leading to a soft tumor	

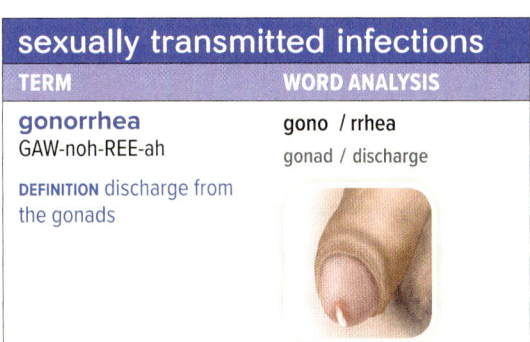

sexually transmitted infections

TERM	WORD ANALYSIS
gonorrhea GAW-noh-REE-ah	gono / rrhea gonad / discharge
DEFINITION discharge from the gonads	

PRONUNCIATION

EXERCISE 1   Indicate which syllable(s) is emphasized when pronounced.

> EXAMPLE: bronchitis bron<u>chi</u>tis

1. orchitis _____

2. testitis _____

3. nephritis _____

4. balanitis _____

5. urethritis _____

6. nephropathy _____

TRANSLATION

EXERCISE 2   Break down the following words into their component parts.

> EXAMPLE: nasopharyngoscope
> *naso | pharyngo | scope*

1. testitis _____

2. nephritis _____

3. gonorrhea _____

4. nephromalacia _____

5. hydronephritis _____

6. urethrocystitis _____

7. pyelonephritis _____

8. nephrolithiasis _____

9. ureteropyelonephritis _____

EXERCISE 3   Underline and define the roots from this chapter in the following terms.

1. prostatitis _____

2. ureteritis _____

3. urethritis _____

4. orchitis _____

5. orchiditis _____

6. balanitis _____

7. cystocele _____

8. pyelopathy _____

9. renal failure _____

10. nephromegaly _____

11. renal cell carcinoma _____

12. testicular carcinoma _____

EXERCISE 4   Match the term on the left with its definition on the right.

_____ 1. urinary tract infection

_____ 2. stress urinary incontinence disease

_____ 3. polycystic kidney disease

_____ 4. hydronephrosis

_____ 5. benign prostate hyperplasia

_____ 6. varicocele

a. disease characterized by the formation of many fluid-filled cysts in the kidneys

b. infection of the urinary tract

c. kidney condition caused by obstruction of urine flow

d. literally, *friendly prostate overformation condition;* noncancerous overdevelopment of the prostate or *enlarged prostate*

e. loss of bladder control caused by the application of external pressure

g. overexpansion of the blood vessels of the testicles, leading to a soft tumor

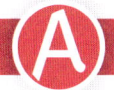

EXERCISE 5 Fill in the blanks.

1. *testitis:* inflammation of the _____

2. *prostatitis:* inflammation of the _____

3. *urethritis:* inflammation of the _____

4. *nephritis:* inflammation of the _____

5. *ureteritis:* inflammation of the _____

6. *orchiditis:* inflammation of the _____

7. *pyelitis:* inflammation of the _____

8. *balanitis:* inflammation of the _____

9. *orchitis:* inflammation of the _____

10. *glomerulonephritis:* inflammation of the
_____ and
_____

11. *urethrocystitis:* inflammation of the
_____ and
_____

12. *pyelonephritis:* inflammation of the
_____ and
_____

13. *ureteropyelonephritis:* inflammation of
the _____,
_____
and _____

EXERCISE 6 Translate the following terms as literally as possible.

> EXAMPLE: nasopharyngoscope *an instrument for looking at the nose and throat*

1. pyelopathy _____

2. gonorrhea _____

3. nephromegaly _____

4. nephrolithiasis _____

5. testicular carcinoma _____

6. benign prostate hyperplasia _____

GENERATION

EXERCISE 7 Build a medical term from the information provided.

> EXAMPLE: inflammation of the sinuses *sinusitis*

1. hernia of the bladder (use *cyst/o*) _____

2. kidney failure (use *ren/o*) _____

3. kidney disease (use *nephr/o*) _____

4. downward displacement of a kidney _____

5. inflammation of the kidneys involving primarily the glomeruli (use *nephr/o*) _____

6. inflammation of the kidney and renal pelvis _____

EXERCISE 8 Multiple-choice questions. Select the correct answer(s).

1. The term *nephropathy* refers to
   a. any cancer of the kidney
   b. any cancer of the urinary tract
   c. any disease of the bladder
   d. any disease of the kidney
   e. any disease of the urinary tract

2. Which of the following statements is true of the term *stress urinary incontinence?*
   a. abbreviated SUI
   b. loss of bladder control caused by the application of external pressure
   c. medical term for loss of bladder control due to excessive laughing, a hard cough, or something like that
   d. would apply to the common phrase "I peed in my pants"
   e. all of these

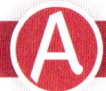

3. A disease characterized by the formation of many fluid-filled cysts in the kidneys is known as
   a. hypernephroma
   b. nephrohypertrophy
   c. nephrolithiasis
   d. polycystic kidney disease
   e. renal cell carcinoma

4. Select all of the choices below that pertain to the term *renal cell carcinoma.*
   a. also known as polycystic kidney disease
   b. benign growth in the kidneys
   c. cancer of the kidneys

P LAN

12.6 Treatments and Therapies

The main medicines used to treat the kidneys and urinary tract are focused on helping the patient urinate more (*diuretic*) or less (*antidiuretic*) often. If urinary control is a problem due to twitching of the muscle that holds back urine flow, an *antispasmodic* may be helpful.

Medicines that are specifically for men are very limited. They include medicine to help correct erectile dysfunction and testosterone, the male hormone, which is used in patients with low levels of the hormone. Patients may also choose to use liquids designed to kill sperm (*spermicides*) as a method of birth control; spermicides are available over the counter.

The most common nonsurgical procedure involving the urinary tract is bladder *catheterization.* A *catheter* is a small tube inserted into the bladder to help with urination or to get a urine sample.

The main nonsurgical treatment for the urinary tract is *dialysis.* Dialysis does the work of the kidneys when they have failed. Dialysis must be done regularly or the patient will die. The two types of dialysis involve either the inner lining of the abdomen (*peritoneal dialysis*) or a machine outside the body (*hemodialysis*). Another nonsurgical treatment in the urinary system is the use of sound waves to break up a stone in the urinary tract (*extracorporeal shock wave lithotripsy*).

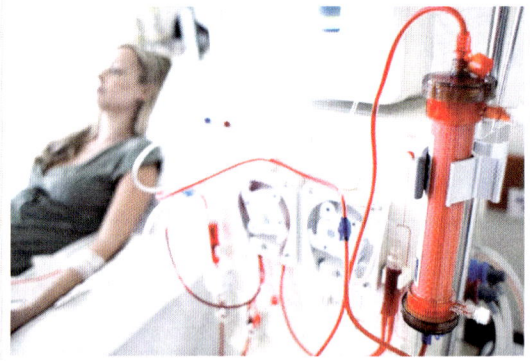

Hemodialysis uses a machine to do the work of kidneys that do not function as they should.
Science Photo Library/Alamy Stock Photo

Often, surgeries of the urinary tract help correct anatomical problems and restore normal urine flow. This can involve direct work on a part of the tract such as the ureter (*ureteroplasty*) or urethra (*urethroplasty*). It could also involve making a new connection between two points in the tract, such as a connection between the kidney and bladder (*nephrocystanastomosis*).

Another surgery of the kidneys is their complete removal (*nephrectomy*), which is often the main

treatment for renal cell carcinoma. In men, the prostate is another organ that can be completely removed (*prostatectomy*) if cancerous. Part of the prostate may be removed through the urethra (*transurethral resection of the prostate*) when the prostate is enlarged and blocking urine flow. Newer, less invasive procedures for this include using a heated needle (*transurethral needle ablation*) to remove part of the prostate.

When a testicle rides high in the scrotum, it may need to be fixed (*orchiopexy*) or removed altogether (*orchiectomy*). When removed, a fake testicle (*testicular prosthesis*) is sometimes placed in the scrotum.

The most common procedure in males is the removal of the foreskin at birth (*circumcision*). While there are small medical benefits, the surgery is generally chosen for cultural or religious reasons. Circumcision is not recommended in patients with hypospadias or epispadias because the foreskin is used to surgically correct those conditions (*balanoplasty*). *Vasectomy* is another very common procedure. In the procedure, a surgeon cuts the vas deferens as a means of birth control. Occasionally, situations change, so a patient may want to reverse the procedure. Doing so is simple—reconnecting the two ends of the vas deferens (*vasovasotomy*).

urinary tract procedures

TERM	WORD ANALYSIS	
cystectomy sis-TEK-toh-mee	cyst / ectomy bladder / removal	
DEFINITION surgical removal of the bladder		
extracorporeal shock wave lithotripsy (ESWL) EKS-trah-cor-POR-ee-al shok wayv LIH-thoh-TRIP-see	extra / corpor / eal outside / body / pertaining to shock wave litho / tripsy shock wave stone / wear down procedure	
DEFINITION breakdown of kidney stones using sound waves generated outside the body		
heminephrectomy HEH-mee-neh-FREK-toh-mee	hemi / nephr / ectomy half / kidney / removal	
DEFINITION surgical removal of half a kidney		

urinary tract procedures *continued*

TERM	WORD ANALYSIS	
hemodialysis HEE-moh-dai-AL-ah-sis	hemo / dia / lysis blood / through / loose	
DEFINITION procedure for removing waste from the bloodstream		
kidney dialysis KID-nee dai-AL-ah-sis	dia / lysis through / loose	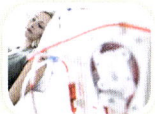
DEFINITION procedure for removing waste from the blood (an alternative name for hemodialysis) NOTE: The name comes from the fact that the procedure separates or loses (*lysis*) blood from waste by passing it through (*dia*) an external filter.		Science Photo Library/ Getty Images
laparonephrectomy LAP-ah-roh-neh-FREK-toh-mee	laparo / nephr / ectomy abdomen / kidney / removal	
DEFINITION surgical removal of a kidney through the abdomen		
lithectomy lih-THEK-toh-mee	lith / ectomy stone / removal	
DEFINITION surgical removal of a stone		
lithotripsy LIH-thoh-TRIP-see	litho / tripsy stone / wear down procedure	
DEFINITION breakdown of a stone		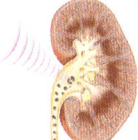
nephrectomy neh-FREK-toh-mee	nephr / ectomy kidney / removal	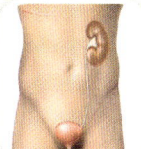
DEFINITION surgical removal of a kidney		

urinary tract procedures *continued*

TERM	WORD ANALYSIS
nephrolithotomy NEH-froh-lih-THAW-toh-mee	nephro / litho / tomy kidney / stone / incision
DEFINITION incision into a kidney to remove a stone 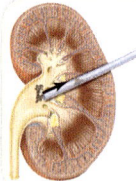	
nephropexy NEH-froh-PEK-see	nephro / pexy kidney / fixation
DEFINITION surgical fixation of a kidney	
nephrostomy neh-FRAW-stoh-mee	nephro / stomy kidney / opening
DEFINITION creation of an opening in a kidney 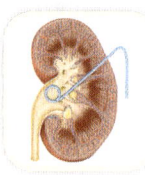	
nephrotomy neh-FRAW-toh-mee	nephro / tomy kidney / incision
DEFINITION incision into a kidney	
nephrotoxin NEH-froh-TOK-sin	nephro / toxin kidney / poison
DEFINITION agent poisonous to the kidney	
pyelolithotomy PAI-el-oh-lih-THAW-toh-mee	pyelo / litho / tomy pelvis / stone / incision
DEFINITION incision into a renal pelvis to remove a stone 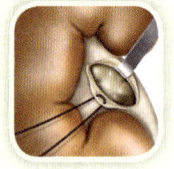	
pyelostomy PAI-el-AW-stoh-mee	pyelo / stomy pelvis / opening
DEFINITION creation of an opening in a renal pelvis	

urinary tract procedures *continued*

TERM	WORD ANALYSIS
ureteroplasty yoo-REE-ter-oh-PLAS-tee	uretero / plasty ureter / reconstruction
DEFINITION surgical recontruction of a ureter	
urinary catheterization YUR-ih-NAR-ee KATH-eh-ter-ih-ZAY-shun	urin / ary urine / pertaining to catheter / ization catheter / procedure
DEFINITION insertion of a catheter into the bladder to drain urine NOTE: The word *catheter* comes from Greek, for *to go inside.* 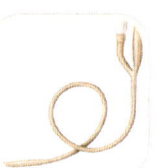	

pharmacology

TERM	WORD ANALYSIS		
antispasmodic AN-tee-spaz-MAW-dik	anti / spasmod / ic against / involuntary contraction / pertaining to		
DEFINITION drug used to prevent spasms			
diuretic DAI-yur-IT-ik	di / uret / ic through / urine / pertaining to		
DEFINITION agent that causes urination			
spermicide SPER-mih-sahyd	spermi / cide sperm / kill		
DEFINITION agent that kills sperm			

male genitalia procedures

TERM	WORD ANALYSIS
circumcision SIR-kum-SIH-zhun	circum / cision around / cut
DEFINITION surgical removal of the foreskin of the penis	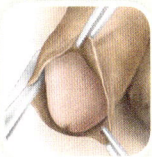
orchidectomy OR-kid-EK-toh-mee	orchid / ectomy testicle / removal
DEFINITION surgical removal of a testicle	
orchidopexy OR-kid-oh-PEK-see	orchido / pexy testicle / fixation
DEFINITION surgical fixation of a testicle	
orchidotomy OR-kid-AW-toh-mee	orchido / tomy testicle / incision
DEFINITION incision into a testicle	
orchiectomy OR-kee-EK-mee	orchi / ectomy testicle / removal
DEFINITION surgical removal of a testicle	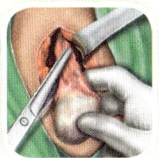
orchiopexy OR-kee-oh-PEK-see	orchio / pexy testicle / fixation
DEFINITION surgical fixation of a testicle	

male genitalia procedures
continued

TERM	WORD ANALYSIS
orchioplasty OR-kee-oh-PLAS-tee	orchio / plasty testicle / reconstruction
DEFINITION surgical reconstruction of a testicle	
prostatectomy PROS-tat-TEK-toh-mee	prostat / ectomy prostate / removal
DEFINITION surgical removal of the prostate	
transurethral resection of the prostate (TURP)	trans / urethr / al through / urethra / pertaining to re / sect / ion back / cut / procedure
DEFINITION procedure of removing all or part of the prostate by the insertion of a resectoscope into the urethra	
vasectomy vah-SEK-toh-mee	vas / ectomy vessel / removal
DEFINITION surgical removal of the vas deferens	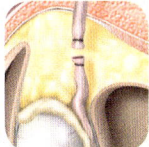
vasovasostomy VAS-oh-vah-SAW-stoh-mee	vaso / vaso / stomy vessel / vessel / opening
DEFINITION creation of an opening between two vessels; this is the technical term for a vasectomy reversal	

TRANSLATION

EXERCISE 1 Break down the following words into their component parts.

> EXAMPLE: nasopharyngoscope
> *naso | pharyngo | scope*

1. nephrotoxin _____

2. orchiopexy _____

3. antispasmodic _____

4. spermicide _____

5. vasovasostomy _____

6. pyelolithotomy _____

7. nephrolithotomy _____

8. heminephrectomy _____

9. laparonephrectomy _____

10. hemodialysis _____

11. circumcision _____

EXERCISE 2 Underline and define the roots from this chapter in the following terms.

1. spermicide _____

2. lithotripsy _____

3. ureteroplasty _____

4. orchioplasty _____

5. nephropexy _____

6. orchidopexy _____

7. nephrostomy _____

8. pyelostomy _____

9. diuretic _____

10. transurethral resection _____

11. urinary catheterization _____

12. extracorporeal shock wave lithotripsy _____

_____

EXERCISE 3   Match the term on the left with its definition on the right.

_____ 1. circumcision

_____ 2. kidney dialysis

_____ 3. urinary catheterization

_____ 4. diuretic

_____ 5. hemodialysis

_____ 6. vasovasostomy

_____ 7. transurethral resection of the prostate

_____ 8. extracorporeal shock wave lithotripsy

a. agent that causes urination

b. insertion of a catheter into the bladder to drain urine

c. procedure for removing waste from the bloodstream

d. procedure for removing waste from the blood (an alternative name for hemodialysis)

e. procedure of removing all or part of the prostate by the insertion of a resectoscope into the urethra

f. surgical removal of the foreskin of the penis

g. breakdown of kidney stones using sound waves generated outside the body

h. creation of an opening between two vessels; the technical term for a vasectomy reversal

EXERCISE 4   Fill in the blanks.

1. *nephrotomy:* incision into _____

_____

2. *orchidotomy:* incision into _____

_____

3. *cystectomy:* surgical removal of the _____

_____

4. *lithectomy:* surgical removal of the _____

_____

5. *nephrectomy:* surgical removal of the _____

_____

6. *orchidectomy:* surgical removal of the _____

_____

7. *orchiectomy:* surgical removal of the _____

_____

8. *prostatectomy:* surgical removal of the _____

_____

9. *vasectomy:* surgical removal of the _____

_____

EXERCISE 5   Translate the following terms as literally as possible.

EXAMPLE: nasopharyngoscope   *an instrument for looking at the nose and throat*

1. vasectomy _____

2. orchidopexy _____

3. pyelostomy _____

4. lithotripsy _____

5. spermicide _____

6. antispasmodic _____

GENERATION

EXERCISE 6 Build a medical term from the information provided.

EXAMPLE: inflammation of the sinuses *sinusitis*

1. incision into a testicle (use *orchid/o*) _____

2. surgical removal of the prostate _____

3. surgical reconstruction of a ureter _____

4. surgical reconstruction of the penis _____

EXERCISE 7 Multiple-choice questions. Select the correct answer(s).

1. The surgical removal of a kidney through the abdomen is known as
   a. abdominonephrectomy
   b. heminephrectomy
   c. laparonephrectomy
   d. meatonephrectomy

2. A *spermicide* is
   a. an agent that assists in conception by making sperm meet with an egg for fertilzation
   b. an agent that assists the testicles in the formation of sperm
   c. an agent that creates sperm
   d. an agent that kills sperm
   e. none of these

3. Which of the following statements is true of the term *kidney dialysis?*
   a. procedure for removing waste from the blood
   b. alternative name for hemodialysis
   c. its name comes from the fact that the procedure separates or looses (*lysis*) blood from waste by passing it through (*dia*) an external filter
   d. all of these
   e. none of these

4. Select all of the following terms that pertain to the urinary tract.
   a. cystectomy   d. orchidectomy
   b. lithectomy   e. prostatectomy
   c. nephrectomy

5. Select all of the following terms that pertain to the male genitalia.
   a. cystectomy   d. orchidectomy
   b. lithectomy   e. prostatectomy
   c. nephrectomy

EXERCISE 8 Briefly describe the difference between each pair of terms.

1. ureteroplasty, orchioplasty _____

2. nephrostomy, nephrotomy _____

3. orchiectomy, orchiopexy _____

4. heminephrectomy, nephrectomy _____

5. nephrolithotomy, pyelolithotomy _____

12.7 Electronic Health Records

Discharge Summary

Patient: Susan Nesbit
Date of Admission: 7/7/2015
Date of Discharge: 7/17/2015

Admission Diagnosis
1. **Dysuria**
2. Fever

Discharge Diagnosis
1. **Pyelonephritis**
2. **Perinephric Abscess**

Discharge Condition: Stable

Consultations
Nephrology
Urology

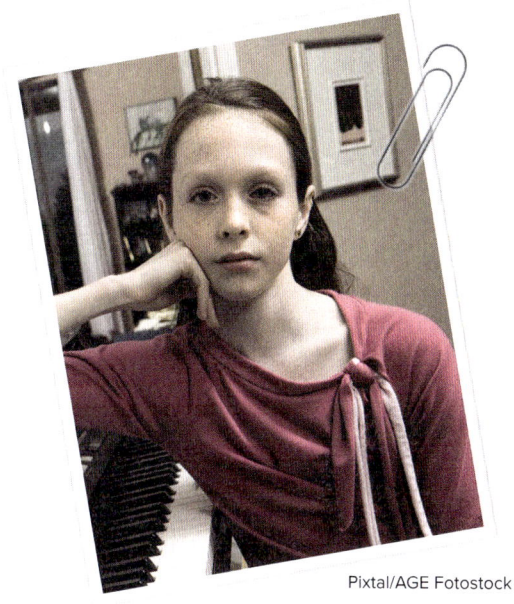
Pixtal/AGE Fotostock

Procedures
1. U/S guided percutaneous **renal** needle aspiration with drain placement.

Labs
Admission labs: UA: **Pyuria:** >20 wbcs; **Hematuria:** 3+ blood; **Albuminuria:** 1+ protein.
Urine culture: *E. coli.*
Blood culture: *E. coli.*
Discharge labs: UA normal. Urine culture normal.

Imaging
VCUG: No **vesicoureteral reflux** noted.
RUS: No **hydronephrosis** noted. Normal.
Spiral CT of kidneys on day 3 of admission revealed perinephric abscess formation of the left kidney.

HPI
Miss Susan Nesbit is a 12-year-old female who first visited her primary care provider for **dysuria.** A **UA** was ordered, but the patient could not urinate in the office. She took the UA cup home but did not return with the sample. The next day, Susan's dysuria worsened, and she developed a fever of 102.3°F, as well as vomiting and **hematuria,** so she returned to the clinic. A urinalysis performed in the office revealed significant **pyuria, hematuria,** and **albuminuria.** Since Susan was not able to keep any fluids down, her primary care provider sent her to the emergency department for evaluation for admission.

Hospital Course

On arrival to the ED, Susan was alert and oriented, but she looked a little pale and tired. She was treated with IVF for dehydration and given antipyretics for her fever. Within an hour, she had improved some, but given her inability to tolerate PO, the pediatric on-call physician recommended that she be admitted. She was admitted for a UTI and treated with IV antibiotics, and a urine culture was sent. On hospital day 2, her fever had improved, and she was looking better overall. Unfortunately, on hospital day 3, Susan's fever returned, and she looked acutely ill.

A spiral CT of Susan's abdomen and pelvis showed a developing perinephric abscess. Both nephrology and urology were consulted at that time, and they both agreed that the best treatment option would be needle aspiration with drain placement. She was taken to the OR, and the drain was placed. Fluid collection from the abscess was sent for culture.

Susan tolerated the procedure well and was admitted to the PICU. She continued IV antibiotics through her PICU course. After 5 days with the drain, the discharge had decreased significantly, so we repeated a spiral CT to confirm clearing of the abscess. The CT was normal, so the drain was removed and Susan was transferred to the regular pediatric wing. A renal ultrasound was also normal, as was a voiding cystourethrogram. Susan switched to oral antibiotics and was discharged home.

Discharge Physical Examination
VS
Temp: 98.6; RR: 24; HR: 86; BP: 100/64.
General: WDWN. Alert.
HEENT: PERRLA, TMs normal. Mucous membranes moist and pink.
CV: RRR.
RESP: CTA.
Abdomen: Soft, nondistended, no CVA tenderness. No suprapubic tenderness.
Skin: Warm, pink.

Activity: No restrictions.

Diet: No restrictions.

Meds: Antibiotics.

Follow-Up Appointments
Primary care provider: 1 week
Urology: 2 weeks
Nephrology: 1 month

—Dictated by Jennifer Wong, DO

EXERCISE 1   Match the term on the left with its definition on the right.

_____ 1. urology   a. bloody urination

_____ 2. nephrology   b. inflammation of the kidney and renal pelvis

_____ 3. dysuria   c. kidney condition caused by the obstruction of urine flow

_____ 4. hematuria   d. painful urination

_____ 5. pyuria   e. protein in the urine

_____ 6. albuminuria   f. pus in the urine

_____ 7. pyelonephritis   g. study of the kidneys

_____ 8. hydronephrosis   h. study of the urinary tract

EXERCISE 2   Fill in the blanks.

1. Admission diagnosis

   a. *Dysuria* (give definition: _____)

2. Discharge diagnosis

   a. *Pyelonephritis* (give definition: _____)

3. Consultations

   a. *Nephrology* (study of the _____)

   b. *Urology* (study of the _____)

4. Labs: UA (give definition for abbreviation: _____)

   a. *pyuria* (_____ in urine)

   b. *hematuria* (_____ in urine)

   c. *albuminuria* (_____ in urine)

EXERCISE 3   True or false questions. Indicate true answers with a T and false answers with an F.

1. Susan's imaging revealed that she has vesicoureteral reflux. _____

2. On arrival to the ED, Susan was treated with intravenous fluids. _____

3. Susan could tolerate oral food and drink upon her arrival to the ED. _____

4. Susan was admitted to the hospital for a urinary tract infection. _____

5. Susan's imaging revealed a kidney condition caused by the obstruction of urine flow. _____

EXERCISE 4   Multiple-choice questions. Select the correct answer(s).

1. According to the in-clinic urinalysis, which of the following was NOT present in Susan's urine?
   a. blood
   b. protein
   c. pus
   d. sugar
   e. all of these were present in Susan's urine

2. According to the discharge diagnosis, Susan had a *perinephric abscess.* Which of the following choices is a correct breakdown of the term *perinephric?*
   a. *peri* (around) + *nephric* (bladder)
   b. *peri* (around) + *nephric* (kidney)
   c. *peri* (inside) + *nephric* (bladder)
   d. *peri* (inside) + *nephric* (kidney)
   e. *peri* (outside) + *nephric* (kidney)

3. The hospital course reports that Susan's *renal ultrasound* was normal. A *renal ultrasound* is an
   a. image of the bladder using high frequency sound waves
   b. image of the kidney using high frequency sound waves
   c. image of the renal pelvis using high frequency sound waves
   d. image of the urinary tract using high frequency sound waves
   e. none of these

Quick Reference

glossary of roots

ROOT	DEFINITION	ROOT	DEFINITION
balan/o	penis	pyel/o	renal pelvis
cyst/o	bladder	ren/o	kidney
epididym/o	epididymis	sperm/o, spermat/o	sperm
glomerul/o	glomerulus	test/o	testicle
lith/o	stone	ur/o, urin/o	urine
nephr/o	kidney	ureter/o	ureter
orch/o, orchi/o, orchid/o	testicle	urethr/o	urethra
prostat/o	prostate	vesic/o	bladder

abbreviations

ABBREVIATION	DEFINITION
BPH	benign prostate hyperplasia
BUN	blood urea nitrogen
cath	catheter
DRE	digital rectal exam
ED	erectile dysfunction
ESWL	extracorporeal shock wave lithotripsy
HD	hemodialysis
I&O	intake and output
IVP	intravenous pyelogram
KUB	kidneys, ureters, bladder
OAB	overactive bladder
PKD	polycystic kidney disease
PSA	prostate-specific antigen
RP	retrograde pyelogram
STD/STI	sexually transmitted disease, sexually transmitted infection
SUI	stress urinary incontinence
TURP	transurethral resection of the prostate
UA	urinalysis
UTI	urinary tract infection
VCUG	voiding cystourethrogram

The Female Reproductive System–Gynecology, Obstetrics, and Neonatology

13

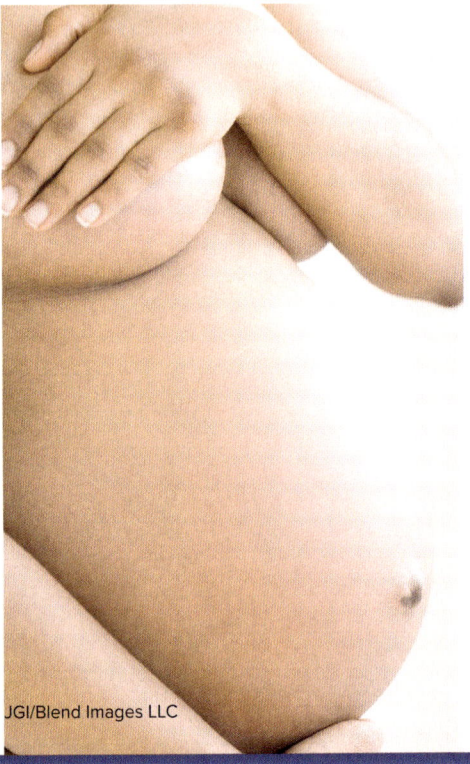

JGI/Blend Images LLC

Introduction and Overview of the Female Reproductive System

With few exceptions, everyone is born with the basic equipment to help bring new life into the world. Both sexes contain reproductive organs that produce half the code for a human life. The female reproductive system is much more active and complex. While the main function of the male reproductive system is the production and the delivery of sperm cells, the female reproductive system is responsible for much more. Females not only provide half the code for a human life, but they also provide the environment and nutrition to sustain and grow that life until birth.

Learning Outcomes

Upon completion of this chapter, you will be able to:

13.1 Identify the **roots/word parts** associated with the **female reproductive system.**

(S) **13.2** Translate the **Subjective** terms associated with the **female reproductive system.**

(O) **13.3** Translate the **Objective** terms associated with the **female reproductive system.**

(A) **13.4** Translate the **Assessment** terms associated with the **female reproductive system.**

(P) **13.5** Translate the **Plan** terms associated with the **female reproductive system.**

13.6 Distinguish terms associated with the **female reproductive system** in the context of **electronic health records.**

13.1 Word Parts of the Female Reproductive System

Gynecology, External

The outer structures of the female reproductive system are collectively known as the *vulva*. The vulva includes the clitoris, the labia majora and labia minora, the urethral meatus, and the vaginal opening.

The *clitoris* is the most sensitive part of a woman's anatomy. In this way, it is similar to the head of a man's penis. The *labia* are the folds of tissue around the opening of the vagina. The outer folds, which are larger, are the *labia majora,* and the inner folds, which are thinner, are the *labia minora.* The urethral opening is located within the labia minora superior to the vaginal opening.

While not directly connected to the rest of the reproductive parts, the *breasts* are a very important outside structure. While they are very sensitive and provide stimulation that plays a part in sexual intercourse, their main purpose is to provide a food supply for a baby.

vulva

ROOTS: *episi/o, vulv/o*

EXAMPLES: episiotomy, vulvodynia

NOTES: *Vulva* is the term for the external genital organs of a female.

perineum

ROOT: *perine/o*

EXAMPLES: perineoplasty, perineorrhaphy

NOTES: *Perineum* is the term for the region between the genital organs and the anus. No one is really sure where the term came from, but one easy way to remember what it means is to think *peri* (*around*) + *anus = region around the anus.* It's not 100 percent accurate, but it's enough to help you remember.

woman

ROOTS: *gynec/o, gyn/o*

EXAMPLES: gynecology, gynecologist

NOTES: This root comes from Greek, for *woman.* If you are afraid of women, you have *gynophobia.* Believe it or not, this root is where the English words *queen* and *goon* come from.

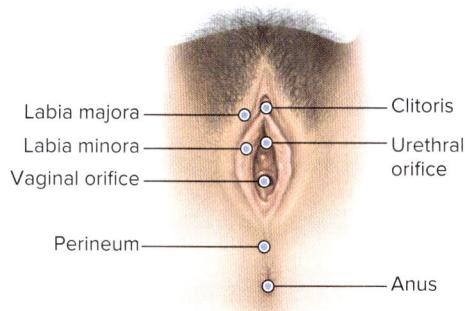

Labia majora — Clitoris
Labia minora — Urethral orifice
Vaginal orifice —
Perineum —
— Anus

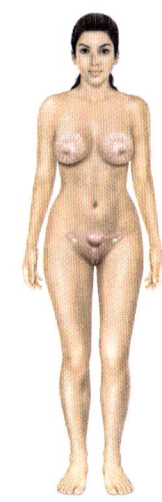

vagina

ROOTS: *colp/o, vagin/o*

EXAMPLES: colposcope, vaginitis

NOTES: The word *vagina* comes from Latin and means the *sheath* or *scabbard of a sword.*

breast

ROOTS: *mast/o, mamm/o*

EXAMPLES: mastopexy, mastectomy, mammogram

NOTES: Believe it or not, the name of the *mastodon,* a long-extinct type of elephant similar to a mammoth, actually breaks down as *mast* (*breast*) and *odon* (*tooth*). The mastodon got its name from a scientist who thought that the animal's molar teeth had nipple-like tops, which gave them the appearance of breasts.

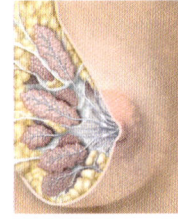

milk

ROOT: *lact/o*

EXAMPLES: lactation, lactorrhea

NOTES: The root for milk, *lacto,* is also the root for the English word *galaxy.* Have you ever looked at the

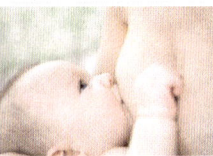

Alik Mulikov/Shutterstock

stars from a really dark spot out in the country? If so, you've seen stars that you'd never be able to see near a city. One thing you can see is the Milky Way, the thick band of stars that makes up our galaxy. It's called the Milky Way because the ancient Greeks thought the dense cloud of stars looked like milk sprayed in the night sky. A Greek myth tells how the hero Hercules, who was breast-fed by the goddess Hera, once bit down so hard that milk sprayed everywhere—creating the Milky Way.

Gynecology, Internal

A woman's inner reproductive system is shaped like a capital "T." On either end of the horizontal part of the "T" rest the ovaries. The *ovaries* hold all of the woman's eggs (*ova*). Roughly every 28 to 30 days during a woman's reproductive years, an ovary will allow an egg to mature and then releases it (*ovulation*). The ova travel along tubes (*fallopian tubes*) to the uterus.

The *uterus* is a pear-shaped organ in the vertical part of the "T," along with the vagina. The uterus is the incubator for growing and developing new life. Every month, the walls of the uterus grow and become rich in blood supply. If the woman's egg is fertilized by a sperm, it travels to the uterus and implants itself in the walls. If a new life is not implanted in the walls of the uterus, the tissues are shed and the process starts all over again. This cycle of building and shedding nutritive tissues in the uterus is known as the *menstrual cycle.* It is driven by the female hormones *estrogen* and *progesterone.* Both of these hormones are made in the ovaries.

At the end of the uterus is a connection to the vagina known as the *cervix.* It is smaller and thicker than the rest of the uterus. Farther down the vertical part of the "T" is the vagina, the reproductive system's main point of contact with the outside world. It is the part of a woman's body that is involved in sexual intercourse. Additionally, the opening of the urethra, which drains the bladder, is found in the anterior wall of the vagina.

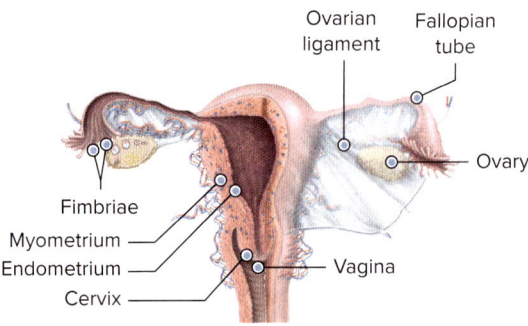

cervix

ROOT: *cervic/o*

EXAMPLES: cervicodynia, cervicitis

NOTES: *Cervix* means *neck* and refers not to the neck connecting your head to your body but to the opening between the uterus and the vagina.

REMEMBER: The letter c changes sounds depending on what vowel follows it. Before e or i, the letter c makes an s sound (cervicitis—**SE**R-vih-**SAI**-tis). Before a, o, or u, the letter c makes a k sound (cervicodynia—**SE**R-vih-**ko**h-DAI-nee-ah).

uterus

ROOTS: *hyster/o, metr/o, uter/o*

EXAMPLES: hysterectomy, endometrium, uterus

NOTES: Break down the word *hysteria* as a medical term. It means a *uterus condition,* right (*hyster* + *ia*)? Believe it or not, that is exactly where the term came from. It was used to refer to a medical condition (usually neurological) occurring in women and caused by a malfunctioning uterus. Think about that the next time you refer to a friend or a movie as "hysterical."

pelvis

ROOT: *pelv/i*

EXAMPLES: pelvimetry, pelvic sonography

NOTES: *Pelvis* comes from a Latin word meaning *basin* or *washtub* and refers to the shape of

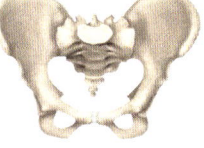

the bones that make up the pelvis. Another root, *pyelo,* also means *pelvis,* but this root is used exclusively for the portion of the kidney called the *renal pelvis.*

ovary

ROOTS: *oophor/o, ovari/o*

EXAMPLES: oophorectomy, ovariocentesis

NOTES: *Oophoro* can be broken down into two words: *oo,* meaning *egg,* and *phor,* meaning *to carry.* Thus, *oophor* literally means *the thing that carries the eggs.*

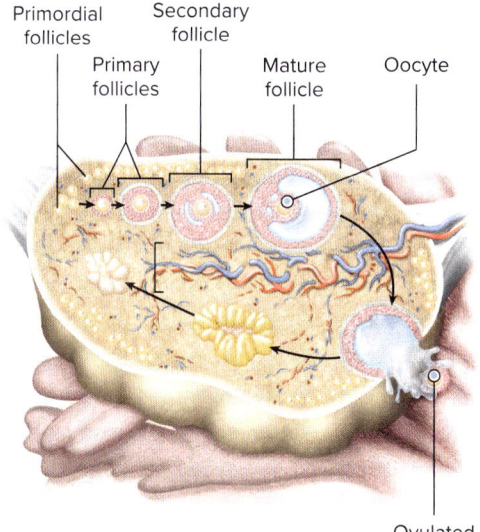

Primordial follicles
Secondary follicle
Primary follicles
Mature follicle
Oocyte
Ovulated oocyte

menstruation

ROOT: *men/o*

EXAMPLES: menorrhea, menopause

NOTES: *Meno* comes from Greek, for *month,* and refers to the standard 28-day recurrence of menstrual cycles. It is no wonder that in ancient Greece, Artemis was both the goddess who watched over young girls entering womanhood and the goddess associated with the moon, which goes through its phases every 28 days.

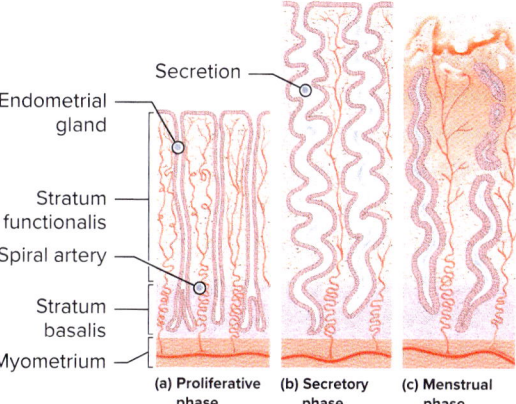

Secretion
Endometrial gland
Stratum functionalis
Spiral artery
Stratum basalis
Myometrium

(a) Proliferative phase (b) Secretory phase (c) Menstrual phase

fallopian tube

ROOT: *salping/o*

EXAMPLES: salpingectomy, salpingoscope

NOTES: *Salpingo* comes from the Latin word for *trumpet.* Four sites in the body use this term due to their resemblance to a long, straight Roman trumpet: the ear canals and the fallopian tubes, which connect the ovaries to the uterus. The fallopian tubes are named for Gabriello Fallopio, an Italian specialist in anatomy who first described them in the 1500s.

REMEMBER: The letter *g* changes sounds depending on what vowel follows it. Before *e* or *i,* the letter *g* makes a *j* sound (salpin**gi**tis—SAL-pin-**JAI**-tis). Before *a, o,* or *u,* the letter *g* makes a *g* sound (salpin**go**scope—sal-PING-**goh**-SKOHP).

Obstetrics

Pregnancy is the amazing process of a human life growing inside a woman. During pregnancy, a baby is called a *fetus.* The fetus grows and develops in the mother's *uterus.* The fetus is connected to the uterus via the *placenta.* The placenta is an important source for feeding the fetus. There, nutrients provided by the mother's blood vessels cross into the blood vessels of the fetus.

The fetus is attached to the placenta through the *umbilical cord,* which is cut at birth. This is where the belly button comes from. The fetus is surrounded by a fluid-filled sac (*amnion* or *amniotic sac*) that helps act as a shock absorber to protect it. Outside the amnion is another membrane, the *chorion,* which helps anchor the baby to the walls of the uterus and provides nutrition.

When the fetus is ready for birth, the woman's body goes through the painful process known as *labor.* During labor, the woman's *cervix* widens and the muscles of the uterus squeeze to push the baby out.

---

amnion

ROOT: **amni/o**

EXAMPLE: amniocentesis

NOTES: The *amnion* is the innermost membrane covering the fetus.

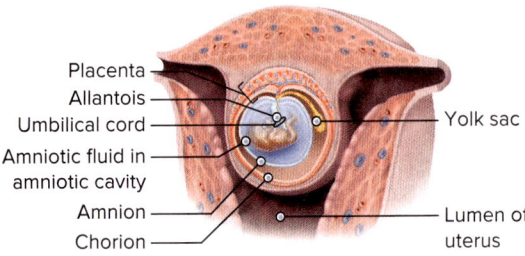

Placenta
Allantois
Umbilical cord
Amniotic fluid in amniotic cavity
Amnion
Chorion
Yolk sac
Lumen of uterus

---

chorion

ROOTS: **chori/o, chorion/o**

EXAMPLE: choriocarcinoma, chorionitis

NOTES: The *chorion* is the outer membrane covering the fetus. It connects the fetus to the wall of the uterus.

---

pregnancy

SUFFIX: **-cyesis**

EXAMPLE: pseudocyesis

NOTES: Although women experience pregnancy firsthand, there is a documented medical condition called Couvade syndrome, or sympathetic pregnancy, in which a man experiences some of the symptoms of pregnancy, including weight gain, morning sickness, and, in some cases, labor "pains."

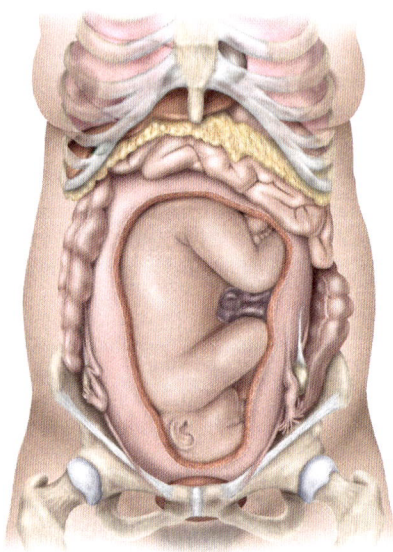

---

labor

ROOT: **toc/o**

EXAMPLES: dystocia, tocograph

NOTES: In the United States, there are more boy babies born than girl babies. For the past 60 years, the ratio has been about the same: 105 male births for every 100 female births. Also, according to some statistics, Tuesday is the most popular day to give birth. One more fun fact: Jimmy Carter was the first U.S. president to be born in a hospital.

(a) Early dilation stage

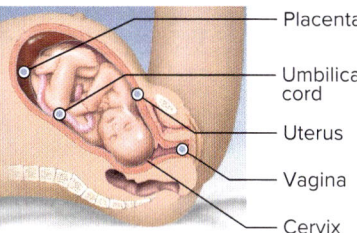

— Placenta
— Umbilical cord
— Uterus
— Vagina
— Cervix

(b) Late dilation stage

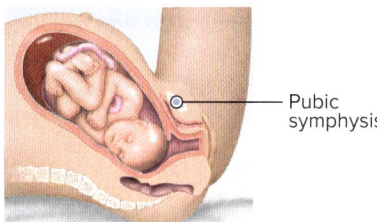

— Pubic symphysis

(c) Expulsion stage

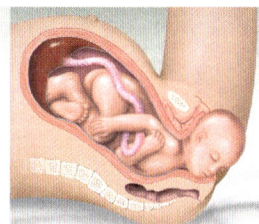

(d) Placental stage

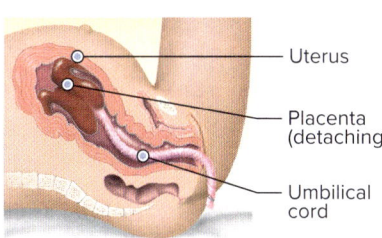

— Uterus
— Placenta (detaching)
— Umbilical cord

fetus

ROOT: *fet/o*
EXAMPLE: fetometry
NOTES: *Fetus* is a Latin word that means *offspring*. The Greek word is *embryo*. In current medical usage, a fetus is an unborn child after the eighth week of pregnancy. Before that time, it is referred to as an embryo. Before the fertilization of an egg, the sperm and egg are called *gametes* (Greek for *husband* and *wife*). Once they join, a separate, distinct, and genetically unique creature is created that is called a *zygote* (Greek for *joined together*). Once the zygote becomes implanted in the wall of the uterus, it is called an embryo.

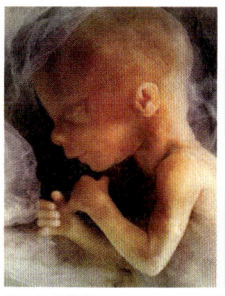

Steve Allen/Getty Images

birth

ROOTS: *part/o, nat/o*
EXAMPLES: postpartum, neonatal
NOTES: Both roots mean *birth,* but their focus is different. *Parto* means more accurately *to give birth* and therefore focuses on the mother. *Nato* means more literally *to be born* and therefore focuses on the baby. Hence, a mother gets *postpartum depression* and a baby is cared for by a *neonatologist.*

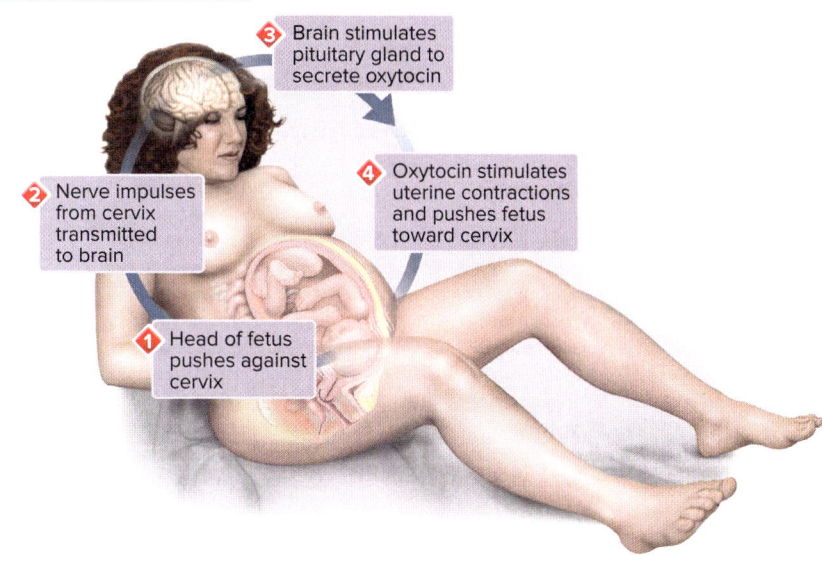

3 Brain stimulates pituitary gland to secrete oxytocin

2 Nerve impulses from cervix transmitted to brain

4 Oxytocin stimulates uterine contractions and pushes fetus toward cervix

1 Head of fetus pushes against cervix

TRANSLATION

EXERCISE 1   Match the root on the left with its definition on the right. Some definitions will be used more than once.

_____ 1. vagin/o
_____ 2. vulv/o
_____ 3. mamm/o
_____ 4. lact/o

a. breast
b. external genital organs of a female
c. milk
d. region between the genital organs and the anus

_____ 5. gynec/o
_____ 6. perine/o
_____ 7. gyn/o
_____ 8. colp/o
_____ 9. episi/o
_____ 10. mast/o

e. vagina
f. woman

EXERCISE 2   Translate the following roots.

1. vagin/o _____
2. vulv/o _____
3. gynec/o _____
4. lact/o _____
5. perine/o _____
6. mamm/o _____
7. gyn/o _____
8. episi/o _____
9. mast/o _____
10. colp/o _____

EXERCISE 3   Underline and define the roots from this chapter in the following terms.

1. vulvitis _____
2. lactation _____
3. perineocele _____
4. colpocystitis _____
5. mammoplasty _____
6. mastoptosis _____

7. episiorrhaphy _____
8. vaginomycosis _____
9. gynecomastia (2 roots) _____
10. vaginoperineorrhaphy (2 roots) _____

EXERCISE 4   Break down the following words into their component parts and translate.

EXAMPLE: sinusitis   _sinus | itis_
inflammation of the sinuses

1. vaginitis _____
2. vulvitis _____
3. mastitis _____
4. colpitis _____
5. gynecologist _____
6. mammogram _____
7. lactogenic _____
8. perineorrhaphy _____
9. episiostenosis _____
10. vulvovaginitis _____

EXERCISE 5   Match the root on the left with its definition on the right. Some definitions will be used more than once.

_____ 1. uter/o
_____ 2. ovari/o
_____ 3. cervic/o

a. fallopian tube
b. menstruation
c. opening between the uterus and the vagina

_____ 4. pelv/i
_____ 5. men/o
_____ 6. hyster/o
_____ 7. metr/o
_____ 8. oophor/o
_____ 9. salping/o

d. ovary
e. pelvis
f. uterus

EXERCISE 6 Translate the following roots.

1. ovari/o _____

2. cervic/o _____

3. pelv/i _____

4. uter/o _____

5. men/o _____

6. hyster/o _____

7. salping/o _____

8. oophor/o _____

9. metr/o _____

9. cephalopelvic disproportion _____

10. metromenorrhagia (2 roots) _____

11. metrocolpocele (2 roots) _____

12. salpingo-oophorectomy (2 roots) _____

_____

13. hysterosalpingectomy (2 roots) _____

_____

EXERCISE 7 Underline and define the roots from this chapter in the following terms.

1. ovariocentesis _____

2. uterine prolapse _____

3. cervical dysplasia _____

4. menorrhagia _____

5. salpingectomy _____

6. endometritis _____

7. hysteroptosis _____

8. oophorocystectomy _____

EXERCISE 8 Break down the following words into their component parts and translate.

EXAMPLE: sinusitis *sinus | itis*
inflammation of the sinuses

1. ovaritis _____

2. cervicography _____

3. hysterography _____

4. oophoroma _____

5. perimetritis _____

6. dysmenorrhea _____

7. hysterosalpingogram _____

8. hysterodynia _____

EXERCISE 9 Match the word part on the left with its definition on the right. Some definitions will be used more than once.

_____ 1. fet/o

_____ 2. nat/o

_____ 3. amni/o

_____ 4. part/o

_____ 5. chorion/o

_____ 6. chori/o

_____ 7. -cyesis

_____ 8. toc/o

a. *to be born;* focus on the baby

b. *to give birth;* focus on the mother

c. innermost membrane covering the fetus

d. labor

e. outer membrane covering the fetus; connects the fetus to the wall of the uterus

f. pregnancy

g. unborn child after the eighth week of pregnancy

EXERCISE 10 Translate the following word parts.

1. amni/o _____

2. chori/o, chorion/o _____

3. fet/o _____

4. nat/o _____

5. part/o _____

6. toc/o _____

7. -cyesis _____

EXERCISE 11 Underline and define the word parts from this chapter in the following terms.

1. fetometry _____

2. amniorrhexis _____

3. choriocarcinoma _____

4. pseudocyesis _____

5. perinatologist _____

6. intrapartum _____

EXERCISE 12 Break down the following words into their component parts and translate.

EXAMPLE: sinusitis   *sinus | itis*
inflammation of the sinuses

1. amnioscopy _____

2. chorioamnionitis _____

3. ovariocyesis _____

4. fetometry _____

5. neonatal _____

6. antepartum _____

7. tocography _____

GENERATION

EXERCISE 13 Identify the roots for the following definitions.

1. perineum _____

2. milk _____

3. woman (2 roots) _____

4. breast (2 roots) _____

5. vagina (2 roots) _____

6. vulva (2 roots) _____

EXERCISE 14 Build a medical term from the information provided.

EXAMPLE: inflammation of the sinuses
sinusitis

1. pain in the vulva (use *vulv/o*) _____

2. surgical removal of a breast (use *mast/o*) _____

3. incision into the vulva (use *episi/o*) _____
_____

4. the discharge of milk (use *-rrhea*) _____
_____

5. surgical reconstruction of a breast (use *mamm/o*) _____

6. surgical reconstruction of the vagina (use *vagin/o*) _____

7. surgical reconstruction of the vagina (use *colp/o*) _____

8. surgical reconstruction of the perineum _____

9. the study of medical issues specific to women _____

10. surgical reconstruction of the vagina and perineum (use *vagin/o*) _____

EXERCISE 15 Identify the roots for the following definitions.

1. cervix _____

2. pelvis _____

3. menstruation _____

4. fallopian tube _____

5. ovary (2 roots) _____

6. uterus (3 roots) _____

EXERCISE 17 Identify the word parts for the following definitions.

1. fetus _____

2. amnion _____

3. pregnancy _____

4. labor _____

5. chorion (2 roots) _____

6. birth (2 roots) _____

EXERCISE 16 Build a medical term from the information provided.

1. instrument for examining the uterus (use *hyster/o*) _____

2. inflammation of an ovary (use *oophor/o*) _____

3. pain in the ovary (use *ovari/o*) _____
   _____

4. inflammation of the cervix _____
   _____

5. procedure for measuring the pelvis _____
   _____

6. inflammation of the fallopian tube _____
   _____

7. inflammation of the fallopian tube and ovary (use *oophor/o*) _____

EXERCISE 18 Build a medical term from the information provided.

1. pertaining to after the birth (use *nat/o*) _____
   _____

2. pertaining to after the birth (use *part/o*) _____
   _____

3. inflammation of the chorion _____
   _____

4. instrument for examining the amnion _____
   _____

5. instrument for recording the strength of labor (contractions) _____
   _____

6. pregnancy in a fallopian tube _____
   _____

ⓈUBJECTIVE

13.2 Patient History, Problems, Complaints

Pain is always a common symptom in medicine, and the female reproductive system is no exception. The nerve fibers of the interior reproductive system share nerves with the lower gastrointestinal tract, so pain originating from this area can be hard to distinguish from gastrointestinal pain.

Pain in the vulva (*vulvodynia*) is often a condition without a known cause. Pain in the vagina (*vaginodynia*) is a common complication of infections, including fungal infections. More commonly, women will present to a medical office with pain that recurs at specific times, such as during menses (*dysmenorrhea*)

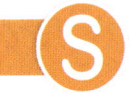

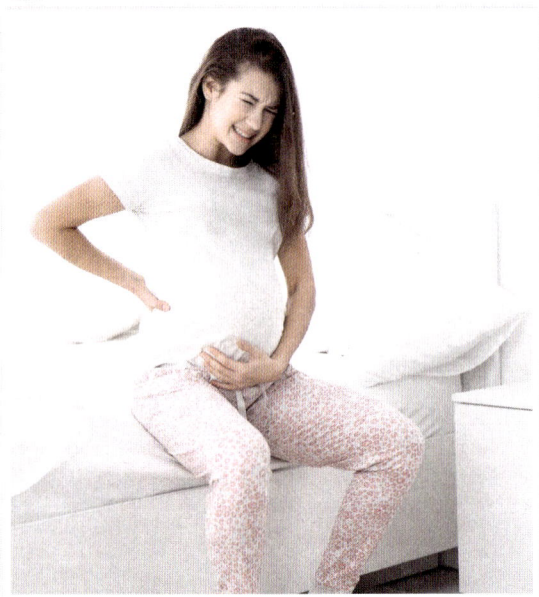

Contractions are a specific type of pain felt during pregnancy.

Africa Studio/Shutterstock

gynecology

TERM	WORD ANALYSIS
amenorrhea AY-men-oh-REE-ah	a / meno / rrhea no / menstruation / discharge
DEFINITION no menstruation	
dysmenorrhea DIS-men-oh-REE-ah	dys / meno / rrhea bad / menstruation / discharge
DEFINITION painful menstruation	
hysteralgia HIS-ter-AL-jah	hyster / algia uterus / pain
DEFINITION pain in the uterus	
hysterodynia HIS-ter-oh-DAI-nee-ah	hystero / dynia uterus / pain
DEFINITION pain in the uterus	
mastalgia mas-TAL-jah	mast / algia breast / pain
DEFINITION breast pain	
mastoptosis MAS-top-TOH-sis	masto / ptosis breast / drooping condition
DEFINITION downward displacement (drooping) of the breast	
menorrhagia MEN-oh-RAY-jah	meno / rrhagia menstruation / excessive discharge
DEFINITION excessive menstrual flow	
menorrhalgia MEN-oh-RAL-jah	meno / rrh / algia uterus / discharge / pain
DEFINITION painful menstruation	

NOTE: The difference between the last two words is only one letter—but that one letter makes a big difference.

or sexual intercourse (*dyspareunia*). Many times, women have both symptoms. These can be complications of *endometriosis* or *pelvic inflammatory disorder.*

Both females and males can present with pain in the breast (*mastalgia*). Women often suffer from this condition during breast-feeding. In males, this usually happens during puberty, when they may develop a small amount of breast tissue (*gynecomastia*).

Women often come to health care providers with problems with menses. Their menses can be too frequent (*metrorrhagia*), too heavy (*menorrhagia*), or both (*metromenorrhagia*). Patients also may experience skipped periods (*oligomenorrhea*) or none at all (*amenorrhea*).

Women may also present with complaints of *abnormal discharge.* The discharge's odor and color can be good indicators of its cause. Sexually transmitted infections, such as *gonorrhea,* are a common cause of abnormal discharge.

During pregnancy, a woman's "water" breaking is also a discharge (*amniorrhea*). It is a good indicator that delivery is near.

gynecology *continued*

TERM	WORD ANALYSIS	
metrorrhagia MEH-troh-RAY-jah	metro uterus	/ rrhagia / excessive discharge
DEFINITION menstrual bleeding at irregular times		
oligomenorrhea AW-lih-goh-MEN-oh-REE-ah	oligo / meno few / menstruation	/ rrhea / discharge
DEFINITION infrequent or light menstrual periods		
ovaralgia OH-var-AL-jah	ovar ovary	/ algia / pain
DEFINITION pain of the ovaries		
ovarialgia oh-VAR-ee-AL-jah	ovari ovary	/ algia / pain
DEFINITION pain of the ovaries NOTE: Both *ovaralgia* and *ovarialgia* are acceptable spellings and mean the same thing.		
vaginodynia VAJ-ih-noh-DAI-nee-ah	vagino vagina	/ dynia / pain
DEFINITION vaginal pain		
vulvodynia VUL-voh-DAI-nee-ah	vulvo vulva	/ dynia / pain
DEFINITION pain in the vulva		

obstetrics

TERM	WORD ANALYSIS
amniorrhea AM-nee-oh-REE-ah	amnio / rrhea amnion / discharge
DEFINITION discharge of amniotic fluid	
amniorrhexis AM-nee-oh-REK-sis	amnio / rrhexis amnion / rupture
DEFINITION rupture of the amniotic sac	
Braxton Hicks contraction BRAKS-ton HIKS con-TRAK-shun	named after John Braxton Hicks, the doctor who first noted them, in 1872
DEFINITION sporadic contractions of the uterine muscles of women not in labor; also known as false labor	
contraction con-TRAK-shun	from Latin, for *to draw together* or *shorten*
DEFINITION shortening or tightening of a muscle; during labor, the uterine muscles contract	

PRONUNCIATION

EXERCISE 1   Indicate which syllable(s) is emphasized when pronounced.

> EXAMPLE: bronchitis bron**chi**tis

1. mastalgia _____

2. contraction _____

3. menorrhagia (2) _____

4. ovaralgia (2) _____

5. amenorrhea (2) _____

TRANSLATION

EXERCISE 2 Break down the following words into their component parts.

> EXAMPLE: nasopharyngoscope
> *naso | pharyngo | scope*

1. ovaralgia _____
2. hysterodynia _____
3. menorrhagia _____
4. menorrhalgia _____
5. amniorrhexis _____
6. mastoptosis _____
7. amenorrhea _____

EXERCISE 3 Underline and define the word parts from this chapter in the following terms.

1. ovarialgia _____
2. vaginodynia _____
3. vulvodynia _____
4. amniorrhea _____
5. hysteralgia _____
6. mastalgia _____
7. metrorrhagia _____
8. dysmenorrhea _____
9. oligomenorrhea _____

EXERCISE 4 Match the term on the left with its definition on the right.

_____ 1. contraction

_____ 2. Braxton Hicks contraction

_____ 3. amenorrhea

_____ 4. amniorrhea

_____ 5. dysmenorrhea

_____ 6. oligomenorrhea

a. discharge of amniotic fluid

b. infrequent or light menstrual periods

c. no menstruation

d. painful menstruation

e. sporadic contraction of the uterine muscles of women not in labor; also known as false labor

f. shortening or tightening of a muscle

EXERCISE 5 Translate the following terms as literally as possible.

> EXAMPLE: nasopharyngoscope *an instrument for looking at the nose and throat*

1. vaginodynia _____
2. vulvodynia _____
3. hysterodynia _____
4. ovaralgia _____
5. hysteralgia _____
6. mastalgia _____
7. amniorrhexis _____
8. metrorrhagia _____
9. oligomenorrhea _____

GENERATION

EXERCISE 6 Build a medical term from the information provided.

> EXAMPLE: inflammation of the sinuses *sinusitis*

1. discharge of amniotic fluid _____

2. no menstruation _____

3. excessive menstrual flow _____

4. painful menstruation _____

5. downward displacement (drooping) of the breast _____

EXERCISE 7 Multiple-choice questions. Select the correct answer.

1. Sporadic contractions of the uterine muscles of women not in labor are known as
   a. Braxton Hicks contractions
   b. dyspareunia
   c. pseudocyesis
   d. hysterodynia

2. Which of the following statements about the term *contraction* is FALSE?
   a. from Greek, for *to ball up*
   b. from Latin, for *to draw together* or *shorten*
   c. means the shortening or tightening of a muscle
   d. occurs during labor

3. Which of the following words is the correct medical term for *pain in the ovaries?*
   a. oopharalgia
   b. oophorodynia
   c. ovarialgia
   d. ovariodynia

OBJECTIVE

13.3 Observation and Discovery

A physical exam of the female reproductive system includes a breast exam, an external genital exam, and a pelvic exam. When examining a patient's breast, the examiner must pay close attention to color changes, skin texture, any lumps in the breast, and the nipple. In an external genital exam, examiners must take into consideration the patient's developmental stage (if she is a child) and the general appearance of the vulvar area.

The most important part of a female reproductive (*gynecologic*) exam is the pelvic exam. This involves placing an instrument called a *speculum* in the opening of the vagina. This instrument spreads open the walls of the vagina to make it easier to visualize the cervix.

An exam of the cervix (*colposcopy*) is a routine exam for all adult females. A critical part of this exam is the Pap smear, which involves removing a sample of tissue from the cervix and examining it with a microscope to screen for cancer.

Feeling the uterus and ovaries requires a *bimanual* exam, which involves placing fingers from one hand inside the vagina and one hand on the abdomen and feeling the structures between both hands. This type of exam aids in detecting any lumps or painful areas.

Finally, the examiner may need to perform a *rectovaginal* exam to best feel the walls of the vagina. The exam involves placing one or two fingers in the patient's rectum and another in her vagina to search for any abnormalities.

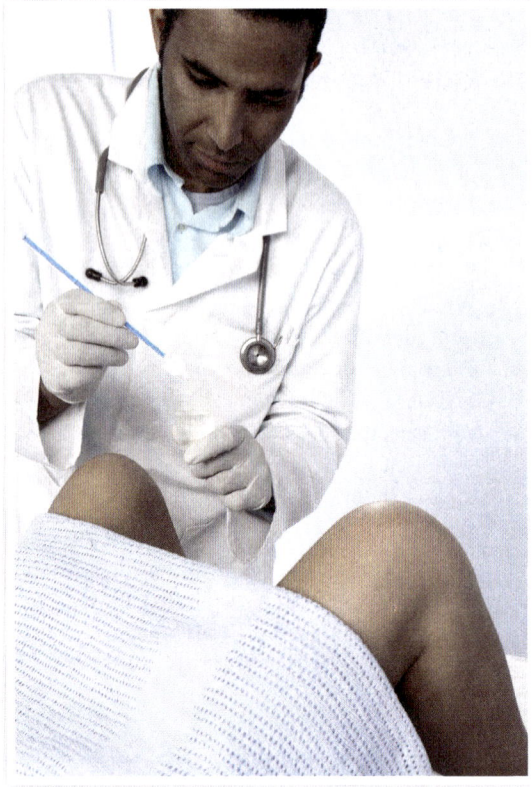

Pelvic exams and mammograms provide vital information for diagnosing gynecological issues.

Adam Gault/SPL/Getty Images

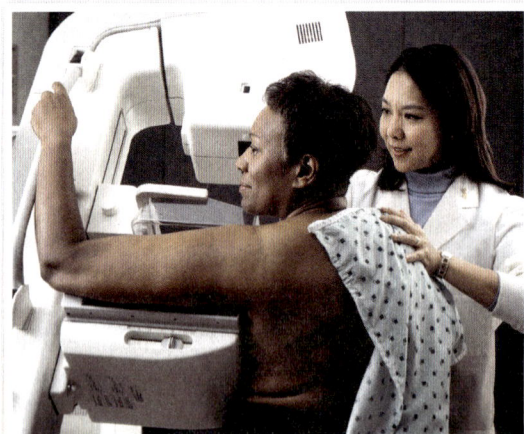

Source: Rhoda Baer/National Cancer Institute (NCI)

Two common types of imaging studies are used to analyze a woman's reproductive system. One is the *mammogram,* a special x-ray that looks for cancer in the breast. The other common image type is an *ultrasound.* An ultrasound placed inside the vagina (*transvaginal ultrasound*) is a common way of looking at the ovaries, uterus, and cervix. During pregnancy, ultrasound is commonly used to screen the health of the uterus and baby (*prenatal ultrasound*). Many times, a more direct visual inspection of a patient's reproductive tract can help a physician determine the nature of a patient's problem. For a more in-depth view of the vulva, vagina, and cervix, the physician may need to use a special magnifying instrument *(colposcope).* This procedure is known as *colposcopy.* Similarly, he or she may use a special device to visualize the inside of the uterus *(hysteroscopy).*

Women frequently see health care providers for *prenatal care* throughout a pregnancy. Just prior to delivery (*antepartum*), it is important to determine how the baby is positioned inside the mother (*presentation*). By the time the baby is ready for delivery, its head should be facing downward (*cephalic*), but at times, a baby's bottom or legs will be near the birth canal (*breech*). Because it is harder to deliver a baby in breech presentation, most obstetricians will choose to deliver the baby surgically (*cesarean section*).

During the antepartum visits, a health care worker will also need to determine the baby's size (*fetometry*), whether or not any birth defects (*congenital anomalies*) are present, and the womb's fluid (*amniotic fluid*) level. A large (*macrocephaly*) or small (*microcephaly*) head could indicate a problem with the brain. Too little amniotic fluid (*oligohydramnios*) generally indicates kidney problems in the baby. Too much fluid (*polyhydramnios*) can have numerous causes, including diabetes in the mother or gastrointestinal or urinary problems in the baby.

During delivery, the goal is a normal, uncomplicated delivery (*eutocia*). However, the delivery can be unusually painful (*dystocia*), perhaps if the baby's head is larger than the delivery canal (*cephalopelvic disproportion*). This condition is another common reason for a cesarean section delivery.

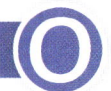

After delivery (*postpartum*), the mother will have follow-up exams to ensure that she is recovering well and to determine whether she has begun producing breast milk (*lactorrhea*). This usually happens by three to four days after delivery.

The laboratory data collected when diagnosing female reproductive problems include results from a test called the *Pap smear,* which screens for cancer. It is among the most common labs specific to females. Another common lab is the wet mount. A *wet mount* involves collecting some vaginal discharge and putting it on a slide to examine with a microscope and look for signs of infection.

Pregnant patients often need lab tests to evaluate the fluid that surrounds the baby (*amniocentesis*). The test's results can reveal information on the baby's lung maturity, the presence of certain birth defects involving the spinal cord, and certain genetic conditions.

gynecology

TERM	WORD ANALYSIS
colpoptosis KOL-pawp-TOH-sis	colpo / ptosis vagina / drooping condition
DEFINITION downward displacement of the vagina	
hypermastia HAI-per-MAS-tee-ah	hyper / mast / ia over / breast / condition
DEFINITION excessively large breasts NOTE: This term can also refer to an abnormal number of breasts.	

gynecology *continued*

TERM	WORD ANALYSIS
hypomastia HAI-poh-MAS-tee-ah	hypo / mast / ia under / breast / condition
DEFINITION abnormally small breasts	
hysteroptosis HIS-ter-awp-TOH-sis	hystero / ptosis uterus / drooping condition
DEFINITION downward displacement of the uterus into the vagina	

gynecology—diagnostic procedures

TERM	WORD ANALYSIS
colposcopy kol-PAW-skoh-pee	colpo / scopy vagina / looking procedure
DEFINITION procedure for examining the vagina	
hysterosalping-ogram HIS-ter-oh-sal-PING-oh-gram	hystero / salpingo / gram uterus / fallopian tube / record
DEFINITION record of the uterus and fallopian tubes	
hysteroscope HIS-ter-oh-SKOHP	hystero / scope uterus / instrument to look
DEFINITION instrument for examining the uterus	
hysteroscopy HIS-ter-AW-skoh-pee	hystero / scopy uterus / looking procedure
DEFINITION procedure for examining the uterus	

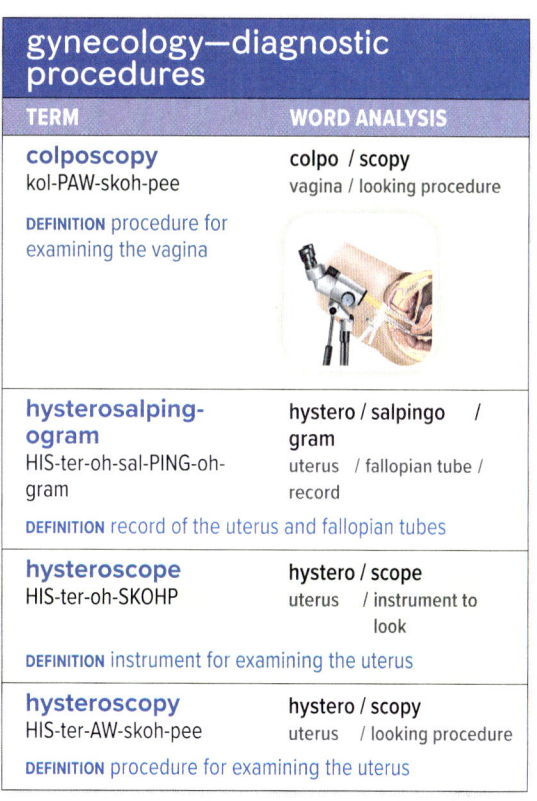

gynecology—diagnostic procedures *continued*

TERM	WORD ANALYSIS
mammogram MAM-oh-GRAM	mammo / gram breast / record
DEFINITION record of a breast exam	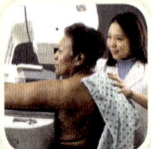 Source: Rhoda Baer/ National Cancer Institute (NCI)
Pap smear PAP SMEER	named after the inventor of the procedure, Dr. Georgios Papanicolaou
DEFINITION test used to detect cancer cells, most commonly in the cervix	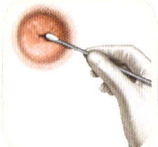
transvaginal sonography TRANZ-VAJ-ih-nal soh-NAW-grah-fee	trans / vagin / al through / vagina / pertaining to sono / graphy sound / writing procedure
DEFINITION imaging procedure using sound waves emitted from a device inserted in the vagina	

gynecology—professional terms

TERM	WORD ANALYSIS
endometrium EN-doh-MEE-tree-um	endo / metr / ium inside / uterus / tissue
DEFINITION inner layer of uterine tissue	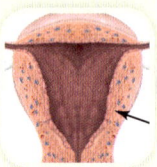
gynecologist GAI-neh-KAW-loh-jist	gyneco / logist woman / specialist
DEFINITION specialist in medical issues specific to women	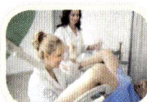 M_a_y_a/Getty Images
gynecology GAI-neh-KAW-loh-jee	gyneco / logy woman / study
DEFINITION study of medical issues specific to women	
myometrium MAI-oh-MEE-tree-um	myo / metr / ium muscle / uterus / tissue
DEFINITION middle layer of uterine muscle tissue	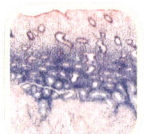 Alvin Telser/McGraw-Hill Education

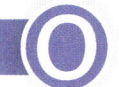

obstetrics

TERM	WORD ANALYSIS
bradytocia BRAY-dih-TOH-shee-ah	brady / toc / ia slow / birth / condition
DEFINITION slow labor	
dystocia dis-TOH-shee-ah	dys / toc / ia bad / birth / condition
DEFINITION difficult labor	
gravida GRAH-vid-ah	gravida heavy
DEFINITION another term for pregnant NOTE: This word, which is also where the word *gravity* comes from, means heavy and is similar to an old expression about pregnancy that a woman is "great with child."	
hysterocele HIS-ter-oh-SEEL	hystero / cele uterus / hernia
DEFINITION hernia of the uterus	
hysterorrhexis HIS-ter-oh-REK-sis	hystero / rrhexis uterus / rupture
DEFINITION rupture of the uterus	

obstetrics—diagnostic procedures

TERM	WORD ANALYSIS
amniocentesis AM-nee-oh-sin-TEE-sis	amnio / centesis amnion / puncture
DEFINITION surgical puncture of the amnion	

obstetrics—diagnostic procedures *continued*

TERM	WORD ANALYSIS
cardiotocograph KAR-dee-oh-TOH-koh-GRAF	cardio / toco / graph heart / birth / instrument to record
DEFINITION instrument for recording the baby's heart rate during contractions; also known as a fetal heart monitor	
fetometry fee-TAW-meh-tree	feto / metry fetus / measuring procedure
DEFINITION procedure for measuring the fetus	
pelvicephalometry PEL-vih-SEF-eh-LAW-meh-tree	pelvi / cephalo / metry pelvis / head / measuring procedure
DEFINITION procedure for measuring the head size of the baby and the pelvis size of the mother	
tocodynagraph TOH-koh-DAI-nah-GRAF	toco / dyna / graph birth / power / instrument to record
DEFINITION instrument for recording the strength of labor contractions	

obstetrics—professional terms

TERM	WORD ANALYSIS
antepartum AN-tee-PAR-tum	ante / partum before / birth
DEFINITION time before birth	
natal NAY-tal	nat / al birth / pertaining to
DEFINITION pertaining to birth	

obstetrics—professional terms *continued*

TERM	WORD ANALYSIS
neonatal NEE-oh-NAY-tal	neo / nat / al new / birth / pertaining to
DEFINITION pertaining to new birth; normally the first 28 days after birth	
neonatologist NEE-oh-nay-TAW-loh-jist	neo / nato / logist new / birth / specialist
DEFINITION specialist in the neonatal period	
neonatology NEE-oh-nay-TAW-loh-jee	neo / nato / logy new / birth / study
DEFINITION study of the neonatal period	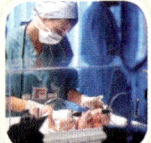 Flying Colours Ltd/Getty Images
obstetrician OB-steh-TRIH-shun	from Latin, for *midwife* or literally *one who stands beside*
DEFINITION specialist in pregnancy, labor, and delivery of newborns	

obstetrics—professional terms *continued*

TERM	WORD ANALYSIS
obstetrics ob-STEH-triks	from Latin, for *midwife* or literally *one who stands beside*
DEFINITION branch of medicine dealing with pregnancy, labor, and delivery of newborns	
postnatal post-NAY-tal	post / nat / al after / birth / pertaining to
DEFINITION pertaining to after birth	
postpartum POST-PAR-tum	post / partum after / birth
DEFINITION pertaining to after birth NOTE: The difference between this word and *postnatal* is the focus. Normally, *nato* words focus on the baby and *partum* words focus on the mother.	
prenatal pree-NAY-tal	pre / nat / al before / birth / pertaining to
DEFINITION pertaining to before birth	

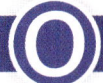

Learning Outcome 13.3 Exercises

TRANSLATION

EXERCISE 1 Break down the following words into their component parts.

> EXAMPLE: **nasopharyngoscope**
> *naso | pharyngo | scope*

1. hysterocele _____
2. gynecology _____
3. neonatal _____
4. postnatal _____
5. dystocia _____
6. amniocentesis _____
7. neonatology _____
8. colpoptosis _____
9. hysteroptosis _____
10. tocodynagraph _____

EXERCISE 2 Underline and define the word parts from this chapter in the following terms.

1. natal _____
2. gynecologist _____

3. mammogram _____

4. prenatal _____

5. postpartum _____

6. cardiotocograph _____

7. hysteroscope _____

8. neonatologist _____

9. antepartum _____

10. bradytocia _____

11. hysterorrhexis _____

12. endometrium _____

13. myometrium _____

14. transvaginal sonography _____

15. pelvicephalometry _____

16. hysterosalpingogram (2 roots) _____

EXERCISE 3   Match the term on the left with its definition on the right.

_____ 1. Pap smear

_____ 2. obstetrics

_____ 3. obstetrician

_____ 4. gravida

a. specialist in pregnancy, labor, and delivery of newborns

b. test used to detect cancer cells, most commonly in the cervix

c. branch of medicine dealing with pregnancy, labor, and delivery of newborns

d. pregnant

EXERCISE 4   Fill in the blanks.

1. *colposcopy:* procedure for examining the

_____

2. *hysteroscopy:* procedure for examining the

_____

3. *mammography:* procedure for imaging the

_____

3. tocodynagraph _____

4. hysterocele _____

5. hypomastia _____

6. amniocentesis _____

7. hysterorrhexis _____

8. colpoptosis _____

9. mammogram _____

10. cardiotocograph _____

11. transvaginal sonography _____

12. pelvicephalometry _____

EXERCISE 5   Translate the following terms as literally as possible.

> EXAMPLE: nasopharyngoscope   *an instrument for looking at the nose and throat*

1. natal _____

2. gynecology _____

GENERATION

EXERCISE 6 Build a medical term from the information provided.

> EXAMPLE: inflammation of the sinuses   *sinusitis*

1. procedure for examining the vagina (use *colp/o*) _____

2. procedure for examining the uterus (use *hyster/o*) _____

3. record of a breast exam (use *mamm/o*) _____

_____

4. procedure for measuring the fetus _____

_____

5. study of the neonatal period _____

_____

6. specialist in medical issues specific to women

_____

7. slow labor _____

8. excessively large breasts _____

9. downward displacement of the uterus _____

_____

10. inner layer of uterine tissue _____

_____

11. record of the uterus and fallopian tubes

_____

EXERCISE 7 Multiple-choice questions. Select the correct answer(s).

1. The middle layer of uterine muscle tissue is the
   a. endometrium
   b. intrametrium
   c. myometrium
   d. perimetrium
   e. none of these

2. Another term for *pregnant* is
   a. amastia
   b. gravida
   c. menarche
   d. prenatal
   e. teratogenic

3. Select all of the following statements that apply to the term *Pap smear.*
   a. a diagnostic procedure used in gynecology
   b. a diagnostic procedure used in obstetrics
   c. a test used to detect cancer cells, most commonly in the cervix
   d. a test used to detect cancer cells, most commonly in the vulva
   e. named after the inventor of the procedure, Dr. Georgios Papanicolaou

4. Select all of the following terms that pertain to obstetrics.
   a. tocodynagraph
   b. vaginoscope
   c. hysteroscope

5. Select all of the following terms that pertain to gynecology.
   a. tocodynagraph
   b. vaginoscope
   c. hysteroscope

EXERCISE 8 Briefly describe the difference between each pair of terms.

1. postnatal, prenatal _____

2. obstetrics, obstetrician _____

_____

3. hypermastia, hypomastia _____

_____

4. antepartum, postpartum _____

_____

5. endometrium, myometrium _____

_____

6. dystocia, bradytocia _____

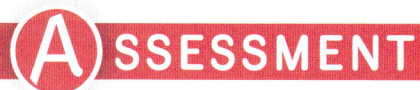

13.4 Diagnosis and Pathology

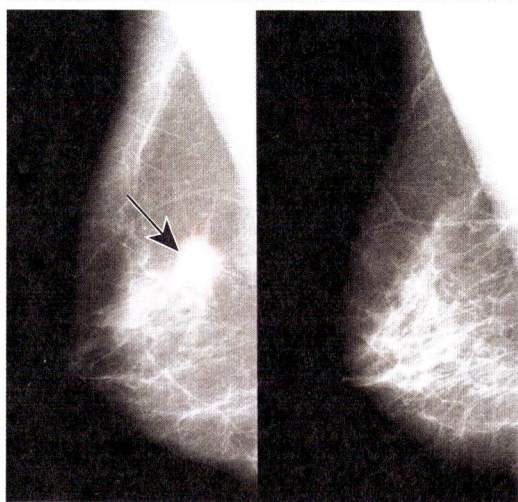

Mammogram of a breast with a tumor at the arrow
(left), compared with the appearance of normal
fibrous connective tissue of the breast (right).
The Image Bank/Getty Images

Problems with periods are very routine causes for
females to seek medical help. The normal range for
a female's first period (*menarche*) is 10 to 16 years of
age. An early or delayed start for periods may indicate an underlying problem. Missing one or more
periods (*amenorrhea*) is a common reason for a medical visit. This can be caused by pregnancy, hormone
problems, or problems with anatomy.

Unfortunately, cancers of the female reproductive
system are common problems. Breast cancer (*adenocarcinoma of the breast*) is the most common cancer
in women. For this reason, routine exams and mammograms are very important in female health care.

The uterus, cervix, and ovaries are also common
areas for cancer. The Pap smear helps detect early
evidence of cancer or precancerous changes in the
cervix (*cervical intraepithelial neoplasia*).

Infection or inflammation of the female reproductive system happens more frequently in the outer
parts of the reproductive system. Irritation of the
vagina (*vaginitis*) or the vagina and its surrounding

area (*vulvovaginitis*) can present with pain and/or
itching. Both bacteria (*bacterial vaginosis*) and fungi
(*vaginomycosis*) are frequent causes.

Many bacterial and viral infections of the female
reproductive tract are spread through sexual intercourse. If infection spreads higher into the reproductive tract, such as to the fallopian tubes (*salpingitis*)
and cervix (*cervicitis*), the patient may become quite
ill; these infections can even lead to scarring and
infertility. Another common infection in females is
infection of the breast (*mastitis*), particularly in nursing mothers. Mastitis can make breast-feeding very
painful.

Pregnancy can cause its own set of medical
issues. A fertilized egg that implants anywhere other
than the uterus is known as an *ectopic pregnancy*.
Examples of ectopic locations include the fallopian
tubes (*salpingocyesis*) and ovaries (*ovariacyesis*). Ectopic pregnancies are not viable, and they can cause
pain and bleeding, infertility, and even death in some
extreme circumstances.

During pregnancy, many women experience nausea and vomiting, a condition commonly known as
morning sickness. In some cases, the vomiting can
become quite severe (*hyperemesis gravidum*) and
need medical treatment.

Another problem encountered by some women
during pregnancy is *preeclampsia*. This condition is
marked by high blood pressure and protein in the
urine. It can progress to include seizures (*eclampsia*).

The connection point between the mother and the
baby (*placenta*) can also be a source of medical problems. A placenta in the wrong position can block the
opening in the uterus (*placenta previa*), making delivery problematic. If the blood supply to the placenta
is interrupted (*abruptio placentae*), the baby may be
at risk of not getting enough blood, and the mother
could suffer severe blood loss.

The membranes of the womb can develop tumors
or infection. Tumors of the womb actually arise
from fetal tissue. Rarely, this can become cancerous (*choriocarcinoma*). Infections in the womb

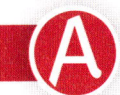

(*chorioamnionitis*) routinely occur just prior to delivery and are treated with antibiotics.

Not every pregnancy produces a baby capable of survival. In fact, upward of 25 percent of all known pregnancies result in the mother's body ending the pregnancy. This is mainly the mother's body's response to a fetus with severe problems that would prevent survival. Commonly known as a *miscarriage,* the medical term is *spontaneous abortion.* This is opposed to common lay use of the term *abortion,* which usually refers to an *induced abortion.* An induced abortion is when a pregnancy is deliberately ended by artificial means. Induced abortions can be performed by taking a medication or via surgery.

gynecology

TERM	WORD ANALYSIS
cervicitis SER-vih-SAI-tis	cervic / itis cervix / inflammation
DEFINITION inflammation of the cervix	
cervicocolpitis SER-vih-koh-kol-PAI-tis	cervico / colp / itis cervix / vagina / inflammation
DEFINITION inflammation of the cervix and vagina	
cystocele SIS-toh-seel	cysto / cele bladder / hernia
DEFINITION hernia of the urinary bladder into the vagina	
endometriosis EN-doh-MEE-tree-OH-sis	endo / metri / osis inside / uterus / condition
DEFINITION condition in which endometrium cells appear and grow outside the uterus	

gynecology *continued*

TERM	WORD ANALYSIS
mastitis mas-TAI-tis	mast / itis breast / inflammation
DEFINITION inflammation of the breast	
menopause MEN-oh-pawz	meno / pause menstruation / stop
DEFINITION cessation of menstruation	
oophoritis OH-aw-for-AI-tis	oophor / itis ovary / inflammation
DEFINITION inflammation of an ovary	
salpingitis SAL-pin-JAI-tis	salping / itis fallopian tube / inflammation
DEFINITION inflammation of a fallopian tube	
salpingocele sal-PING-goh-seel	salpingo / cele fallopian tube / hernia
DEFINITION hernia of a fallopian tube	

gynecology *continued*

TERM	WORD ANALYSIS
urethrocele yur-EE-throh-seel	urethro / cele urethra / pouch / hernia
DEFINITION hernia or prolapse of the urethra into the vagina	
vaginitis VAJ-ih-NAI-tis	vagin / itis vagina / inflammation
DEFINITION inflammation of the vagina	
vesicovaginal fistula VES-ih-koh-VAJ-ih-nal FIS-tyoo-lah	vesico / vagin / al bladder / vagina / pertaining to fistula pipe
DEFINITION abnormal opening between the urinary bladder and the vagina	
vulvitis vul-VAI-tis	vulv / itis vulva / inflammation
DEFINITION inflammation of the vulva	

obstetrics

TERM	WORD ANALYSIS
abortion ah-BOR-shun	from Latin, for *an untimely birth or miscarriage*
DEFINITION termination of pregnancy NOTE: There are two general categories of abortion: *spontaneous* (when the body does it of its own accord) and *induced* (when there is an external cause). Outside the medical world, many people commonly use the terms *miscarriage* to refer to a spontaneous abortion and *abortion* to refer exclusively to an induced abortion.	

obstetrics *continued*

TERM	WORD ANALYSIS
abruptio placentae ah-BRUP-shee-oh plah-SIN-tee	abruptio placentae tear away placenta
DEFINITION separation of the placenta from the wall of the uterus	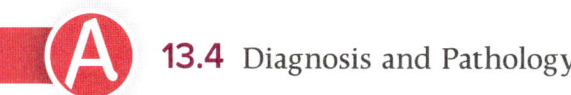
eclampsia eh-KLAMP-see-ah	from Greek, for *to shine or lightning*
DEFINITION severe, life-threatening complication of pregnancy characterized by seizures NOTE: The term probably comes from the fact that seizures strike suddenly, like lightning.	
ectopic pregnancy ek-TOP-ik PREG-nan-see	ec / top / ic outside / place / pertaining to pregnancy pregnancy
DEFINITION implantation of a fertilized egg in a place other than the uterus	
hyperemesis gravidarum HAI-per-eh-MEE-sis GRAV-ih-DAR-um	hyper / emesis gravidarum over / vomit pregnancy
DEFINITION pregnancy-related vomiting; an extreme form of the more common *morning sickness*	
hysterorrhexis HIS-ter-oh-REK-sis	hystero / rrhexis uterus / rupture
DEFINITION rupture of the uterus	
ovariocyesis oh-VAR-ee-oh-sai-EE-sis	ovario / cyesis ovary / pregnancy
DEFINITION ectopic pregnancy in an ovary	

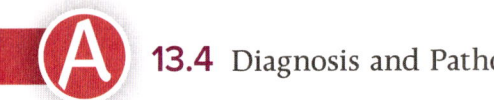

obstetrics *continued*

TERM	WORD ANALYSIS
placenta previa plah-SIN-tah PREE-vee-ah	placenta previa placenta first
DEFINITION condition in which the placenta is attached to the uterus near the cervix	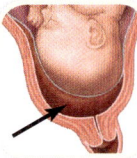
preeclampsia PREE-eh-KLAMP-see-ah	pre / eclampsia before / eclampsia
DEFINITION condition characterized by high blood pressure and high protein in the urine NOTE: See *eclampsia* for the origin of the term. The term comes from the fact that without proper treatment, a patient will develop eclampsia.	

obstetrics *continued*

TERM	WORD ANALYSIS
pseudocyesis SOO-doh-sai-EE-sis	pseudo / cyesis false / pregnancy
DEFINITION false pregnancy	
salpingocyesis sal-PING-goh-sai-EE-sis	salpingo / cyesis fallopian tube / pregnancy
DEFINITION ectopic pregnancy in a fallopian tube	
spontaneous abortion spawn-TAY-nee-is ah-BOR-shun	
DEFINITION naturally occurring termination of pregnancy; also known as a *miscarriage* NOTE: See *abortion* for the origin of the term.	

A Learning Outcome 13.4 Exercises

TRANSLATION

EXERCISE 1 Break down the following words into their component parts.

EXAMPLE: nasopharyngoscope
naso | pharyngo | scope

1. cystocele _____
2. rectocele _____
3. urethrocele _____
4. pseudocyesis _____
5. hysterorrhexis _____

EXERCISE 2 Underline and define the word parts from this chapter in the following terms.

1. menopause _____
2. salpingocele _____
3. endometriosis _____
4. vesicovaginal fistula _____
5. ovariocyesis (2 word parts) _____
6. salpingocyesis (2 word parts) _____

EXERCISE 3   Match the term on the left with its definition on the right.

_____   1. abortion

_____   2. spontaneous abortion

_____   3. ectopic pregnancy

_____   4. abruptio placentae

_____   5. placenta previa

_____   6. eclampsia

_____   7. hyperemesis gravidarum

_____   8. preeclampsia

a.   condition characterized by high blood pressure and high level of protein in the urine

b.   condition in which the placenta is attached to the uterus near the cervix

c.   characterized by seizures

d.   pregnancy-related vomiting; an extreme form of the more common *morning sickness*

e.   implantation of a fertilized egg in a place other than the uterus

f.   termination of pregnancy

g.   naturally occurring termination of pregnancy; also known as a *miscarriage*

h.   separation of the placenta from the wall of the uterus

EXERCISE 4   Fill in the blanks.

1. *vaginitis:* inflammation of the _____

_____

2. *vulvitis:* inflammation of the   _____

_____

3. *cervicitis:* inflammation of the   _____

_____

4. *mastitis:* inflammation of the   _____

_____

5. *oophoritis:* inflammation of the   _____

_____

6. *salpingitis:* inflammation of the   _____

_____

7. *cervicolpitis:* inflammation of the

_____ and

_____

EXERCISE 5   Translate the following terms as literally as possible.

EXAMPLE:	nasopharyngoscope *an instrument for looking at the nose and throat*

1. oophoritis   _____

2. salpingitis   _____

3. menopause   _____

4. cervicocolpitis   _____

GENERATION

EXERCISE 6 Build a medical term from the information provided.

> EXAMPLE: inflammation of the sinuses   *sinusitis*

1. inflammation of the vagina (use *vagin/o*) _____

   _____

2. inflammation of the vulva (use *vulv/o*) _____

   _____

3. inflammation of the cervix   _____

   _____

4. false pregnancy _____

5. rupture of the uterus _____

6. hernia of a fallopian tube _____

EXERCISE 7 Multiple-choice questions. Select the correct answer(s).

1. The implantation of a fertilized egg in a place other than the uterus is called a(n)
   a. ectopic pregnancy
   b. ovariocyesis
   c. pseudocyesis
   d. salpingocyesis
   e. none of these

2. Which of the following options is the correct breakdown of the term *hyperemesis gravidarum?*
   a. over (*hyper*) + throw up (*emesis*) + pregnancy (*gravidarum*)
   b. under (*hyper*) + throw up (*emesis*) + pregnancy (*gravidarum*)
   c. over (*hyper*) + grow (*emesis*) + pregnancy (*gravidarum*)
   d. under (*hyper*) + grow (*emesis*) + pregnancy (*gravidarum*)
   e. none of these

3. Which of the following statements is the correct definition of *endometriosis?*
   a. a condition in which endometrium cells appear and grow outside the uterus
   b. condition of the inside of the cervix
   c. inflammation of the endometrium
   d. inflammation of the inside of the cervix
   e. none of these

4. Which of the following statements is the correct definition of the term *vesicovaginal fistula?*
   a. an abnormal opening between the urinary bladder and the vagina
   b. hernia of the uterus and prolapse into the vagina
   c. an abnormal opening between the uterus and the vagina
   d. hernia of the urinary bladder into the vagina
   e. none of these

EXERCISE 8 Briefly describe the difference between each pair of terms.

1. induced abortion, spontaneous abortion _____

   _____

2. ovariocyesis, salpingocyesis _____

   _____

3. cystocele, urethrocele _____

   _____

4. eclampsia, preeclampsia _____

   _____

5. abruptio placentae, placenta previa _____

   _____

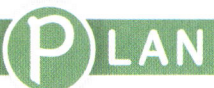

13.5 Treatments and Therapies

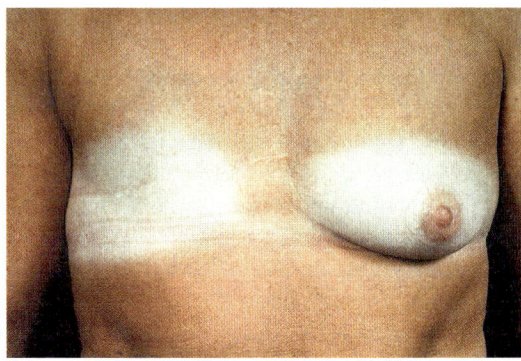

Breast cancer is a common reason a doctor might recommend a mastectomy.

Biophoto Associates/Science Source

One unique attribute of physicians trained in obstetrics and gynecology is that they are primary care providers for many women's health issues, but they are also surgeons. *Gynecologic surgeries* involve the interior structures of the female reproductive tract, such as the ovaries, fallopian tubes, and uterus. Ovarian surgeries can include the removal of an ovary (*oophorectomy*) to treat ovarian cancer or just the removal of a cyst on the ovary (*ovarian cystectomy*). At times, a fallopian tube is removed along with an ovary (*salpingo-oophorectomy*).

The fallopian tubes are common sites for ectopic pregnancies, and their standard treatment involves surgically opening the fallopian tube (*salpingotomy*) and removing the developing embryo. This procedure can maintain fertility and proper function of the reproductive system, but sometimes, as with a ruptured ectopic pregnancy, the tube must be removed altogether (*salpingectomy*). Another procedure involving the fallopian tubes involves blocking them (*tubal ligation*) as a means of preventing future pregnancies (*sterilization*).

Among the most frequently performed surgeries in gynecology is removal of the uterus (*hysterectomy*). Numerous medical problems are treated with hysterectomy, including cancer, fibroid tumors, and endometriosis. Prolapse of the uterus can be treated by surgically securing the uterus to another structure (*hysteropexy* or *colpopexy*).

Another very common procedure involving the uterus is *dilation and curettage* (commonly referred to as *D&C*). In this procedure, the opening of the cervix is gradually dilated with special instruments. Then, tissues lining the uterus are removed. D&C is commonly used to evaluate and treat problems of the uterus, such as abnormal bleeding. This may be due to benign problems, such as polyps, or fibroid tumors, which can be removed by cutting them out of the muscular wall of the uterus (*myomectomy.*) D&C is also utilized following a miscarriage when the uterus fails to fully shed the nonviable tissue.

Defects of the vagina, whether they originate from birth or from abuse, can be corrected by a plastic surgeon (*vaginoplasty*).

Surgeries involving the breast are much more common procedures, with breast cancer being the leading reason. In some instances, the breast can be spared and just the cancer is removed (*mastotomy* with *lumpectomy*). Many times, the entire breast is removed (*mastectomy*). In these cases, breast reconstruction surgery can help restore the normal appearance of the breast. Other breast surgeries include breast reduction (*mammoplasty*) and breast lift (*mastopexy*).

The science of obstetrics is focused on keeping both mother and baby healthy during pregnancy. One important aspect is making sure that the mother avoids substances that can harm the growth of the baby (*teratogen*).

In a healthy pregnancy, delivery involves the muscles of the uterus squeezing to push the baby through the canal. If her contractions come too early, before her baby is ready to be born, a patient can take medicines that can help stop them (*tocolytic*). There are also medicines, such as oxytocin, that can be used to bring on contractions and induce labor.

Once it is time for delivery, there are two possibilities. The most common is a vaginal delivery, which involves delivering the baby naturally through the birth canal. It may be necessary to make a small cut in the mother's perineum (*episiotomy*) to help

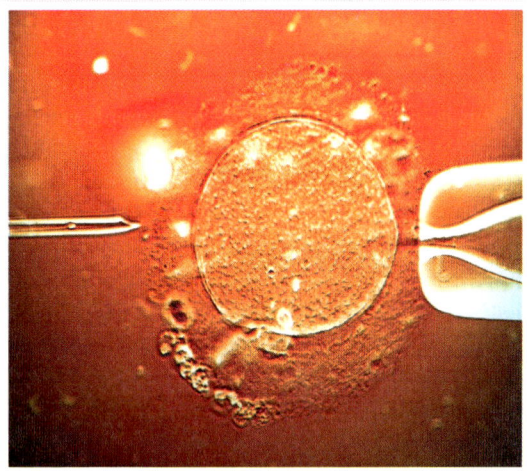

For couples struggling with fertility issues, in vitro fertilization provides possibility.

Zephyr/Science Source

prevent tearing of skin during delivery. In cases in which a baby is positioned in the wrong direction or is not moving quickly through the birth canal, the baby might need to be delivered surgically (*cesarean section*). This surgery, the most common one in medicine, involves first cutting the abdomen of the mother (*laparotomy*) and then cutting open her uterus (*hysterotomy*) to gain access to the baby.

Another procedure unique to women's health is in vitro fertilization, the fertilization of a female's egg by a male's sperm outside the body (*in vitro*). After the fertilization is complete, the *zygote* is then transferred into the woman's uterus.

gynecology

TERM	WORD ANALYSIS
episiorrhaphy eh-PEE-zee-OR-ah-fee	episio / rrhaphy vulva / suture
DEFINITION suture of the vulva	
hysterectomy HIS-ter-EK-toh-mee	hyster / ectomy uterus / removal
DEFINITION surgical removal of the uterus	
hysteropexy HIS-ter-oh-PEK-see	hystero / pexy uterus / fixation
DEFINITION surgical fixation of the uterus	
hysterosalping-ectomy HIS-ter-oh-SAL-pin-JEK-toh-mee	hystero / salping / ectomy uterus / tube / removal
DEFINITION surgical removal of the uterus and fallopian tube(s)	

gynecology *continued*

TERM	WORD ANALYSIS
mammoplasty MAM-oh-PLAS-tee	mammo / plasty breast / reconstruction
DEFINITION surgical reconstruction of a breast	

Biophoto Associates/Science Source

mastectomy mas-TEK-toh-mee	mast / ectomy breast / removal
DEFINITION surgical removal of a breast	
mastopexy MAS-toh-PEK-see	masto / pexy breast / fixation
DEFINITION surgical fixation of a breast	
myomectomy MAI-oh-MEK-toh-mee	my / om / ectomy muscle / tumor / removal
DEFINITION surgical removal of a tumor in the muscle (usually refers to the muscle of the uterine wall)	
oophorectomy OH-aw-for-EK-toh-mee	oophor / ectomy ovary / removal
DEFINITION surgical removal of an ovary	

13.5 Treatments and Therapies

gynecology *continued*

TERM	WORD ANALYSIS
ovariocentesis oh-VAW-ree-oh-sin-TEE-sis	ovario / centesis ovary / puncture
DEFINITION surgical puncture of an ovary	
perineoplasty PER-ih-NEE-oh-PLAS-tee	perineo / plasty perineum / reconstruction
DEFINITION surgical reconstruction of the perineum	
perineorrhaphy PER-ih-nee-OR-ah-fee	perineo / rrhaphy perineum / suture
DEFINITION suture of the perineum	
salpingectomy SAL-pin-JEK-toh-mee	salping / ectomy fallopian tube / removal
DEFINITION surgical removal of a fallopian tube	
salpingo-oophorectomy sal-PING-goh-OH-aw-for-EK-toh-mee	salpingo / oophor / ectomy fallopian tube / ovary / removal
DEFINITION surgical removal of a fallopian tube and ovary	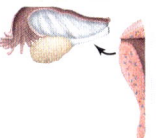
vaginoplasty vah-JI-noh-PLAS-tee	vagino / plasty vagina / reconstruction
DEFINITION surgical reconstruction of the vagina	

obstetrics

TERM	WORD ANALYSIS
cesarean section sih-SER-ee-an SEK-shun	cesarean section
DEFINITION delivery of a baby through an incision made in the uterus NOTE: This term does *not* refer to Julius Caesar's method of delivery. Rather, it refers to an ancient Roman law that required a child to be cut from a mother's womb if the mother died in childbirth.	

obstetrics *continued*

TERM	WORD ANALYSIS
episiotomy eh-PEE-zee-AW-toh-mee	episio / tomy vulva / incision
DEFINITION incision into the vulva	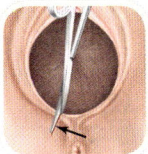
in vitro fertilization in VEE-troh FER-tih-lih-ZAY-shun	in vitro fertilization in glass fertilization
DEFINITION fertilization of an egg done in a test tube	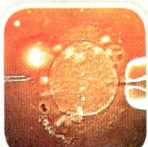 Zephyr/Science Source
induced abortion in-DOOST ah-BOR-shun	
DEFINITION intentional termination of pregnancy	

pharmacology

TERM	WORD ANALYSIS
abortifacient ah-BOR-tih-FAY-shunt	aborti / facient abortion / do
DEFINITION drug or device that causes the termination of pregnancy	
oxytocin OK-see-TOH-sin	oxy / toc / in swift / birth / agent
DEFINITION agent that stimulates uterine contractions and accelerates labor	
tocolytic TOH-koh-LIH-tik	toco / lyt / ic labor / loosing / agent
DEFINITION agent that stops or delays premature labor and contractions	

PRONUNCIATION

EXERCISE 1   Indicate which syllable(s) are emphasized when pronounced.

EXAMPLE: bronchitis bron<u>chi</u>tis

1. mammoplasty (2) _____

2. salpingectomy (2) _____

3. oxytocin (2) _____

TRANSLATION

EXERCISE 2   Break down the following words into their component parts.

EXAMPLE: nasopharyngoscope
            naso | pharyngo | scope

1. mammoplasty _____

2. ovariocentesis _____

3. episiorrhaphy _____

EXERCISE 3   Underline and define the word parts from this chapter in the following terms.

1. vaginoplasty _____

2. perineoplasty _____

3. episiotomy _____

4. hysteropexy _____

5. mastopexy _____

EXERCISE 4   Match the term on the left with its definition on the right.

_____ 1. cesarean section

_____ 2. in vitro fertilization

_____ 3. induced abortion

_____ 4. perineorrhaphy

_____ 5. abortifacient

_____ 6. oxytocin

a. drug or device that causes the termination of a pregnancy

b. agent that stimulates uterine contractions and accelerates labor

c. delivery of a baby through an incision made in the uterus

d. fertilization of an egg done in a test tube

e. suture of the perineum

f. intentional termination of pregnancy

EXERCISE 5   Fill in the blanks.

1. *hysterectomy:* surgical removal of the _____

2. *mastectomy:* surgical removal of a(n) _____

3. *oophorectomy:* surgical removal of a(n) _____

4. *salpingectomy:* surgical removal of a(n) _____

5. *salpingo-oophorectomy:* surgical removal of a(n) _____ and _____

6. *hysterosalpingectomy:* surgical removal of the _____ and _____

7. *myomectomy:* surgical removal of a(n) _____

EXERCISE 6 Translate the following terms as literally as possible.

EXAMPLE: nasopharyngoscope *an instrument for looking at the nose and throat*

1. vaginoplasty _____

2. perineoplasty _____

3. episiotomy _____

4. mastectomy _____

5. ovariocentesis _____

6. hysteropexy _____

7. myomectomy _____

8. in vitro fertilization _____

GENERATION

EXERCISE 7 Build a medical term from the information provided.

EXAMPLE: inflammation of the sinuses *sinusitis*

1. surgical removal of the uterus (use *hyster/o*) _____

2. surgical removal of an ovary (use *oophor/o*) _____

3. surgical removal of the fallopian tube _____

4. surgical reconstruction of a breast (use *mamm/o*) _____

5. surgical fixation of a breast (use *mast/o*) _____

6. suture of the vulva (use *episi/o*) _____

_____

7. suture of the perineum _____

_____

8. surgical removal of a fallopian tube and ovary _____

9. surgical removal of the uterus and fallopian tube _____

EXERCISE 8 Multiple-choice questions. Select the correct answer(s).

1. A drug or device that causes the termination of a pregnancy is called a(n)
   a. abortifacient
   b. oxytocin
   c. amniotomy
   d. cesarean section
   e. episiorrhaphy

2. An *induced abortion* is
   a. the intentional termination of pregnancy
   b. the naturally occurring termination of pregnancy
   c. a drug or device that causes the termination of a pregnancy
   d. the separation of the placenta from the wall of the uterus
   e. none of these

3. Select all of the following statements that apply to the term *cesarean section.*
   a. a term common in obstetrics
   b. delivery of a baby through an incision in the perineum
   c. delivery of a baby through an incision made in the uterus
   d. refers to an ancient Roman law that required a child to be cut from its mother's womb if the mother died in childbirth
   e. the way in which Julius Caesar was delivered

13.6 Electronic Health Records

Postoperative Note

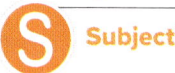

Subjective

Preoperative Diagnosis:

1. **Abruptio placentae**
2. **Chorioamnionitis**
3. **Fetal distress**

Postoperative Diagnosis:

1. Abruptio placentae
2. Chorioamnionitis
3. Fetal distress

Procedure: Emergency cesarean section

Anesthesia: General

Estimated blood loss: 750 mL

Complications: None

Findings: Male infant with cephalic presentation. Normal uterus, fallopian tubes, and ovaries.

Indications: The patient, Mrs. Jenna Friedman, is a 23-year-old **gravida** 2 **para** 1 female who presents at 37 4/7 weeks' **gestation** with *bleeding* and painful **uterine contractions** for 4 hours. An emergent ultrasound was performed to rule out **placenta previa**. The ultrasound showed a **retroplacental** hematoma. She was admitted for evaluation and treatment for **abruptio placentae**. Her physical exam on admission was significant for fever to 101.2°F, as well as abdominal and uterine tenderness.

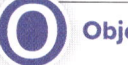

Objective

She was 3 cm *dilated and effaced*. Initial lab work included a CBC that showed an elevated white blood cell count but no anemia. Fibrinogen and PT/PTT were all normal, which reassured us that she did not have DIC or a coagulopathy. The patient was placed on IV fluids and antibiotics for presumed **chorioamnionitis** and was placed under continuous monitoring. Two hours after admission, fetal heart rate monitors alerted us to **fetal bradycardia** and late decelerations. The decision was made to proceed with **emergency cesarean section**.

Input: 2 L normal saline via peripheral IV.
Output: 750 mL blood, 500 mL urine.

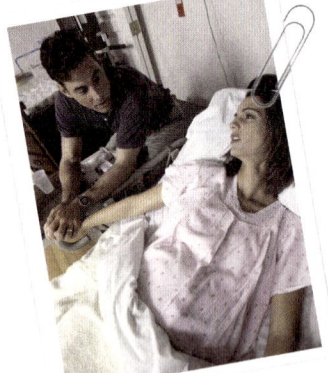

Purestock/Getty Images

Postoperative Note (*continued*)

HR: 76; RR: 22; BP: 102/72.

General: Sedated. Nasal cannula O_2 at 0.5 lpm.

HEENT: PERRLA. Mucous membranes moist and pink. Nares patent. No nasal flaring.

CV: RRR with murmur.

Resp: CTA.

Abd: Midline surgical wound. Dressing is clean, dry, and intact.

GU: Grossly normal, no bleeding.

(A) Assessment

1. Postop cesarean section—stable.
2. Chorioamnionitis.
3. Abruptio placentae—resolved. Hemodynamically stable.

(P) Plan

1. Continue IV fluids and progress to PO as patient becomes more alert.
2. Continue IV antibiotics.
3. Monitor blood pressure. Follow-up CBC.

—Patricia Collingsworth, PA

Learning Outcome 13.6 Exercises

EXERCISE 1   Match the term on the left with its definition on the right.

_____ 1. cesarean section	a. condition in which the placenta is attached to the uterus near the cervix
_____ 2. contraction	b. another term for pregnant
_____ 3. choriamnionitis	c. delivery of a baby through an incision made in the uterus
_____ 4. abruptio placentae	d. inflammation of the chorion and amnion
_____ 5. placenta previa	e. separation of the placenta from the wall of the uterus
_____ 6. gravida	f. shortening or tightening of a muscle

EXERCISE 2 Fill in the blanks.

1. Using the data recorded at the patient's physical examination, fill in the following blanks.

   a. Mrs. Friedman's heart rate:

   _____

   b. Mrs. Friedman's respiratory rate:

   _____

   c. Mrs. Friedman's blood pressure:

   _____

2. Preoperative diagnois:

   a. *Abruptio placentae*–give definition:

   _____

   _____

   b. _____: inflammation of the chorion
   and amnion

   c. *Fetal distress:* presence of signs in a pregnant woman either *prepartum* (give definition:

   _____)

   or *intrapartum* (give definition: _____)
   that suggest the fetus may not be well.

3. Plan:

   a. Continue IV fluids (give definition for abbreviation: _____)
   and progress to _____
   (*per os*–give definition: _____)
   as patient becomes more alert.

   b. Continue _____ (intravenous) antibiotics.

   c. Monitor BP (give definition for abbreviation: _____).
   Follow-up _____ (complete
   blood count).

EXERCISE 3 True or false questions. Indicate true answers with a T and false answers with an F.

1. Mrs. Friedman is a 23-year-old pregnant woman. _____

2. Mrs. Friedman is afebrile. _____

3. Mrs. Friedman has placenta previa. _____

4. Mrs. Friedman was placed on intravenous antibiotics. _____

5. Mrs. Friedman had a vaginal birth. _____

6. Mrs. Friedman was given 2 L of saline through an IV. _____

EXERCISE 4   Multiple-choice questions. Select the correct answer.

1. The ultrasound performed on Mrs. Friedman showed *retroplacental hematoma*. Which of the following options is the correct breakdown of this term?
   a. *retro* (behind) + *placental* (placenta) + *hemat* (blood) + *oma* (tumor)
   b. *retro* (behind) + *placental* (position) + *hemat* (blood) + *oma* (tumor)
   c. *retro* (behind) + *placental* (position) + *hemat* (urine) + *oma* (tumor)
   d. *retro* (behind) + *placental* (uterus) + *hemat* (blood) + *oma* (hole)
   e. *retro* (behind) + *placental* (uterus) + *hemat* (urine) + *oma* (hole)

2. Two hours after admission, heart rate monitors alerted the medical staff to *fetal bradycardia*. Which of the following options is the correct breakdown of this term?
   a. *fetal* (pertaining to the fetus) + *brady* (fast) + *cardia* (blood flow)
   b. *fetal* (pertaining to the fetus) + *brady* (fast) + *cardia* (heartbeat)
   c. *fetal* (pertaining to the fetus) + *brady* (slow) + *cardia* (heartbeat)
   d. *fetal* (pertaining to the uterus) + *brady* (fast) + *cardia* (blood flow)
   e. *fetal* (pertaining to the uterus) + *brady* (slow) + *cardia* (heartbeat)

3. Which of the following options is the correct abbreviation for *cesarean section?*
   a. CS
   b. C-sec
   c. C-section
   d. CS and C-sec
   e. CS and C-section

Quick Reference

glossary of roots

ROOT	DEFINITION	ROOT	DEFINITION
amni/o	amnion	men/o	menstruation
cervic/o	cervix	metr/o	uterus
chori/o	chorion	nat/o	birth
chorion/o	chorion	oophor/o	ovary
colp/o	vagina	ovari/o	ovary
-cyesis	pregnancy	part/o	birth
episi/o	vulva	pelv/i	pelvis
fet/o	fetus	perine/o	perineum
gyn/o	woman	salping/o	fallopian tube
gynec/o	woman	toc/o	labor
hyster/o	uterus	uter/o	uterus
lact/o	milk	vagin/o	vagina
mamm/o	breast	vulv/o	vulva
mast/o	breast		

gynecology

ABBREVIATION	DEFINITION
CIPP	chronic idiopathic pelvic pain
Cx	cervix
GYN	gynecology
HPV	human papillomavirus
HRT	hormone replacement therapy
HSG	hysterosalpingogram
PID	pelvic inflammatory disease
PMS	premenstrual syndrome
STD/STI	sexually transmitted disease/infection
TAH/BSO	total abdominal hysterectomy/bilateral salpingo-oophorectomy
TSS	toxic shock syndrome

obstetrics

ABBREVIATION	DEFINITION
CPD	cephalopelvic disproportion
CS, C-section	cesarean section Martin Valigursky/Shutterstock
DOB	date of birth
EDD	expected date of delivery
FOB	father of the baby (or fecal occult blood)
G	gravida
IVF	in vitro fertilization
LGA	large for gestational age
LMP	last menstrual period
P	births (comes from the word *para*, which means *birth)* ERproductions Ltd/Getty Images
RDS	respiratory distress syndrome
SGA	small for gestational age

A

abdominocentesis (ab-DAW-min-oh-sin-TEE-sis) puncture of the abdomen (usually for the purpose of withdrawing fluid)

abortifacient (ah-BOR-tih-FAY-shunt) drug or device that causes the termination of a pregnancy

abortion (ah-BOR-shun) termination of pregnancy

abrasion (ah-BRAY-zhun) a scraping away of skin

abruptio placentae (ah-BRUP-shee-oh plah-SIN-tee) separation of the placenta from the wall of the uterus

abscess (AB-ses) a localized collection of pus in the body

acne vulgaris (AK-nee vul-GAR-is) common acne; an inflammation of the skin follicles

acoustic neuroma (ah-KOO-stik nir-OH-mah) a tumor on the acoustic nerve

acromegaly (AK-roh-MEH-gah-lee) abnormal enlargement of the extremities

acrophobia (AK-roh-FOH-bee-ah) fear of heights

adenectomy (AD-en-EK-toh-mee) removal of a gland

adenitis (AD-en-AI-tis) inflammation of a gland

adenoma (AD-eh-NOH-mah) glandular tumor

adipocele (a-dih-poh-SEEL) hernia filled with fatty tissue

adrenal virilism (a-DREE-nal VIR-il-izm) development of male secondary sexual characteristics caused by excessive secretion of the adrenal gland

adrenalectomy (a-DREE-nal-EK-toh-mee) removal of the adrenal gland

adrenaline (a-DREN-ah-lin) hormone secreted by the adrenal gland (from Latin; see also *epinephrine*)

adrenalitis (a-DREE-nah-LAI-tis) inflammation of the adrenal gland

aerotitis (AIR-oh-TAI-tis) inflammation of the ear caused by air

afferent nerve (A-fir-ent nirv) a nerve that carries impulses toward the central nervous system

agoraphobia (ah-GOR-ah-FOH-bee-ah) fear of outdoor spaces

albinism (AL-bin-ism) lack of pigment in skin causing the patient to look white

albino (al-BAY-noh) a person afflicted with albinism

albuminuria (al-byoo-mih-NUR-ee-ah) protein in the urine

allograft (A-loh-GRAFT) see *homograft*

alopecia (a-loh-PEE-sha) baldness

amblyopia (AM-blih-OH-pee-ah) decreased vision (when it occurs in one eye, it is referred to as lazy eye)

amenorrhea (AY-men-oh-REE-ah) no menstruation

amniocentesis (AM-nee-oh-sin-TEE-sis) surgical puncture of the amnion

amniorrhea (AM-nee-oh-REE-ah) discharge of amniotic fluid

amniorrhexis (AM-nee-oh-REK-sis) rupture of the amniotic sac

amniotomy (AM-nee-AW-toh-mee) incision into the amnion

analgesic (an-al-JEE-zik) a drug that relieves pain

anastomosis (ah-NAS-toh-moh-sis) creation of an opening; a surgical procedure connecting two previously unconnected hollow tubes.

anemia (ah-NEE-mee-ah) reduction of red blood cells noticed by the patient as weakness and fatigue

anesthetic (an-es-THET-ik) a drug that causes loss of sensation

aneurysm (AN-yir-IZ-um) bulge in a blood vessel

angina pectoris (an-JAI-nah PEK-tor-is) oppressive pain in the chest caused by irregular blood flow to the heart

angiogram (AN-jee-oh-GRAM) record of the blood vessels

angiography (AN-jee-AW-grah-fee) procedure to describe the blood vessels

angioma (AN-jee-OH-mah) blood vessel tumor

angioplasty (AN-jee-oh-PLAS-tee) surgical reconstruction of a vessel

angiorrhaphy (AN-jee-OR-ah-fee) suture of a vessel

anhidrosis (an-hi-DROH-sis) lack of sweating

anorchidism (an-OR-kih-DIZ-um) absence of a testicle

anorexia (a-noh-REK-see-ah) an eating disorder characterized by the patient's refusal to eat

antacid (ant-AS-id) agent that neutralizes acid

antepartum (AN-tee-PAR-tum) time before birth

antianginal (AN-tee-AN-jih-nal) a drug that prevents or relieves the symptoms of angina pectoris

antiarrhythmic (AN-tee-a-RITH-mik) a drug that opposes an irregular heartbeat

antiarthritic (AN-tee-ar-THRIH-tik) a drug that opposes joint inflammation

antibiotic (an-tai-bai-OH-tik) a drug that destroys or opposes the growth of microorganisms

anticoagulant (AN-tee-coh-AG-yoo-lant) drug that prevents the coagulation of blood

anticonvulsant (AN-tee-kon-VUL-sant) a drug that opposes convulsions

antiemetic (AN-tee-EE-met-ik) agent that prevents/relieves nausea or vomiting

antihistamine (an-tee-HIS-tah-meen) a drug that opposes the effects of histamine

antihypertensive (AN-tee-HAI-per-TEN-siv) drug that opposes high blood pressure

anti-inflammatory (AN-tee-in-FLA-mah-TOR-ee) a drug that opposes inflammation

antipruritic (an-tee-pruh-RIH-tik) a drug that prevents or relieves itching

antispasmodic (AN-tee-spaz-MAW-dik) drug used to prevent spasms

antitussive (an-tee-TUSS-iv) a drug that prevents coughing

anuria (an-YUR-ee-ah) lack of urination

anxiolytic (ANG-zee-oh-LIH-tik) a drug that lessens anxiety

aortalgia (AY-or-TAL-jah) pain in the aorta

aortic stenosis (ay-OR-tik stih-NOH-sis) narrowing of the aorta

aortorrhaphy (ay-or-TOR-ah-fee) suture of the aorta

aphagia (ah-FAY-jah) inability to eat

aphakia (ah-FAY-kee-ia) absence of a lens

aphasia (ah-FAY-zhah) inability to speak

apheresis (AH-fer-EE-sis) general term for a process, similar to dialysis, that draws blood, removes something from it, then returns the rest of the blood to the patient

aplastic anemia (AY-plas-tik ah-NEE-mee-ah) anemia caused by red blood cells not being formed in sufficient quantities

apnea (AP-nee-yah) cessation of breathing

arrhythmia (ay-RITH-mee-ah) irregular heartbeat

arteriogram (ar-TER-ee-oh-GRAM) record of an artery

arteriolith (ar-TER-ee-oh-LITH) stone in an artery

arteriopathy (ar-TER-ee-AW-pah-thee) disease of the arteries

arteriorrhaphy (ar-TER-ee-OR-ah-fee) suture of an artery

arteriorrhexis (ar-TER-ee-oh-REK-sis) rupture of an artery

arteriosclerosis (ar-TER-ee-oh-skleh-ROH-sis) hardening of an artery

arteritis (AR-ter-AI-tis) inflammation of the arteries

arthralgia (ar-THRAL-jah) joint pain

arthritis (ar-THRAI-tis) joint inflammation

arthrocentesis (ar-throh-sin-TEE-sis) puncture of a joint

arthrodynia (ar-throh-DAI-nee-ah) joint pain

arthrogram (AR-throh-gram) visual record of a joint

arthropathy (ar-THRAW-pah-thee) joint disease

arthroplasty (AR-throh-PLAS-tee) reconstruction of a joint

arthroscope (AR-throh-skohp) instrument for looking into a joint

arthroscopy (ar-THRAW-skoh-pee) procedure of looking into a joint

arthrotomy (ar-THRAW-toh-mee) incision into a joint

ascites (ah-SAI-teez) retention of fluid in the peritoneum

aspermia (ay-SPER-mee-ah) condition characterized by a lack of sperm

asthma (AZ-ma) a disease caused by episodic narrowing and inflammation of the airway

astigmatism (ah-STIG-mah-TIZ-um) vision problem caused by the fact that light rays entering the eye aren't focused on a single point in the back of the eye

atelectasis (ah-tel-EK-ta-sis) incomplete expansion

atherectomy (A-ther-EK-toh-mee) surgical removal of fatty plaque within an artery

atherogenesis (A-ther-oh-JIN-eh-sis) formation of fatty plaque on the wall of an artery

atherosclerosis (A-ther-oh-skleh-ROH-sis) hardening of an artery due to buildup of fatty plaque

atrial septal defect (AY-tree-al SEP-tal DEE-fekt) flaw in the septum that divides the two atria of the heart

atrophy (A-troh-fee) underdevelopment, decrease, or loss of muscle tissue

audiogram (AW-dee-oh-GRAM) record produced by an audiometer

audiologist (aw-dee-AW-loh-jist) hearing specialist

audiometer (aw-dee-AW-meh-ter) instrument for measuring hearing

audiometry (aw-dee-AW-meh-tree) procedure for measuring hearing

aural (AW-ral) pertaining to the ear

auscultation (ah-skul-TAY-shun) from the Latin word *ausculto,* meaning *to listen;* a doctor using a stethoscope is performing an auscultation

autism (AW-tiz-um) a psychiatric disorder characterized by the withdrawal from communication with others. The patient is focused only on the self

autograft (AW-toh-GRAFT) skin transplant taken from a different place on the patient's body

azoturia (AZ-oh-TUR-ee-ah) excess nitrogen in the urine

B

balanitis (bal-ah-NAI-tis) inflammation of the penis

balanorrhea (BAL-ah-noh-REE-ah) discharge from the penis

bariatrics (BAR-ee-ah-triks) branch of medicine dealing with weight issues

benign prostate hyperplasia (beh-NAIN PROS-tayt HAI-per-PLAY-zhah) noncancerous overdevelopment of the prostate; also known as enlarged prostate

biopsy (BAI-op-see) removal of tissue in order to examine it

blepharitis (BLEF-ah-RAI-tis) eyelid inflammation

blepharoplasty (BLEF-ah-roh-PLAS-tee) surgical reconstruction of the eyelid

blepharoplegia (BLEF-ah-roh-PLEE-jah) paralysis of the eyelid

blepharoptosis (BLEF-ar-awp-TOH-sis) drooping eyelid

blepharospasm (BLEF-ah-roh-SPAZ-um) involuntary contraction of an eyelid

blepharotomy (BLEF-ah-RAW-toh-mee) incision into the eyelid

blood pressure (blud PRESH-ir) force exerted by blood on the walls of blood vessels

blood urea nitrogen (BUN) (blud yoo-REE-ah NAI-troh-jun) nitrogen in the blood in the form of urea; it is the product of the breakdown of amino acids for energy

bradycardia (BRAY-dih-KAR-dee-ah) slow heartbeat

bradykinesia (bray-dih-kih-NEE-zhah) slow movement

bradypnea (brad-ip-NEE-ah) slow breathing

bradytocia (BRAY-dih-TOH-shee-ah) slow labor

Braxton Hicks contraction (BRAKS-ton HIKS con-TRAK-shun) sporadic contractions of the uterine muscles of women not in labor; also known as false labor

bronchiectasis (bron-key-EK-ta-sis) expansion of the bronchi

bronchiogenic carcinoma (bron-kee-oh-JEN-ic car-si-NO-ma) a cancerous tumor originating in the bronchi

bronchiolitis (bron-kee-yo-LAI-tis) inflammation of the bronchiole

bronchitis (bron-KAI-tis) inflammation of the bronchi

bronchodilator (bron-koh-DAI-lay-tor) a drug that expands the walls of the bronchi

bronchoplasty (bron-koh-PLAS-tee) reconstruction of a bronchus

bronchoscopy (bron-KOS-koh-pee) a procedure to look inside the bronchi

bulimia (boo-LEE-mee-ah) an eating disorder characterized by overeating and usually followed by forced vomiting

bulla (BUL-lah) from Latin, for *bubble;* a large blister

bursitis (bur-SAI-tis) inflammation of the bursa

C

capnography (cap-NAH-gra-fee) a procedure to record carbon dioxide levels

capnometer (cap-NOM-eh-ter) instrument to measure carbon dioxide levels

cardiac arrest (KAR-dee-ak ah-REST) cessation of functional circulation

cardiac catheterization (KAR-dee-ak KATH-eh-ter-ih-ZAY-shun) the process of inserting a tube (catheter) into the heart

cardiologist (KAR-dee-AW-loh-jist) heart specialist

cardiology (KAR-dee-AW-loh-jee) branch of medicine dealing with the heart

cardiomegaly (KAR-dee-oh-MEH-gah-lee) enlarged heart

cardiomyopathy (KAR-dee-oh-mai-AW-pah-thee) disease of the heart muscle

cardiopulmonary bypass (KAR-dee-oh-PUL-mon-AR-ee BAI-pas) procedure that temporarily circulates and oxygenates a patient's blood during a portion of heart surgery where the heart is stopped

cardiopulmonary resuscitation (CPR) (KAR-dee-oh-PUL-mon-air-ee ree-sus-ih-TAY-shun) a method of artificially maintaining blood flow and airflow when breathing and pulse have stopped

cardiotocograph (KAR-dee-oh-TOH-koh-GRAF) instrument for recording the fetal heart rate during labor

cardiovascular (KAR-dee-oh-VAS-kyoo-lar) pertaining to the heart and blood vessels

cardioversion (KAR-dee-oh-VER-zhun) returning a heart to normal rhythm

carpectomy (kar-PEK-toh-mee) removal of all or part of the wrist

cataract (KAT-ah-RAKT) opacity (cloudiness) of the lens of the eye (from Latin, for *waterfall*)

cathartic (kah-THAR-tik) agent that produces bowel movements

cephalalgia (SEH-ful-AL-jah) head pain

cerebral angiography (seih-REE-bral AN-jee-AW-grah-fee) procedure used to examine blood vessels in the brain

cerebral palsy (seh-REE-bral PAL-zee) paralysis caused by damage to the area of the brain responsible for movement

cerebrovascular accident (CVA) (seh-REE-broh-VAS-kyoo-lar AK-sih-dent) an accident involving the blood vessels of the brain

cerumen impaction (SEH-roo-men im-PAK-shun) buildup of ear wax blocking the ear canal

ceruminolytic (seh-ROO-min-oh-LIH-tik) drug that aids in the breakdown of ear wax

ceruminosis (seh-ROO-min-OH-sis) excessive formation of ear wax

cervicectomy (SER-vih-SEK-toh-mee) surgical removal of the cervix

cervicitis (SER-vih-SAI-tis) inflammation of the cervix

cervicocolpitis (SER-vih-koh-kol-PAI-tis) inflammation of the cervix and vagina

cervicodynia (sir-vih-koh-DAI-nee-ah) neck pain

cesarean section (sih-SER-ee-an SEK-shun) delivery of a baby through an incision made in the uterus

chemotherapy (KEE-moh-THER-ah-pee) treatment using chemicals

cholangiogram (koh-LAN-jee-oh-gram) record of the bile vessels (ducts)

cholangiography (koh-LAN-jee-AW-grah-fee) procedure for mapping the bile vessels (ducts)

cholangiopancreatography (koh-LAN-jee-oh-PAN-kree-ah-TAW-grah-fee) procedure for mapping the bile vessels (ducts) and pancreas

cholangitis (KOH-lan-JAI-tis) inflammation of the bile vessels (ducts)

cholecystectomy (KOH-lay-sis-TEK-toh-me) surgical removal of the bile (gall) bladder

cholecystitis (KOH-lay-sis-TAI-tis) inflammation of the bile (gall) bladder

choledocholithectomy (KOH-ley-DOH-koh-lih-THEK-toh-mee) surgical removal of a stone from the (common) bile duct

choledocholithiasis (koh-lay-DOH-koh-lith-AI-ah-sis) presence of a stone in the (common) bile duct

cholelith (KOH-lay-lith) gallstone; literally, a stone in the bile

cholelithiasis (KOH-lay-lih-THAI-ah-sis) presence of a gallstone

cholelithotripsy (KOH-lay-lih-THOH-trip-see) crushing of bile (gall) stones

chondrectomy (kawn-DREK-toh-mee) removal of cartilage

chondroma (kawn-DROH-mah) a tumor-like growth of cartilage tissue

chronic obstructive pulmonary disease (COPD) (KRON-ik ob-STRUKT-iv pul-mon-AIR-ee dih-ZEEZ) a lung disease caused by the continual blockage of lung passages

cicatrix (plural cicatrices) (SIK-ah-triks) from Latin, for *scar;* a scar

circulation (SIR-kyoo-LAY-shun) moving of blood from the heart through the vessels and back to the heart

circumcision (SIR-kum-SIH-zhun) surgical removal of the foreskin of the penis

cirrhosis (sir-OH-sis) liver disease named for the change of color in the liver

cochlear implant (KOH-klee-ar IM-plant) electronic device that stimulates the cochlea; it can give the sense of sound to those who are profoundly deaf

colitis (coh-LAI-tis) inflammation of the colon

colonoscopy (COH-lon-AW-skoh-pee) procedure for looking at the colon

colorectal carcinoma (COH-loh-REK-tal KAR-sih-NOH-mah) cancerous tumor of the colon or rectum

colostomy (koh-LAW-stoh-mee) creation of an opening in the colon

colpopexy (KOL-poh-PEK-see) surgical fixation of the vagina

colpoplasty (KOL-poh-PLAS-tee) surgical reconstruction of the vagina

colpoptosis (KOL-pawp-TOH-sis) downward placement of the vagina

colposcopy (kol-PAW-skoh-pee) procedure for examining the vagina

computed axial tomography (CAT or CT) (kom-PYOO-ted AK-see-al taw-MAW-grah-fee) imaging procedure using a computer to produce cross sections along an axis

computed tomography (kom-PYOO-ted tom-O-grah-fee) an imaging procedure using a computer to "cut" or view "slices" of a patient's organs

conductive hearing loss (con-DUK-tiv HEER-ing loss) sound does not get to the middle/inner ear (due to blockages)

congenital heart defect (con-JEN-ih-tal HART DEE-fekt) flaw in the structure of the heart, present at birth

congestive heart failure (con-JES-tiv HART FAYL-yir) heart failure characterized by the heart cavity being unable to pump all the blood out of it (congestive)

conjunctivitis (con-JUNK-tih-VAI-tis) inflammation of the conjunctiva (also known as pink eye)

contraction (con-TRAK-shun) shortening or tightening of a muscle (during labor, uterine muscles contract)

corneal abrasion (KOR-nee-al a-BRAY-zhun) scratch on the cornea

corneal transplant (KOR-nee-al TRANZ-plant) replacement of damaged cornea with donated tissue

coronary artery bypass graft (CABG) (KOR-ah-NAR-ee AR-ter-ee BAI-pas GRAFT) borrowed piece of blood vessel used to bypass a blocked artery in the heart

coronary artery bypass surgery (KOR-ah-NAR-ee AR-ter-ee BAI-pas SIR-jir-ee) surgery to bypass a blocked artery in the heart

corticotropin (KOR-tih-koh-TROH-pin) shorter name for adrenocorticotropic hormone (ACTH)

costalgia (kaws-TAL-jah) rib pain

costectomy (kaws-TEK-toh-mee) removal of a rib

costochondritis (KAW-stoh-kawn-DRAI-tis) inflammation of the cartilage of the rib

craniectomy (KRAY-nee-EK-toh-mee) removal of a portion of the skull (bone is not replaced)

craniotomy (KRAY-nee-AW-toh-mee) removal of a portion of the skull (bone is later replaced)

crust (krust) dried substance (i.e., blood, pus) on the skin

cryosurgery (KRAI-oh-SIR-juh-ree) destruction of tissue through freezing

cryptorchidism (krip-TOR-kih-DIZ-um) hidden testicle

culture & sensitivity (KUL-chur and sin-sih-TIH-vih-tee) growing microorganisms in isolation in order to determine which drugs it might respond to

cyanosis (SAI-ah-NOH-sis) a bluish appearance to the skin; a sign that the tissue isn't receiving enough oxygen

cystectomy (sis-TEK-toh-mee) surgical removal of the bladder

cystocele (SIS-toh-seel) hernia of the bladder

cystodynia (SIS-toh-DAI-nee-ah) pain in the bladder

cystogram (SIS-toh-gram) image of the bladder

cystography (sis-TAW-grah-fee) process for recording/imaging the bladder

cystoplegia (SIS-toh-PLEE-jah) bladder paralysis

cystorrhexis (SIS-toh-REK-sis) rupture of the bladder

cystoscopy (sis-TAWS-koh-pee) process for examining the bladder

cytapheresis (SAI-tah-fer-EE-sis) apheresis to remove cellular material

D

decubitus ulcer (deh-KYOO-bih-tus UL-sir) bed sore

deep vein thrombosis (DEEP VAYN throm-BOH-sis) the formation of a blood clot deep in the body, most commonly in the leg

dementia (da-MEN-chah) loss/decline in mental function

dentalgia (den-TAL-jah) tooth pain

dentifrice (DEN-ti-fris) toothpaste

dentist (DEN-tist) specialist in teeth

dentistry (DEN-tis-tree) branch of medicine dealing with teeth

dermabrasion (der-mah-BRAY-zhun) rubbing or scraping away the outer surface of skin

dermatalgia (der-mah-TAL-jah) skin pain

dermatitis (der-mah-TAI-tis) inflammation of the skin

dermatoconiosis (der-ma-toh-COH-nee-oh-sis) a skin condition caused by dirt

dermatodynia (der-MA-toh-DAI-nee-ah) skin pain

dermatomycosis (der-mah-toh-mai-KOH-sis) a fungal skin condition

dermatosis (der-mah-TOH-sis) skin condition

dermopathy (der-MAW-pa-thee) skin disease

diabetes mellitus (DAI-ah-BEE-teez MEH-lih-tis) metabolic disease characterized by excessive urination and hyperglycemia

diaphoresis (DAI-ah-for-EE-sis) profuse sweating

diarrhea (DAI-ah-REE-ah) passing of fluid or unformed feces

digital rectal exam (DIJ-ih-tal REK-tal ek-ZAM) examination of the prostate using a finger inserted into the rectum

dipsogenic (DIP-soh-JIN-ik) creating thirst

diuresis (DAI-yur-EE-sis) excessive urination

diuretic (DAI-yur-IT-ik) agent that causes urination

duodenectomy (doo-AW-den-EK-toh-mee) surgical removal of the duodenum

duodenitis (doo-AH-den-AI-tis) inflammation of the duodenum

dysentery (DIS-en-TER-ee) another name for diarrhea

dyskinesia (dis-kih-NEE-zhah) inability to control movement

dysmenorrhea (DIS-men-oh-REE-ah) painful menstruation

dyspepsia (dis-PEP-see-ah) bad digestion

dysphasia (dis-FAY-zhah) difficulty speaking

dyspnea (disp-NEE-ah) difficulty breathing

dysrhythmia (dis-RITH-mee-ah) irregular heartbeat

dystaxia (dis-TAK-see-ah) poor coordination

dystocia (dis-TOH-shee-ah) difficult labor

dystonia (dis-TOH-nee-ah) poor muscle tone

dysuria (dis-YUR-ee-ah) painful urination

E

ear lavage (ee-ir lah-VAJ) rinsing/washing the external ear canal (usually to remove ear wax); from Latin, for *to wash, bathe*

ecchymosis (eh-kih-MOH-sis) from Greek, for *to pour out;* a larger bruise

echocardiogram (EK-oh-KAR-dee-oh-GRAM) image of the heart produced using sound waves; it is the same procedure as an ultrasound performed on a pregnant woman, but done on the heart

echocardiography (EK-oh-KAR-dee-AW-grah-fee) use of sound waves to produce an image of the heart

eclampsia (eh-KLAMP-see-ah) severe, life-threatening complication of pregnancy characterized by seizures

ectopic pregnancy (ek-TOP-ik PREG-nan-see) implantation of a fertilized egg in a place other than the uterus

eczema (EK-zeh-mah) from Greek, for *to boil over;* a red, itchy rash that may weep or ooze, then become crusted and scaly

efferent nerve (EH-fir-ent nirv) a nerve that carries impulses away from the central nervous system

electrocardiogram (eh-LEK-troh-KAR-dee-oh-GRAM) record of the electrical currents of the heart

electrocardiography (eh-LEK-troh-KAR-dee-AW-grah-fee) procedure for recording the electrical currents of the heart

electroencephalography (eh-LEK-troh-in-SEH-fah-LAW-grah-fee) procedure used to examine the electrical activity of the brain

embolism (EM-boh-LIZ-um) blockage in a blood vessel caused by an embolus

embolus (EM-boh-lus) mass of matter present in the blood

emphysema (em-fi-ZEE-ma) a disease that causes the alveoli to lose their elasticity; patients can inhale but have difficulty exhaling

encephalitis (en-SEF-ah-LAI-tis) inflammation of the brain

encephalocele (en-SEF-ah-loh-SEEL) hernia of the brain (normally through a defect in the skull)

encephalopathy (en-SEF-ah-LAW-pah-thee) disease of the brain

endarterectomy (END-ar-ter-EK-toh-me) surgical removal of the inside of an artery

endocarditis (EN-doh-kar-DAI-tis) inflammation of the tissue lining the inside of the heart

endocardium (EN-doh-KAR-dee-um) tissue lining the inside of the heart

endocrine (EN-doh-krin) secrete internally (i.e., into the bloodstream)

endocrinologist (EN-doh-krih-NAW-loh-jist) specialist in internal secretions

endometriosis (EN-doh-MEE-tree-OH-sis) condition in which endometrium cells appear and grow outside the uterus

endometrium (EN-doh-MEE-tree-um) inner layer of uterine tissue

endoscopy (en-DAW-skoh-pee) procedure of looking inside

endotracheal intubation (en-doh-TRAY-kee-al in-too-BAY-shun) insertion of a tube inside the trachea

enuresis (EN-yur-EE-sis) involuntary urination

epicardium (EH-pee-KAR-dee-um) tissue lining the outside of the heart

epidermal (eh-pi-DER-mal) pertaining to the skin

epidural hematoma (EH-pi-DIR-al HEE-mah-TOH-mah) a hematoma located on top of the dura

epilepsy (eh-pih-LEP-see) a disease marked by seizures

epinephrine (EH-pee-NEF-rin) hormone secreted by the adrenal gland (from Greek; see also *adrenaline*)

episiorrhaphy (eh-PEE-zee-OR-ah-fee) suture of the vulva

episiotomy (eh-PEE-zee-AW-toh-mee) incision into the vulva

epistaxis (ep-ee-STAKS-is) nosebleed

erythema (eh-rih-THEE-ma) from Greek, for *redness;* redness

erythrocyanosis (eh-RITH-roh-SAI-an-OH-sis) a red and/or blue discoloration of the skin

erythrocyte (eh-RIH-throh-SAIT) red blood cell

erythroderma (eh-RIH-throh-DER-ma) red skin

esophagitis (eh-SAWF-ah-JAI-tis) inflammation of the esophagus

esophagogastroduodenoscopy (eh-SAWF-ah-goh-GAS-stroh-DOO-aw-den-AW-skoh-pee) procedure for looking inside the esophagus, stomach, and duodenum

esophagoscopy (eh-SAW-fah-GAW-skoh-pee) procedure for looking inside the esophagus

esotropia (AY-soh-TROH-pee-ah) inward turning of the eye, toward the nose

euglycemia (YOO-glai-SEE-mee-ah) good blood sugar

eupnea (YOOP-nee-yah) good/normal breathing

euthyroid (YOO-thai-royd) a normal functioning thyroid

exophthalmos (EKS-of-THAL-mus) protrusion of the eye out of the eye socket

exotropia (EKS-oh-TROH-pee-ah) outward turning of the eye, away from the nose

expectorant (eks-PEK-tor-ant) a drug that encourages expulsion of material from the lungs

expectoration (eks-pec-tor-A-shun) coughing or spitting material out of the lungs

extracorporeal shock wave lithotripsy (ESWL) (EKS-trah-cor-POR-ee-al shok wayv LIH-thoh-TRIP-see) breakdown of kidney stones using sound waves generated outside the body

F

fecal occult blood test (FOBT) (FEE-kal ah-KULT blud test) test of feces to discover blood not visibly apparent

fetometry (fee-TAW-meh-tree) procedure for measuring the fetus

fissure (FIH-zhur) from Latin, for a *split* or *divide;* a crack in the skin

fistula (FIS-tyoo-la) any abnormal passageway in the body that shouldn't be there

flatus (FLAH-tus) medical term for passing gas

fracture (FRAK-shur) from Latin, for *break;* a bone break

G

gastralgia (gas-TRAL-jah) stomach pain

gastrectomy (gas-TREK-toh-mee) surgical removal of the stomach

gastritis (gas-TRAI-tis) inflammation of the stomach

gastroduodenostomy (GAS-troh-doo-AH-den-AW-stoh-mee) creation of an opening between the stomach and the duodenum

gastrodynia (GAS-troh-DAI-nee-ah) stomach pain

gastroenteritis (GAS-troh-EN-ter-AI-tis) inflammation of the stomach and intestines

gastroenterologist (GAS-troh-EN-ter-AW-loh-jist) specialist in the stomach and intestines

gastroenterology (GAS-troh-EN-ter-AW-loh-jee) study of the stomach and intestines

gastroesophageal reflux disease (GERD) (GAS-troh-eh-SOF-ah-JEE-al REE-fluks dih-ZEEZ) disease in which acid comes up from the stomach and damages the esophagus

gastroscopy (gas-TRAW-skoh-pee) procedure for looking at the stomach

gingivitis (JIN-jih-VAI-tis) inflammation of the gums

gingivostomatitis (JIN-jih-voh-STOH-mah-TAI-tis) inflammation of the mouth and gums

glomerulonephritis (gloh-MER-yoo-loh-neh-FRAI-tis) inflammation of the kidneys involving primarily the glomeruli

glossorrhaphy (glaws-OR-ah-fee) suture of the tongue

glucosuria (GLOO-koh-SOO-ree-ah) sugar in the urine

goiter (GOY-ter) swollen thyroid gland

gonadotropin (goh-NAD-oh-TROH-pin) hormone that stimulates the gonads

gonads (GOH-nadz) the pair of organs used for sexual reproduction; testicles in males and ovaries in females

gonorrhea (GAW-noh-REE-ah) discharge from the gonads

gravida (GRAH-vid-ah) another term for pregnant

gynecologist (GAI-neh-KAW-loh-jist) specialist in medical issues specific to women

gynecology (GAI-neh-KAW-loh-jee) study of medical issues specific to women

H

hematemesis (HEM-at-EM-eh-sis) vomiting blood

hematocrit (hee-MAT-oh-krit) test to judge or separate the blood; used to determine the ratio of red blood cells to total blood volume

hematology (HEE-mah-TAW-loh-jee) study of the blood

hematoma (HEE-mah-TOH-mah) mass of blood within an organ, cavity, or tissue

hematopoiesis (heh-MAH-toh-poh-EE-sis) formation of blood cells

hematuria (HEE-mah-TUR-ee-ah) bloody urination

heminephrectomy (HEH-mee-neh-FREK-toh-mee) surgical removal of half a kidney

hemodialysis (HEE-moh-dai-AL-ah-sis) procedure for removing waste from the bloodstream

hemolysis (hee-MAW-lih-sis) breakdown of blood cells

hemolytic anemia (HEE-moh-LIH-tik ah-NEE-mee-ah) anemia caused by the destruction of red blood cells

hemophilia (HEE-moh-FEE-lee-ah) condition in which the blood doesn't clot, thus causing excessive bleeding

hemoptysis (heem-op-TIS-is) coughing up blood

hemorrhage (HEM-oh-RIJ) excessive blood loss

hemorrhoid (HEM-oh-ROID) inflammation of the veins surrounding the anus

hemorrhoidectomy (HEM-oh-roi-DEK-toh-mee) surgical removal of hemorrhoids

hemothorax (heem-oh-THOR-aks) blood in the chest

hepatitis (HEH-pah-TAI-tis) inflammation of the liver

hepatomegaly (heh-PAT-oh-MEG-ah-lee) enlargement of the liver

hepatosplenomegaly (heh-PAT-oh-SPLEE-noh-MEH-gah-lee) enlargement of the liver and spleen

hernia (HER-nee-ah) rupture or protrusion of an organ through the wall that normally contains it

herniorrhaphy (her-nee-OR-ah-fee) suture of a hernia

heterograft (HEH-ter-oh-GRAFT) skin transplant taken from a species other than the patient's

hidradenitis (hih-dra-deh-NAI-tis) inflammation of the sweat glands

hidradenoma (hih-drad-eh-NOH-mah) tumor of the sweat gland

hidropoiesis (hih-droh-poh-EE-sis) the formation of sweat

homograft (HOH-moh-GRAFT) skin transplant taken from another member of the patient's species

hydrarthrosis (hai-drar-THROH-sis) water (fluid) in a joint

hydrocele (HAI-droh-SEEL) fluid-filled mass in a testicle

hydrocephaly (HAI-droh-SEH-fah-lee) abnormal accumulation of spinal fluid in the brain

hydronephrosis (HAI-droh-neh-FROH-sis) kidney condition caused by the obstruction of urine flow

hydrophobia (HAI-droh-FOH-bee-ah) fear of water

hypercapnia (hai-per-CAP-nee-yah) condition of having excessive carbon dioxide in the blood

hypercarbia (hai-per-CAR-bee-yah) excessive carbon dioxide

hyperemesis (HAI-per-EM-eh-sis) excessive vomiting

hyperemesis gravidarum (HAI-per-eh-MEE-sis GRAV-ih-DAR-um) excessive pregnancy-related vomiting; an extreme form of the more common morning sickness

hyperglycemia (HAI-per-glai-SEE-mee-ah) high blood sugar

hyperhidrosis (hai-per-hih-DROH-sis) excessive sweating

hyperkeratosis (hai-per-ker-ah-TOH-sis) excessive growth of horny skin

hyperkinesia (hai-per-kih-NEE-zhah) increase in muscle movement or activity

hyperlipidemia (HAI-per-lih-pih-DEE-mee-ah) excessive fat in the blood

hypermelanosis (hai-per-mel-an-OH-sis) excessive melanin in the skin

hyperopia (HAI-per-OH-pee-ah) farsightedness

hyperparathyroidism (HAI-per-PAR-ah-THAI-roid-IZM) overproduction by the parathyroid glands

hyperpigmentation (hai-per-pig-men-TAY-shun) excessive pigment in the skin

hyperpituitarism (HAI-per-pih-TOO-ih-tar-IZM) over-functioning of the pituitary gland

hyperpnea (hai-perp-NEE-ah) heavy breathing

hypertension (HAI-per-TEN-shun) high blood pressure

hyperthyroidism (HAI-per-THAI-roid-IZM) overproduction by the thyroid

hypertrichosis (HAI-per-trih-KOH-sis) excessive growth of hair

hypertrophy (hai-PER-troh-fee) overdevelopment of muscle tissue

hyperventilation (hai-per-ven-ti-LAY-shun) over-breathing; condition of having too much air flowing into and out of the lungs; leads to hypocapnia

hypocapnia (hai-poh-CAP-nee-yah) insufficient carbon dioxide

hypocarbia (hai-poh-CAR-bee-yah) insufficient carbon dioxide

hypodermic (hai-poh-DER-mik) pertaining to beneath the skin

hypoglycemia (HAI-poh-glai-SEE-mee-ah) low blood sugar

hypoglycemic (HAI-poh-glai-SEE-mik) pertaining to low blood sugar

hypohidrosis (hai-poh-hih-DROH-sis) diminished sweating

hypomagnesemia (HAI-poh-MAG-nee-SEE-mee-ah) deficient magnesium in the blood

hypomelanosis (hai-poh-mel-an-OH-sis) diminished melanin in the skin

hypoparathyroidism (HAI-poh-PAR-ah-THAI-roid-IZM) underproduction by the parathyroid

hypophysectomy (hai-POF-is-EK-toh-mee) removal of the pituitary gland

hypopigmentation (hai-poh-pig-men-TAY-shun) diminished pigment in the skin

hypopituitarism (HAI-poh-pih-TOO-ih-tar-IZM) condition caused by the undersecretion of the pituitary gland

hypopnea (hai-POP-nee-ah) shallow breathing

hypospadias (HAI-poh-SPAY-dee-as) birth defect in which the opening of the urethra is on the underside, instead of the end, of the penis

hypotension (HAI-poh-TEN-shun) low blood pressure

hypothyroidism (HAI-poh-THAI-roid-IZM) underproduction by the thyroid

hypotonia (hai-poh-TOH-nee-yah) decrease in muscle tone or tightness

hypoventilation (hai-poh-ven-ti-LAY-shun) under-breathing; condition of having too little air flowing into and out of the lungs; leads to hypercapnia

hypoxemia (hai-poks-EEM-ee-yah) insufficient oxygen in the blood

hypoxia (hai-POKS-ee-yah) insufficient oxygen

hysteralgia (HIS-ter-AL-jah) pain in the uterus

hysterectomy (HIS-ter-EK-toh-mee) surgical removal of the uterus

hysterocele (HIS-ter-oh-SEEL) hernia of the uterus

hysterodynia (HIS-ter-oh-DAI-nee-ah) pain in the uterus

hysteropexy (HIS-ter-oh-PEK-see) surgical fixation of the uterus

hysteroptosis (HIS-ter-awp-TOH-sis) downward displacement of the uterus into the vagina

hysterorrhexis (HIS-ter-oh-REK-sis) rupture of the uterus

hysterosalpingectomy (HIS-ter-oh-SAL-pin-JEK-toh-mee) surgical removal of the uterus and fallopian tube

hysterosalpingogram (HIS-ter-oh-sal-PIN-goh-gram) record of the uterus and fallopian tubes

hysteroscope (HIS-ter-oh-SKOHP) instrument for examining the uterus

hysteroscopy (HIS-ter-AW-skoh-pee) procedure for examining the uterus

hysterotomy (HIS-ter-AW-toh-mee) incision into the uterus

I

ichthyosis (ik-thee-OH-sis) a condition in which the skin is dry and scaly, resembling fish scales

icterus (IK-ter-us) see *jaundice*

ileostomy (IH-lee-AW-stoh-mee) creation of an opening in the ileum

immunocompromised (ih-MYOO-noh-COM-proh-MAIZD) having an immune system incapable of responding normally and completely to a pathogen or disease

immunodeficiency (ih-MYOO-noh-deh-FIH-shin-see) immune system with decreased or compromised response to disease-causing organisms

immunosuppression (ih-MYOO-noh-suh-PREH-shun) reduction in the activity of the body's immune system

impetigo (im-peh-TAI-goh) from Latin, for *to attack;* a highly contagious bacterial infection of the skin

in vitro fertilization (in VEE-troh FER-tih-lih-ZAY-shun) fertilization of an egg done in a test tube

incision and drainage (I&D) (in-SIH-zhun and DRAY-nij) to cut into a wound to allow trapped infected liquid to drain

incontinence (in-CON-tih-nentz) inability to control urination

induced abortion (in-DOOST ah-BOR-shun) the intentional termination of pregnancy

inferior vena cava (in-FEER-ee-or VEE-nah CAY-vah) portion of the vena cava that gathers blood from the lower portion of the body

insulin (IN-suh-lin) hormone secreted by the pancreas that controls the metabolism and uptake of sugar and fats

insulinoma (IN-suh-lin-OH-mah) tumor that secretes insulin (found in the insulin-producing cells in the pancreas)

intracerebral hematoma (IN-trah-seh-REE-bral HEE-mah-TOH-mah) a hematoma located inside the brain

intradermal (in-trah-DER-mal) pertaining to inside the skin

intraocular lens implant (IN-trah-AW-kyoo-lar lenz IM-plant) insertion of a new lens inside the eye

intravitreal antibiotic (IN-trah-VEE-tree-al AN-tai-bai-AW-tik) antibiotic administered directly into the vitreous gel liquid

iridectomy (EAR-id-EK-toh-mee) removal of the iris

iridopathy (EAR-ih-DOP-ah-thee) disease of the iris

iridotomy (EAR-id-AW-toh-mee) incision into the iris

iritis (ai-RAI-tis) inflammation of the iris

iron deficiency anemia (AI-ern deh-FIH-shin-see ah-NEE-mee-ah) anemia caused by inadequate iron intake

ischemia (ih-SKEE-mee-ah) blockage of blood flow to an organ

J

jaundice (JAWN-dis) yellowing of skin, tissue, and fluids caused by increased levels of bilirubin in the blood

jejunostomy (JE-joo-NAW-stoh-mee) creation of an opening in the jejunum

K

keloid (KEE-loid) overgrowth of scar tissue

keratalgia (KEH-rah-TAL-jah) pain in the cornea

keratogenic (keh-RA-toh-jen-ik) causing horny tissue development

keratopathy (KEH-ra-TOP-ah-thee) disease of the cornea

keratoplasty (ker-A-toh-PLAS-tee) surgical reconstruction of the cornea

keratosis (keh-rah-TOH-sis) horny tissue condition

keratotomy (KER-ah-TAW-toh-mee) incision into the cornea

kidney dialysis (KID-nee dai-AL-ah-sis) procedure for removing waste from the blood (an alternative name for hemodialysis)

kleptomania (KLEP-toh-MAY-nee-ah) desire to steal

kyphosis (kai-FOH-sis) humped back—abnormal forward curvature of the upper spine

L

laparocele (LAP-ar-oh-seel) abdominal hernia

laparonephrectomy (LAP-ah-roh-neh-FREK-toh-mee) surgical removal of a kidney through the abdomen

laparoscope (LAP-ar-oh-skohp) instrument for looking inside the abdomen

laparoscopic surgery (LAP-rah-SKAW-pik SIR-jir-ee) use of a laparoscope to perform minimally invasive surgery

laparoscopy (LAP-ar-AW-skoh-pee) procedure for looking inside the abdomen

laryngectomy (la-rin-JEK-toe-mee) removal of the larynx

laryngitis (la-rin-JAI-tis) inflammation of the larynx

laryngotracheobronchitis (la-rin-go-tray-key-o-bron-KAI-tis) inflammation of the larynx, trachea, and bronchi

leukemia (loo-KEE-mee-ah) cancer of the blood or bone marrow characterized by the abnormal increase in white blood cells

leukocyte (LOO-koh-sait) white blood cell

leukoderma (loo-koh-DER-mah) white skin

leukopenia (LOO-koh-PEE-nee-ah) deficiency in white blood cells

lipectomy (lih-PEK-toh-mee) removal of fatty tissue

liposuction (LAI-poh-SUK-shun) removal of fatty tissue using a vacuum

lithectomy (lih-THEK-toh-mee) surgical removal of a stone in the bladder

lithotripsy (LIH-thoh-TRIP-see) breakdown of a stone

lobectomy (loh-BEK-toh-mee) removal of a lobe

lordosis (lor-DOH-sis) swayback—abnormal forward curvature of the lower spine

lumbar puncture (LP) (LUM-bar PUNK-chir) inserting a needle into the lumbar region of the spine in order to collect spinal fluid

lymphadenectomy (lim-FAD-eh-NEK-toh-mee) surgical removal of a lymph gland (node)

lymphadenitis (LIM-fad-eh-NAI-tis) inflammation of a lymph gland (node)

lymphadenopathy (lim-FAD-eh-NAW-pah-thee) any disease of a lymph gland (node); used to refer to noticeably swollen lymph nodes, especially in the neck

lymphadenotomy (lim-FAD-eh-NAW-toh-mee) incision into a lymph gland (node)

lymphangiography (lim-FAN-jee-AW-grah-fee) procedure to study the lymph vessels

lymphangitis (LIM-fan-JAI-tis) inflammation of the lymph vessels

lymphedema (LIMF-ah-DEE-mah) swelling caused by abnormal accumulation of lymph

lymphocyte (LIM-foh-SAIT) lymph cell

lymphoma (lim-FOH-mah) tumor originating in lymphocytes

M

macule (MA-kyool) from Latin, for *spot* or *stain;* small, flat, discolored area (freckle)

malignant melanoma (ma-LIG-nant meh-lah-NOH-mah) a harmful tumor of melanin cells

mammogram (MAM-oh-GRAM) record of a breast exam

mammoplasty (MAM-oh-PLAS-tee) surgical reconstruction of a breast

mastalgia (mas-TAL-jah) breast pain

mastectomy (mas-TEK-toh-mee) surgical removal of a breast

mastitis (mas-TAI-tis) inflammation of the breast

mastopexy (MAS-toh-PEK-see) surgical fixation of a breast

mastoptosis (MAS-top-TOH-sis) downward displacement (drooping) of the breast

meningitis (MEH-nin-JAI-tus) inflammation of the meninges

meningocele (meh-NIN-goh-seel) a hernia of the meninges

menopause (MEN-oh-pawz) cessation of menstruation

menorrhagia (MEN-oh-RAY-jah) excessive menstrual flow

menorrhalgia (MEN-oh-RAL-jah) painful menstruation

metrorrhagia (MEH-troh-RAY-jah) menstrual bleeding at irregular times

miosis (mai-OH-sis) abnormal contraction of the pupil (from Greek, for *to lessen*)

miotic (mai-AW-tik) drug that causes the abnormal contraction of the pupil

mononucleosis (MAW-noh-NOO-klee-OH-sis) condition characterized by an abnormally large number of mononuclear leukocytes

mucolytic (myoo-koh-LIT-ik) a drug that aids in the breakdown of mucus

murmur (MIR-mir) abnormal heart sound

muscular dystrophy (MUS-kyoo-lar DIS-troh-fee) disorder characterized by poor muscle development

myalgia (mai-AL-jah) muscle pain

mycodermatitis (mai-koh-der-mah-TAI-tis) inflammation of the skin caused by fungus

mydriasis (mi-DRAI-ah-sis) abnormal dilation of the pupil

mydriatic (MID-ree-AT-ik) drug that causes the abnormal dilation of the pupil

myectomy (mai-EK-toh-mee) removal of muscle

myelitis (MAI-el-AI-tis) inflammation of the spinal cord

myelogram (MAI-el-oh-gram) image of the spinal cord, usually done using x-ray

myeloma (MAI-eh-LOH-mah) cancerous tumor of the bone marrow

myocardial infarction (MAI-oh-KAR-dee-al in-FARK-shun) death of heart muscle tissue

myocardial ischemia (MAI-oh-KAR-dee-al ih-SKEE-mee-ah) blockage of blood to the heart muscle

myocarditis (MAI-oh-kar-DAI-tis) inflammation of the heart muscle

myocardium (MAI-oh-KAR-dee-um) heart muscle tissue

myolysis (mai-AW-lih-sis) loss of muscle tissue

myoma (mai-OH-mah) a muscle tumor

myomectomy (MAI-oh-MEK-toh-mee) surgical removal of a tumor in the muscle (usually refers to the muscle of the uterine wall)

myometrium (MAI-oh-MEE-tree-um) the middle layer of uterine muscle tissue

myopathy (mai-AW-pah-thee) muscle disease

myopia (mai-OH-pee-ah) nearsightedness

myoplasty (MAI-oh-PLAS-tee) muscle reconstruction

myorrhaphy (mai-OR-ah-fee) muscle suture

myosarcoma (MAI-oh-sar-KOH-mah) a cancerous muscle tumor

myositis (MAI-oh-SAI-tis) muscle inflammation

myotomy (mai-AW-toh-mee) incision into muscle

myringitis (MIR-in-JAI-tis) inflammation of the eardrum

myringomycosis (mir-IN-goh-mai-KOH-sis) fungal condition of the eardrum

myringoplasty (mir-IN-goh-PLAS-tee) surgical reconstruction of the eardrum

myringotomy (mir-in-GAW-toh-mee) incision into the eardrum

myxedema (MIX-eh-DEE-mah) swelling of the skin caused by deposits under the skin

N

narcolepsy (NAR-coh-LEP-see) a disease characterized by sudden, uncontrolled sleepiness

nasogastric tube (NAY-soh-GAS-trik TOOB) tube inserted through the nose into the stomach

nasolacrimal (NAY-zoh-LAH-krih-mal) pertaining to the nose and tear system

natal (NAY-tal) pertaining to birth

nebulizer (neh-byoo-LAI-zir) a machine that administers respiratory medication by creating a "cloud" or mist that is inhaled by the patient

necrosis (neh-KROH-sis) tissue death

neonatal (NEE-oh-NAY-tal) pertaining to new birth (normally the first 28 days after birth)

neonatologist (NEE-oh-nay-TAW-loh-jist) specialist in the neonatal period

neonatology (NEE-oh-nay-TAW-loh-jee) study of the neonatal period

nephralgia (neh-FRAL-jah) pain in the kidney

nephrectomy (neh-FREK-toh-mee) surgical removal of a kidney

nephritis (neh-FRAI-tis) inflammation of the kidney

nephrolithiasis (NEH-froh-lih-THAI-ah-sis) the presence of stones in the kidney

nephrolithotomy (NEH-froh-lih-THAW-toh-mee) incision into a kidney to remove a stone

nephrologist (neh-FRAW-loh-jist) specialist in the kidneys

nephrology (neh-FRAW-loh-jee) study of the kidneys

nephromalacia (NEH-froh-mah-LAY-shah) abnormal softening of a kidney

nephromegaly (NEH-froh-MEG-ah-lee) abnormal enlargement of a kidney

nephropathy (neh-FRAW-pah-thee) any kidney disease

nephropexy (NEH-froh-PEK-see) surgical fixation of a kidney

nephroptosis (nef-rop-TOH-sis) downward displacement of a kidney

nephroscopy (ne-FRAW-skoh-pee) procedure for examining a kidney

nephrosis (neh-FROH-sis) kidney condition

nephrosonography (NEF-roh-soh-NAW-grah-fee) procedure for imaging a kidney using sound waves

nephrosplenopexy (NEF-roh-SPLEE-noh-PEK-see) surgical fixation of the spleen and a kidney

nephrostomy (neh-FRAW-stoh-mee) creation of an opening in a kidney

nephrotomy (neh-FRAW-toh-mee) incision into a kidney to remove a stone

nephrotoxin (NEH-froh-TOK-sin) an agent poisonous to the kidney

neuralgia (nur-AL-jah) nerve pain

neurectomy (nir-EK-toh-mee) removal of a nerve

neuritis (nir-AI-tis) nerve inflammation

neurolysis (nir-AW-lih-sis) destruction of nerve tissue

neuropathy (nir-AW-pah-thee) disease of the nervous system

neuroplasty (NIR-oh-PLAS-tee) reconstruction of a nerve

neurorrhaphy (nir-OR-ah-fee) suturing of a nerve (often the severed ends of a nerve)

neurosis (neh-ROH-sis) a nerve condition

nevus (NEE-vus) from Latin, for *birthmark* or *mole;* a mole

nodule (NAWD-jyool) a solid mass that extends deep into the skin

nystagmus (nih-STAG-mus) involuntary back-and-forth movement of the eyes (from Greek, for *to nod*)

O

obstetrician (OB-steh-TRIH-shun) specialist in pregnancy, labor, and delivery of newborns

obstetrics (ob-STEH-triks) branch of medicine dealing with pregnancy, labor, and delivery of newborns

occlusion (oh-KLOO-zhun) closing or blockage of a passage

oculopathy (AW-kyoo-LAW-pah-thee) disease of the eye

odontalgia (OH-dawn-TAL-jah) tooth pain

odontectomy (oh-dawn-TEK-toh-mee) surgical removal of a tooth

odontodynia (oh-DAWN-toh-DAI-nee-ah) tooth pain

oligomenorrhea (AW-lih-goh-MEN-oh-REE-ah) infrequent or light menstrual periods

oliguria (aw-lih-GYIR-ee-ah) low urine output

onychectomy (aw-nik-EK-toh-mee) removal of a nail

onychia (oh-NIK-ee-ah) a nail condition

onychocryptosis (AW-nih-koh-krip-TOH-sis) an ingrown nail

onychomycosis (AW-nih-koh-mai-KOH-sis) a fungal condition of the nail

onychopathy (aw-nik-AW-pah-thee) nail disease

onychotomy (aw-ni-KAW-toh-mee) incision into a nail

oophorectomy (OH-aw-for-EK-toh-mee) surgical removal of an ovary

oophoritis (OH-aw-for-AI-tis) inflammation of an ovary

oophorocystectomy (oh-AW-for-oh-sis-TEK-toh-mee) surgical removal of an ovarian cyst

oophorotomy (oh-AW-for-AW-toh-mee) incision into an ovary

ophthalmalgia (awf-thal-MAL-jah) eye pain

ophthalmitis (AWF-thal-MAI-tis) inflammation of the eye

ophthalmologist (AWF-thal-MAW-loh-jist) eye specialist

ophthalmopathy (AWF-thal-MOH-pah-thee) eye disease

ophthalmoplegia (off-THAL-moh-PLEE-jah) eye paralysis

ophthalmoscope (awf-THAL-mah-SKOHP) instrument for looking at the eye

optic (AWP-tik) pertaining to the eye

optometrist (awp-TAW-meh-trist) specialist in measuring the eye

orchialgia (OR-kee-AL-jah) testicle pain

orchichorhea (OR-kee-kor-EE-ah) involuntary jerking movement of the testicles

orchidectomy (OR-kid-EK-toh-mee) surgical removal of a testicle

orchiditis (OR-kih-DAI-tis) inflammation of the testicles and epididymis

orchidopexy (OR-kid-oh-PEK-see) surgical fixation of a testicle

orchidoptosis (OR-kih-dop-TOH-sis) downward displacement of a testicle

orchidotomy (OR-kid-AW-toh-mee) incision into a testicle

orchiectomy (OR-kee-EK-toh-mee) surgical removal of a testicle

orchiodynia (OR-kee-oh-DAI-nee-ah) testicle pain

orchiopexy (OR-kee-oh-PEK-see) surgical fixation of a testicle

orchioplasty (OR-kee-oh-PLAS-tee) surgical reconstruction of a testicle

orchitis (or-KAI-tis) inflammation of the testicles and epididymis

orthodontics (or-thoh-DAWN-tiks) branch of medicine dealing with the straightening of teeth

orthodontist (or-thoh-DAWN-tist) specialist in straightening teeth

orthopnea (or-thop-NEE-ah) able to breathe only in an upright position

ostealgia (aw-stee-AL-jah) bone pain

osteitis (AW-stee-AI-tis) bone inflammation

osteoarthritis (AW-stee-oh-ar-THRAI-tis) inflammation of the joints, specifically those that bear weight

osteochondritis (AW-stee-oh-kon-DRAI-tis) inflammation of bone and cartilage

osteochondroma (AW-stee-oh-kon-DROH-mah) a tumor made up of bone and cartilage

osteodynia (aw-stee-oh-DAI-nee-ah) bone pain

osteodystrophy (aw-stee-oh-DIH-stroh-fee) poor bone development

osteomalacia (AW-stee-oh-mah-LAY-shah) softening of the bone

osteomyelitis (AW-stee-oh-MAI-eh-LAI-tis) inflammation of the bone and bone marrow

osteopenia (AW-stee-oh-PEE-nee-yah) reduction in bone volume

osteoporosis (AW-stee-oh-por-OH-sis) loss of bone density

otalgia (oh-TAL-jah) ear pain

otitis externa (oh-TAI-tis eks-TERN-nah) inflammation of the outer ear

otitis media (oh-TAI-tis MEH-dee-ah) inflammation of the middle ear

otolaryngologist (OH-toh-LAH-rin-GAW-loh-jist) specialist in the ear and throat

otomycosis (oh-toh-mai-KOH-sis) a fungal ear condition

otoneurologist (OH-toh-nih-RAW-loh-jist) specialist in the nerve connections between the ear and brain

otoplasty (OH-toh-PLAS-tee) surgical reconstruction of the ear

otorhinolaryngologist (OH-toh-RAI-noh-LAH-rin-GAW-loh-jist) specialist in the ear, nose, and throat

otosclerosis (oh-toh-skleh-ROH-sis) hearing loss caused by the hardening of the bones of the middle ear

otoscope (OH-toh-SKOHP) instrument for looking in the ear

otoscopy (oh-TAW-skoh-pee) procedure for looking in the ear

ototoxic (OH-toh-TOK-sik) drug that is damaging to the ear/hearing

ovaralgia (OH-var-AL-jah) pain in the ovaries

ovarialgia (oh-VAR-ee-AL-jah) pain in the ovaries

ovarian cystectomy (oh-VAR-ee-an sis-TEK-toh-mee) surgical removal of an ovarian cyst

ovariocyesis (oh-VAR-ee-oh-sai-EE-sis) ectopic pregnancy in an ovary

ovariorrhexis (oh-VAR-ee-oh-REK-sis) rupture of an ovary

ovariostomy (oh-VAR-ee-AW-stoh-me) creation of an opening into an ovary

oximetry (ok-SIM-ah-tree) a procedure to measure oxygen levels

oxytocin (OK-see-TOH-sin) agent that stimulates uterine contractions and accelerates labor

P

palpitation (PAL-pih-TAY-shun) rapid or irregular beating of the heart

pancreatectomy (PAN-kree-ah-TEK-toh-mee) surgical removal of the pancreas

pancreatitis (PAN-kree-ah-TAI-tis) inflammation of the pancreas

pancreatography (PAN-kree-ah-TAW-graw-FEE) procedure for mapping the pancreas

pancreatolith (PAN-kree-AT-oh-lith) stone in the pancreas

pancreatolithiasis (PAN-kree-at-oh-lih-THAI-ah-sis) presence of a stone in the pancreas

panhypopituitarism (PAN-HAI-poh-pih-TOO-ih-tar-IZM) defective or absent function of the entire pituitary gland

pansinusitis (pan-sai-nus-AI-tis) inflammation of all sinuses

Pap (Papanicolaou) smear (PAP SMEER) test used to detect cancer cells, most commonly in the cervix

papule (PA-pyool) from Latin, for *pimple;* a small, solid mass

paralysis (puh-RAH-lu-sis) complete loss of sensation and motor function

parathyroidectomy (PAR-ah-THAI-roid EK-toh-mee) removal of the parathyroid

paresis (puh-REE-sis) partial paralysis characterized by varying degrees of sensation and motor function

patch (pach) large, flat discolored area

pectoralgia (PEK-tor-AL-jah) chest pain

pectus carinatum (PEK-tus car-ee-NAH-tum) a chest that protrudes like the keel of a ship

pelvicephalometry (PEL-vih-SEF-eh-LAW-meh-tree) procedure for measuring the head size of the baby and the pelvis size of the mother

percutaneous (per-kyoo-TAY-nee-us) pertaining to through the skin

percutaneous coronary intervention (PER-kyoo-TAY-nee-us KOR-ah-NAR-ee IN-ter-VEN-shun) alternative treatment for the coronary artery that passes instruments up a patient's blood vessels into the heart

pericarditis (PER-ee-kar-DAI-tis) inflammation of the tissue around the heart

pericardium (PER-ee- KAR-dee-um) tissue around the heart

perineoplasty (PER-ih-NEE-oh-PLAS-tee) surgical reconstruction of the perineum

perineorrhaphy (PER-ih-nee-OR-ah-fee) suture of the perineum

perineotomy (PER-ih-nee-AW-toh-mee) incision into the perineum

peritonitis (PER-ih-toh-NAI-tis) inflammation of the peritoneum

petechia (puh-TEE-kee-yah) small bruise

phacoemulsification (FAY-koh-ee-MUL-sih-fih-KAY-shun) fragmentation of an existing lens in order to remove and replace it

phimosis (fih-MOH-sis) contraction of the foreskin of the penis, preventing it from being retracted

phlebalgia (fleh-BAL-jah) pain in a vein

phlebectomy (fleb-EK-toh-mee) surgical removal of a vein

phlebitis (fleh-BAI-tis) inflammation of the veins

phlebotomist (fleh-BAW-toh-mist) specialist in drawing blood

phlebotomy (fleh-BAW-toh-mee) incision into a vein (another name for drawing blood)

phrenoplegia (fre-no-PLEE-jah) paralysis of the diaphragm

phrenospasm (fre-no-SPAZ-um) involuntary contraction of the diaphragm

pituitary dwarfism (pih-TOO-ih-TER-ee DWAR-fizm) abnormally short height caused by undersecretions of growth hormone from the pituitary gland

pituitary gigantism (pih-TOO-ih-TER-ee jai-GAN-tizm) abnormally tall height caused by oversecretion of growth hormone from the pituitary gland

placenta previa (plah-SIN-tah PREE-vee-ah) condition in which the placenta is attached to the uterus near the cervix

plaque (PLAK) a solid mass on the surface of the skin

plasmapheresis (PLAZ-mah-fer-EE-sis) apheresis to remove plasma

plateletpheresis (PLAYT-let-fer-EE-sis) apheresis to remove platelets (for the purpose of donating them to patients in need of platelets)

pleural effusion (PLUR-al ef-YOO-zhun) fluid pouring out into the pleura

pleuralgia (plur-AL-jah) pain in the pleura

pleurisy (PLUR-ih-see) inflammation of the pleura; another word for pleuritis

pleuritis (plur-AI-tis) inflammation of the pleura

pleurodynia (plur-oh-DAI-nee-ah) pain in the pleura

pleuropexy (ploo-rah-PEK-see) reattachment of the pleura

pneumoconiosis (new-moh-con-i-OH-sis) a lung condition caused by dust

pneumohemothorax (new-moh-hee-moh-THOR-aks) air and blood in the chest

pneumonectomy (new-mon-EK-toe-mee) removal of a lung

pneumonia (new-MOH-nee-yah) a lung condition

pneumonitis (new-moh-NAI-tis) inflammation of the lung

pneumothorax (new-moh-THOR-aks) air in the chest

poliomyelitis (POH-lee-oh-MAI-el-AI-tis) inflammation of the gray matter of the spinal cord

polycystic kidney disease (PAW-lee-SIS-tik KID-nee dih-ZEEZ) disease characterized by the formation of many fluid-filled cysts in the kidneys

polydipsia (PAW-lee-DIP-see-ah) excessive thirst

polysomnography (paw-lee-som-NAH-gra-fee) recording multiple aspects of sleep

polyuria (PAW-lee-YOO-ree-ah) excessive urination

positron emission tomography (PET) scan (PAWZ-ih-trawn ee-MISH-un taw-MAW-gra-fee skan) an imaging procedure that uses radiation (positrons) to produce cross sections of the brain

postnatal (post-NAY-tal) pertaining to after birth

postpartum (post-PAR-tum) pertaining to after birth

preeclampsia (PREE-eh-KLAMP-see-ah) condition characterized by high blood pressure and high levels of protein in the urine

prenatal (pree-NAY-tal) pertaining to before birth

presbycusis (PREZ-bih-KOO-sis) loss of hearing in old age

presbyopia (PREZ-bee-OH-pee-ah) decreased vision caused by old age

priapism (PREE-ap-izm) persistent and painful erection

proctologist (prok-TAW-loh-jist) specialist in the anus, rectum, and colon

proctology (prok-TAW-loh-jee) branch of medicine dealing with the anus, rectum, and colon

proctoscope (PROK-toh-skohp) instrument for looking at the anus and rectum

proctoscopy (prok-TAW-skoh-pee) procedure for looking at the anus and rectum

prostatectomy (PROS-tat-TEK-toh-mee) surgical removal of the prostate

prostatitis (PROS-tah-TAI-tis) inflammation of the prostate

prostatomegaly (PROS-ta-toh-MEH-gah-lee) abnormal enlargement of the prostate

pruritus (prur-AI-tis) from Latin, for *burning nettle;* swollen, raised, itchy areas of the skin

pseudocyesis (SOO-doh-sai-EE-sis) false pregnancy

psychiatrist (sai-KAI-ah-trist) doctor who specializes in treatment of the mind

psychiatry (sai-KAI-ah-tree) branch of medicine that focuses on the treatment of the mind

psychologist (sai-KAW-loh-jist) doctor who specializes in the study of the mind

psychology (sai-KAW-loh-jee) branch of medicine that focuses on the study of the mind

psychosis (sai-KOH-sis) a mind condition (involves some sort of break with reality interfering with rational thought or daily functioning)

psychosomatic (SAI-koh-soh-MA-tik) pertaining to the relationship between the body and the mind

pterygium (ter-IH-jee-um) winglike growth of conjunctival tissue extending to the cornea (from Greek, for *wing*)

pulmonary angiography (pul-mon-AIR-ee an-jee-AH-grah-fee) an imaging procedure for recording pulmonary blood vessel activity

pulmonary edema (pul-mon-AIR-ee ah-DEE-ma) swelling in the lungs

pulmonary embolism (pul-mon-AIR-ee em-bol-IZ-um) blockage in the pulmonary blood supply

pulmonary function testing (pul-mon-AIR-ee funk-shun TES-ting) a group of tests used to evaluate the condition of the lungs

pustule (PUS-tyool) from Latin, for *little blister;* a pus-filled blister

pyelitis (PAI-el-AI-tis) inflammation of the renal pelvis

pyelogram (PAI-el-oh-GRAM) image of the renal pelvis

pyelolithotomy (PAI-el-oh-lih-THAW-toh-mee) incision into a renal pelvis to remove a stone

pyelonephritis (PAI-el-oh-neh-FRAI-tis) inflammation of the kidney and renal pelvis

pyelopathy (PAI-el-AW-pah-thee) disease of the renal pelvis

pyelostomy (PAI-el-AW-stoh-mee) creation of an opening in a renal pelvis

pyromania (PAI-roh-MAY-nee-ah) desire to set fires

pyuria (pai-YUR-ee-ah) pus in the urine

R

renal angiography (REE-nal AN-jee-AW-grah-fee) process of imaging a kidney blood vessel

renal cell carcinoma (REE-nal SELL KAR-sih-NOH-mah) cancer of the kidneys; also known as hypernephroma

renal failure (REE-nal FAY-el-yur) kidney failure

retinal (REH-tih-nal) pertaining to the retina

retinopathy (REH-tih-NOP-ah-thee) disease of the retina

retinopexy (reh-TIH-noh-PEK-see) surgical fixation (reattachment) of a retina

retrograde pyelogram (REH-troh-grayd PAI-el-oh-GRAM) image of the renal pelvis produced by injecting a contrast dye from the bladder to the kidney

rheumatoid arthritis (ROO-mah-toyd ar-THRAI-tis) inflammation of the joint; called rheumatoid because its symptoms resemble those of rheumatic fever

rhinitis (rai-NAI-tis) inflammation of the nasal passages

rhinorrhea (rai-no-REE-yah) runny nose

S

salpingectomy (SAL-pin-JEK-toh-mee) surgical removal of a fallopian tube

salpingitis (SAL-pin-JAI-tis) inflammation of a fallopian tube

salpingocele (sal-PING-goh-seel) hernia of a fallopian tube

salpingocyesis (sal-PING-goh-sai-EE-sis) ectopic pregnancy in a fallopian tube

salpingo-oophorectomy (sal-PING-goh-OH-aw-for-EK-toh-mee) surgical removal of a fallopian tube and ovary

salpingopexy (sal-PING-goh-PEK-see) surgical fixation of a fallopian tube

scale (SKAYL) skin flaking off

schizophrenia (SKIT-zoh-FREH-nee-ah) a mental illness characterized by delusions, hallucinations, and disordered speech

sclerodermatitis (skleh-roh-der-mah-TAI-tis) inflammation of the skin accompanied by thickening and hardening

scleronychia (skleh-raw-NIH-kee-ah) thickening and hardening of the nails

scoliosis (SKOH-lee-OH-sis) crooked back, or abnormal lateral curvature of the spine

sensorineural hearing loss (SEN-sor-ee-NIR-al HEER-ing loss) sound is not transmitted from the inner ear to the brain (due to problems with the sense organs or nerves)

septicemia (SEP-tih-SEE-mee-ah) presence of disease-causing microorganisms in the blood

sialoadenectomy (sai-AL-oh-AD-en-EK-toh-mee) surgical removal of a salivary gland

sialoadenitis (sai-AL-oh-AD-en-AI-tis) inflammation of the salivary glands

sialolith (sai-AL-oh-lith) stone in the saliva

sialolithiasis (sai-AL-oh-lih-THAI-ah-sis) presence of salivary stones

sigmoidoscopy (sig-moy-DAW-skoh-pee) procedure for looking at the sigmoid colon

sinusitis (sai-nus-AI-tis) inflammation of the sinus

sleep apnea (sleep AP-nee-ah) a condition where the patient ceases to breathe while asleep

spermatogenesis (sper-MAT-oh-JIN-eh-sis) creation of sperm

spermicide (SPER-mih-sahyd) agent that kills sperm

sphygmomanometer (SFIG-moh-mah-NAW-meh-ter) fancy name for the device used to measure blood pressure

spirometry (speer-AH-me-tree) a procedure to measure breathing

splenalgia (splee-NAL-jah) pain in the spleen

splenectomy (spleh-NEK-toh-mee) surgical removal of the spleen

splenitis (splee-NAI-tis) inflammation of the spleen

splenodynia (SPLEE-noh-DAI-nee-ah) pain in the spleen

splenomegaly (SPLEE-noh-MEH-gah-lee) enlargement of the spleen

splenorrhexis (SPLEE-noh-REK-sis) rupture of the spleen

spondylitis (spawn-dih-LAI-tis) inflammation of the vertebra

spondylodynia (spawn-dih-loh-DAI-nee-ah) vertebra pain

spondylolisthesis (SPAWN-dih-loh-lis-THEE-sis) the slipping or dislocation of a vertebra

spondylomalacia (spawn-dih-loh-mah-LAY-shah) softening of the vertebra

spondylosis (SPAWN-dih-LOH-sis) vertebra condition

spondylosyndesis (SPAWN-dih-loh-sin-DEE-sis) fusing together of multiple vertebrae

spontaneous abortion (spawn-TAY-nee-is ah-BOR-shun) the naturally occurring termination of pregnancy; also known as a miscarriage.

sputum (SPYOO-tum) mucus discharged from the lungs by coughing

steatitis (stay-ah-TAI-tis) inflammation of fat tissue

steatoma (STAY-ah-TOH-ma) a fatty tumor

sternotomy (stir-NAW-toh-mee) incision into the sternum

stomatitis (STOH-mah-TAI-tis) inflammation of the mouth

stomatogastric (stoh-MAT-oh-GAS-trik) pertaining to the mouth and stomach

strabismus (struh-BIZ-mus) condition where the eyes deviate when looking at the same object (from Latin, for *to squint*)

stress urinary incontinence (SUI) (stress YUR-ih-NAR-ee in-CON-tih-nentz) loss of bladder control caused by the application of external pressure

stroke (STROHK) loss of brain function caused by interruption of blood flow/supply to the brain

subcutaneous (sub-kyoo-TAY-nee-us) pertaining to beneath the skin

subdural hematoma (sub-DIR-al HEE-mah-TOH-mah) a hematoma located beneath the dura

syncope (SIN-koh-pee) fainting; losing consciousness due to temporary loss of blood flow to the brain

T

tachycardia (TAK-ih-KAR-dee-ah) rapid heartbeat

tachypnea (ta-KIP-nee-yah) rapid breathing

tarsoptosis (tar-sawp-TOH-sis) flat feet

tenalgia (ten-AL-jah) tendon pain

tendonitis (TEN-dah-NAI-tis) tendon inflammation

tenorrhaphy (ten-OR-ah-fee) suture of a tendon

testicular carcinoma (tes-TIK-yoo-lar KAR-sih-NOH-mah) testicular cancer

testitis (tes-TAI-tis) inflammation of the testicles and epididymis

thoracalgia (thor-a-KAL-jah) chest pain

thoracentesis (thor-a-sin-TEE-sis) puncture of the chest

thoracocentesis (thor-a-koh-sin-TEE-sis) puncture of the chest

thoracoscopy (thor-a-KOS-koh-pee) examination of the chest

thoracostomy (thor-a-KOS-toe-mee) creation of an opening in the chest

thoracotomy (thor-a-KAH-toe-mee) incision into the chest

thrombocyte (THROM-boh-sait) cell that helps blood clot (also known as a platelet)

thromboembolism (THROM-boh-EM-boh-LIZ-um) blockage of a vessel (embolism) caused by a clot that has broken off from where it formed

thrombolytic (THROM-boh-LIH-tik) drug that breaks down blood clots

thrombophlebitis (THROM-boh-fleh-BAI-tis) inflammation of a vein caused by a clot

thrombosis (throm-BOH-sis) formation of a blood clot

thrombus (THROM-bus) blood clot

thymectomy (thai-MEK-toh-mee) surgical removal of the thymus

thyroid function tests (THAI-roid FUNK-shun TESTS) tests performed to evaluate the function of the thyroid

thyroidectomy (THAI-roid-EK-toh-mee) removal of the thyroid

thyroiditis (THAI-roid-AI-tis) inflammation of the thyroid

thyroidotomy (THAI-roid-AW-toh-mee) incision into the thyroid

thyroidotoxin (thai-ROI-doh-TOK-sin) substance poisonous to the thyroid gland

thyrotoxicosis (THAI-roh-TOKS-ih-KOH-sis) condition caused by the exposure of body tissue to excessive levels of thyroid hormone (an extreme version of this is known as a thyroid storm)

thyrotropin (THAI-roh-TROH-pin) hormone that stimulates the thyroid

tibialgia (tih-bee-AL-ja) tibia (shin) pain

tinnitus (tih-NAI-tis) ringing in the ears (from Latin, for *to ring* or *jingle*)

tocodynagraph (TOH-koh-DAI-nah-GRAF) instrument for recording the strength of labor contractions

tocolytic (TOH-koh-LIH-tik) agent that stops or delays premature labor and contractions

tonometer (TOH-naw-MEE-tir) instrument for measuring tension or pressure in the eye (intraocular pressure)

tonsillectomy (TON-sil-EK-toh-mee) surgical removal of a tonsil

tonsillitis (TON-sil-AI-tis) inflammation of a tonsil

tracheostomy (tray-kee-AH-stoh-mee) creation of an opening in the trachea

tracheotomy (tray-kee-AH-toe-mee) incision into the trachea

transdermal (trans-DER-mal) pertaining to through the skin

transesophageal electrocardiogram (TRANZ-eh-SOF-ah-JEE-al eh-LEK-troh-KAR-dee-oh-GRAM) record of the heart using sound waves performed by inserting a sonograph into the esophagus

transfusion (tranz-FYOO-zhun) infusion into a patient of blood from another source

transient ischemic attack (TIA) (TRAN-zee-ent ih-SKEE-mik ah-TAK) a mini-stroke caused by the blockage of a blood vessel that resolves (goes away) within 24 hours

transrectal ultrasonography (TRANZ-REK-tal UL-trah-soh-NAW-grah-fee) procedure involving a probe inserted into the rectum using high-frequency sound

waves to scan through the rectum to nearby tissue (most commonly, the prostate)

transurethral resection of the prostate (TURP) (TRANS-yoo-REE-thral ree-SEK-shun of the PROS-tayt) procedure of removing all or part of the prostate by the insertion of a resectoscope into the urethra

transvaginal sonography (TRANZ-VAJ-ih-nal soh-NAW-grah-fee) imaging procedure using sound waves emitted from a device inserted in the vagina

trichomegaly (tri-koh-MEG-ah-lee) abnormally thick hair

trichomycosis (trik-koh-mai-KOH-sis) a fungal condition of the hair

tumor (TOO-mur) a large solid mass

tympanocentesis (tim-PAN-oh-sin-TEE-sis) puncture of the eardrum

tympanoplasty (tim-PAN-oh-PLAS-tee) surgical reconstruction of the eardrum

tympanostomy (TIM-pan-AW-stoh-mee) creation of an opening in the eardrum

U

ulcer (UL-sir) from Latin, for *sore;* a sore

ultrasonography (UL-trah-soh-NAW-grah-fee) imaging procedure using high-frequency sound waves

uremia (yoo-REE-mee-ah) presence of urinary waste in the blood

ureteritis (yoo-REE-ter-AI-tis) inflammation of a ureter

ureteroplasty (yoo-REE-ter-oh-PLAS-tee) surgical reconstruction of a ureter

ureteropyelonephritis (yoo-REE-ter-oh-PAI-el-oh-neh-FRAI-tis) inflammation of a kidney, renal pelvis, and ureter

urethritis (yoo-ree-THRAI-tis) inflammation of the urethra

urethrocele (yoo-REE-throh-seel) hernia or prolapse of the urethra into the vagina

urethrocystitis (yoo-REE-throh-sis-TAI-tis) inflammation of the urethra and bladder

urethrodynia (yoo-REE-throh-DAI-nee-ah) pain in the urethra

urethrorrhea (yoo-REE-throh-REE-ah) discharge from the urethra

urethroscopy (yoo-ree-THRAW-skoh-pee) process of examining the urethra

urethrostenosis (yoo-REE-throh-steh-NOH-sis) narrowing of the urethra

urinalysis (YUR-ih-NAL-ih-sis) analysis of the urine

urinary catheterization (YUR-ih-NAR-ee KATH-eh-ter-ih-ZAY-shun) insertion of a catheter into the bladder to drain urine

urinary tract infection (UTI) (YUR-ih-NAR-ee trakt in-FEK-shun) infection of the urinary tract

urodynia (YUR-oh-DAI-nee-ah) painful urination

urologist (yur-AW-loh-jist) specialist in the urinary tract

urology (yur-AW-loh-jee) study of the urinary tract

urticaria (ur-tih-KAR-ee-ah) swollen raised itchy areas of the skin

V

vaginitis (VAJ-ih-NAI-tis) inflammation of the vagina

vaginodynia (VAJ-ih-noh-DAI-nee-ah) vaginal pain

vaginoperineoplasty (VAJ-ih-noh-PER-ih-NEE-oh-PLAS-tee) suture of the vagina and perineum

vaginoperineorrhaphy (VAJ-ih-noh-PER-ih-nee-OR-ah-fee) suture of the vagina and perineum

vaginoperineotomy (VAJ-ih-noh-PER-ih-nee-AW-toh-mee) incision into the vagina and perineum

vaginoplasty (vah-JI-noh-PLAS-tee) surgical reconstruction of the vagina

valvotomy (val-VAW-toh-mee) incision into a heart valve

valvuloplasty (VAL-vyoo-loh-PLAS-tee) surgical reconstruction of a heart valve

varicocele (VAR-ih-koh-SEEL) overexpansion of the blood vessels of the testicles, leading to a soft tumor

varicose veins (VAR-ih-kohs VAYNS) enlarged, dilated vein toward the surface of the skin

vasectomy (vah-SEK-toh-mee) surgical removal of the vas deferens

vasoconstrictor (VAS-oh-kin-STRIK-tor) drug that constricts or narrows the diameter of a blood vessel

vasodilator (VAS-oh-DAI-lay-tor) drug that causes the relaxation or expansion of a blood vessel

vasovasostomy (VAS-oh-vah-SAW-stoh-mee) creation of an opening between two vessels; technical term for a vasectomy reversal

vena cava (VEE-nah CAY-vah) large-diameter vein that gathers blood from the body and returns it to the heart

venogram (VEE-noh-gram) record of a vein

ventilation–perfusion scan (ven-ti-LAY-shun–per-FYOO-shun skan) a scan that tests whether a problem in the lungs is caused by airflow (ventilation) or blood flow (perfusion)

ventricular septal defect (VSD) (ven-TRIK-yoo-lar SEP-tal DEE-fekt) defect/flaw in the septum that divides the two ventricles of the heart

verruca (vah-ROO-kah) from Latin, for *wart;* a wart

vertigo (VER-tih-goh) sensation of moving through space (while stationary); from Latin, for *to whirl around*

vesicle (VEH-sih-kul) from Latin, for *little bladder;* a small blister

vesicovaginal fistula (VES-ih-koh-VAJ-ih-nal FIS-tyoo-lah) abnormal opening between the urinary bladder and the vagina

vitiligo (vih-tih-LAI-goh) see *patch*

voiding cystourethrogram (VOI-ding SIS-toh-yoo-REE-throh-GRAM) imaging procedure of the bladder and urethra produced during urination

vulvitis (vul-VAI-tis) inflammation of the vulva

vulvodynia (VUL-voh-DAI-nee-ah) pain in the vulva

X

xanthoderma (zan-thoh-DER-mah) yellow skin

xanthoma (zan-THOH-mah) a yellow tumor

xanthosis (zan-THOH-sis) yellowing of the skin

xenograft (ZEE-noh-graft) see *heterograft*

xeroderma (zeh-roh-DER-mah) dry skin

xerophthalmia (ZER-off-THAL-mee-ah) dry eyes

xerosis (ze-ROH-sis) condition of dryness

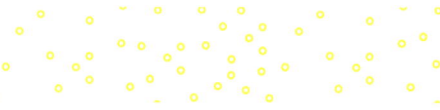

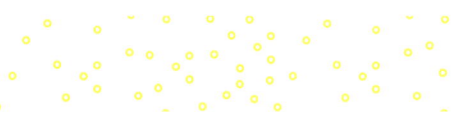

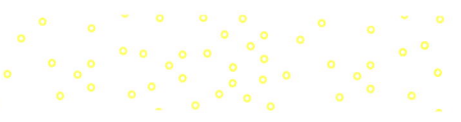

Heart—*Cont.*
  diagnostic procedures for, 213–214,
      217–218, 222
  function of, 204
  infections of, 222
  inflammation of, 222, 223
  objective terms describing, 213–221
  records and notes on, 232–233
  structure and function of, 205–206
  subjective terms describing, 210–213
  treatments and therapies for, 226–231
  valves of
      anatomy and function of, 205–206
      imaging of, 214
      sounds of, 214
      treatments and therapies for, 228
      word parts associated with, 205
  word parts associated with, 205–206, 235
Heart attack, 222, 223
Heart defect, congenital, 222, 223
Heart failure, congestive, 222, 223
Heart murmurs, 214, 215
Heart rate, 213–214
Heart sounds, 214
Heart surgery, 226–229
Hematemesis, 276
Hematocrit, 190
Hematology, 177–203
  abbreviations in, 203
  assessment (diagnosis) in, 193–196
  definition of, 190
  diagnostic procedures in, 187–188
  objective terms in, 187–192
  overview of, 177
  professional terms in, 190–191
  records and notes in, 200–202
  subjective terms in, 184–187
  treatment and therapies in, 197–199
  word parts associated with, 178–179, 202
Hematoma
  definition of, 110, 184
  epidural, 110
  intracerebral, 110
  periorbital, 61
  subdural, 110
Hematopoiesis, 188
Hemat/o (root), 10, 178, 179
Hematuria, 200, 306, 310
  gross, 310
  microscopic, 310
Hemianopsia, 132
Hemicrania, 77, 101
Heminephrectomy, 325
Hemiparesis, 120
Hemispheres, of brain, 100
Hemodialysis, 324, 325

Hemoglobin, 178, 193, 200
Hemolysis, 188
  microangiopathic, 200
Hemolytic anemia, 193, 194
Hemophilia, 184
Hemoptysis, 200, 243, 244
Hem/o (root), 10, 178, 179
Hemorrhage, 184, 211
Hemorrhagic stroke, 113
Hemorrhoid, 276
Hemorrhoidectomy, 290
Hemothorax, 247
Hepatic/o (root), 269, 295
Hepatitis, 284, 286
Hepatomegaly, 278–280
Hepat/o (root), 263, 269, 295
Hepatosplenomegaly, 189
Hereditary, definition of, 39
Hernia, 279, 310
Herniorrhaphy, 290
Heterograft, skin, 69
Hidradenitis, 66
Hidropoiesis, 58
Hidr/o (root), 54, 74
Hippocrates, 4
Hippocratic Oath, 4
Hip replacement, 93
Hirsutism, 163
History
  cardiovascular, 210–213
  dermatologic, 58–60
  endocrine, 162–165
  family, 34
  female reproductive system, 345–349
  gastrointestinal, 275–278
  hematologic and immunologic, 184–187
  musculoskeletal, 82–84
  nervous system, 105–108
  past medical, 34
  past surgical, 34
  present illness, 34
  respiratory, 243–246
  sensory system, 132–135
  social, 34
  urinary system and male reproductive
      system, 306–309
Hives (urticaria), 58, 59
Homograft, 69
Hormone replacement therapy, 172
Hormones, 154
  assessment of disorders, 169–171
  insufficient, 169
  measuring levels of, 165–166
  objective terms describing, 165–168
  receptors for, 154
  releasing, 155, 156

secretion of, 154, 158–160
  stimulating, 160, 166
  subjective terms describing, 162–165
  treatments affecting, 172–173
  word roots associated with, 158–160, 176
Horniness of skin, 55
Humerus, 76
Humors, 56
Hydrocele, 310, 313
Hydrocephalus, 117
Hydrocephaly, 114
Hydronephrosis, 319
Hydrophobia, 106
Hydr/o (root), 11
Hyperacusis, 132
Hyperbilirubinemia, 200
Hypercapnia, 240, 248
Hypercarbia, 248
Hypercoagulability, 193
Hyperemesis, 276
Hyperemesis gravidarum, 357, 359
Hyperglycemia, 159, 166
Hypergonadism, 163
Hyperhidrosis, 58
Hyperkalemia, 310
Hyperkeratosis, 58, 72
Hyperkinesia, 82
Hyperlipidemia, 193, 194
Hypermagnesemia, 166
Hypermastia, 351
Hypermelanosis, 58
Hyperopia, 132, 133
Hyperparathyroidism, 170
Hyperpigmentation, 58, 72
Hyperpituitarism, 170
Hyperplasia, 27
Hyperpnea, 244
Hyper- (prefix), 166, 169
Hypersomnolence, 120
Hypersplenism, 193
Hypertension, 214, 224
  renovascular, 318
Hyperthyroidism, 136, 158, 162, 169, 170
Hypertrichosis, 58, 67
Hypertrophic cardiomyopathy, 222
Hypertrophy, 82, 87
Hyperventilation, 240, 243, 244
Hypoacusis, 132
Hypocalcemia, 174
Hypocapnia, 248
Hypocarbia, 240, 248
Hypochondriacs, 78
Hypodermic, definition of, 69
Hypodermic needle, 69
Hypodermis, 54
Hypoglycemia, 159, 166

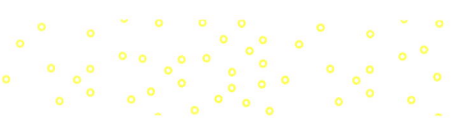

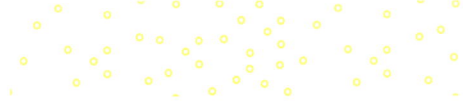

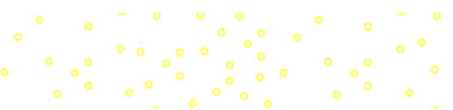

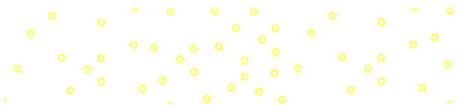